A Fatal Inheritance

A Fatal Inheritance

HOW A FAMILY MISFORTUNE REVEALED
A DEADLY MEDICAL MYSTERY

Lawrence Ingrassia

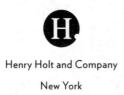

Henry Holt and Company

New York

Henry Holt and Company
Publishers since 1866
120 Broadway
New York, NY 10271
www.henryholt.com

Henry Holt ® and ⓗ ® are registered trademarks of Macmillan Publishing Group, LLC.

Distributed in Canada by Raincoast Book Distribution Limited

Library of Congress Cataloging-in-Publication Data

Names: Ingrassia, Lawrence, author.
Title: A fatal inheritance : how a family misfortune revealed a deadly
    medical mystery / Lawrence Ingrassia.
Description: First edition. | New York : Henry Holt and Company, 2024. |
    Includes bibliographical references and index.
Identifiers: LCCN 2023055907 | ISBN 9781250837226 (hardcover) |
    ISBN 9781250837219 (ebook)
Subjects: LCSH: p53 antioncogene—Popular works. | p53
    antioncogene—Patients—United States—Popular works. | p53
    antioncogene—Patients—United States—Biography. | Cancer—Genetic
    aspects—Research—History—Popular works. | Fraumeni, Joseph F. | Li,
    Frederick P. | Ingrassia, Lawrence. | Ingrassia, Lawrence—Family.
Classification: LCC RC268.44.P16 I54 2024 | DDC 616.99/4042092
    [B]—dc23/eng/20231227
LC record available at https://lccn.loc.gov/2023055907

Our books may be purchased in bulk for promotional, educational, or business use. Please
contact your local bookseller or the Macmillan Corporate and Premium Sales Department at
(800) 221-7945, extension 5442, or by e-mail at MacmillanSpecialMarkets@macmillan.com.

First Edition 2024

Designed by Gabriel Guma

Printed in the United States of America

10 9 8 7 6 5 4 3 2 1

To my mother Regina, my brother Paul, my sisters
Gina and Angela, and my nephew Charlie, gone too soon.

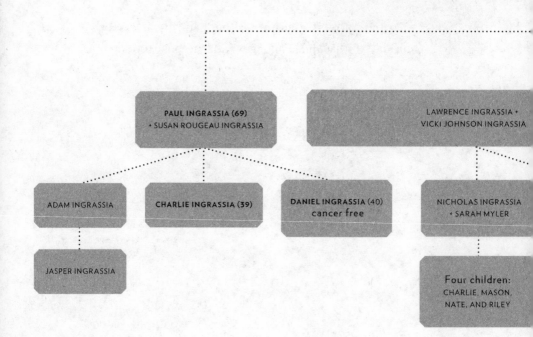

Six other children:
GRACE, ANDREW,
ANTHONY, JOSEPH,
NANCY (74), AND MARION

PAUL INGRASSIA (69)
+ SUSAN ROUGEAU INGRASSIA

LAWRENCE INGRASSIA +
VICKI JOHNSON INGRASSIA

ADAM INGRASSIA

CHARLIE INGRASSIA (39)

DANIEL INGRASSIA (40)
cancer free

NICHOLAS INGRASSIA
+ SARAH MYLER

JASPER INGRASSIA

Four children:
CHARLIE, MASON,
NATE, AND RILEY

INGRASSIA-IACONO FAMILY TREE

Parentheses in chart denote age of death for family members with
cancer; bold type denotes known or presumed p53 mutation

SOURCE: Lawrence Ingrassia

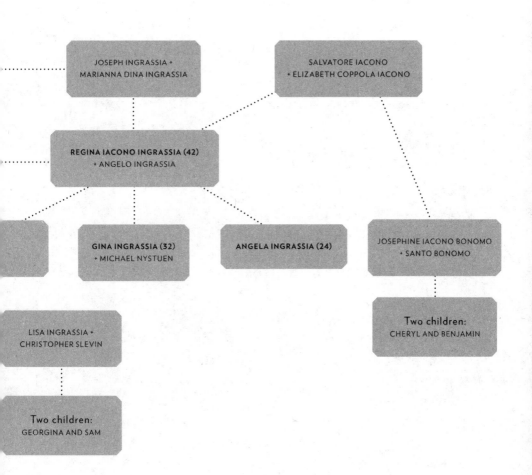

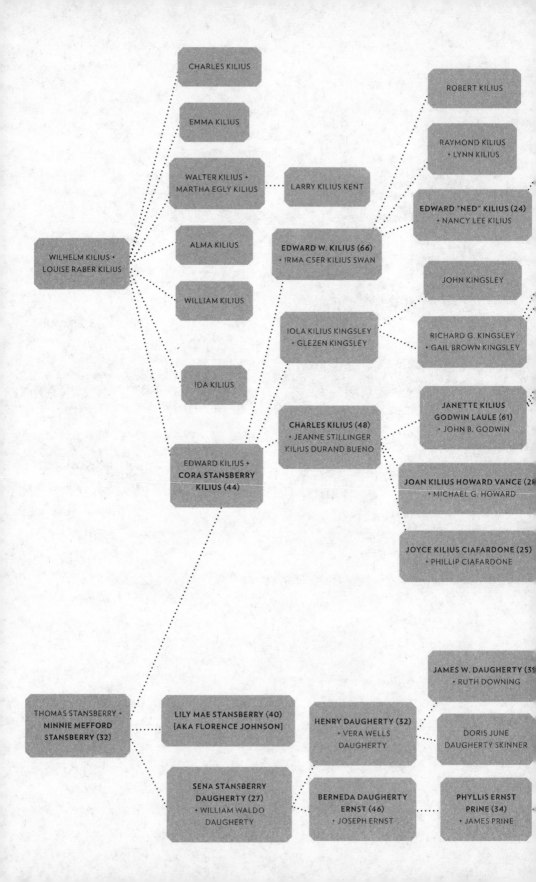

"FAMILY A": EXTENDED KILIUS-STANSBERRY FAMILY TREE

- Parentheses denote age of death for family members with cancer; bold type denotes presumed or known p53 mutation
- West Coast branch of family at top; Midwest branch of family below

DARREL KILIUS (29)
+ KELLY KIRKPATRICK

WENDY KINGSLEY NORMAN
+ WILLIAM NORMAN

RICHARD S. KINGSLEY
+ JOAN KINGSLEY

JILL GODWIN (45)

JENNIFER GODWIN RIVAS ········· RUDY RIVAS

JOHN C. GODWIN (3)

MICHAEL C. HOWARD (2)

JEREMY HOWARD (10)

GRACEE FINNELL

GERALD "JERRY" HOWARD (32)
+ DONNA CRAGER HOWARD

JAIMEE HOWARD FINNELL
+ SEAN FINNELL

TAYLIN FINNELL

DARREN DELIN +
DEENA DELIN

JED DELIN

TAMERA "TAMMY" HOWARD DELIN (40) + PATRICK DELIN

REMY DELIN

RONALD VANCE JR.

DIANE SMELCER

JESSICA HOPE

MONTANA DELIN

LYNDSEY RENEE
ARMOUR DAVIS

DEBRA DAUGHERTY ARMOUR (23)
+ GEORGE ROBERT ARMOUR

WESTON CARRINGTON

BETHANY ANN ARMOUR
CARRINGTON + NATHAN
CARRINGTON

STEPHEN SKINNER

HAYDEN CARRINGTON

THOMAS PRINE (24)
+ NANCY PRINE

SOURCES: Members of the extended Kilius-Stansberry family, Dana-Farber Cancer Institute records, state death certificates, and obituaries

A Fatal Inheritance

1

M Y MOST ENDURING CHILDHOOD MEMORIES OF MY MOM ARE OF HER BEING
sick. Of visiting her in the hospital with my older brother and two
younger sisters. Of our grandmother coming to stay with us while our
mom recuperated from breast cancer surgery. Of seeing her in bed at
home with a soulful, sad look on her face as she tried to smile.

She had been ill, sometimes gravely, off and on while I was growing
up. I'm pretty sure she first had breast cancer as early as 1958, when she
was just thirty-two, though my memory is vague because I was only six
then.

At the time, we were living in Laurel, Mississippi, far from where my
parents grew up. My mom, Regina, the elder of two girls, was raised in
modest circumstances in Norwalk, Connecticut, the daughter of a seam-
stress and a hospital orderly who had come to the United States from
southern Italy in the early twentieth century. My dad, Angelo, five years
older than my mom, was the eldest of seven children, and the son of Italian immigrants as well. According to family lore, his father had fled Sic-
ily after a dispute with a local mafioso. After living for a brief period in
the tenements of New York City, the family settled in the Catskills, on
the outskirts of Middletown, New York, on a road populated by so many

members of the close-knit extended family that it came to be named Ingrassia Road.

Starting as sharecroppers in the 1920s, they all toiled long hours—the children, too, including my dad, his siblings, and his cousins—before saving enough by the 1930s to collectively purchase what they called a small "truck" farm (as the celery, onions, lettuce, and spinach they grew were hauled to markets in trucks). Some winters, part of the family would travel to Florida—not for vacation, but to earn money by harvesting oranges and grapefruit. As one of my dad's cousins put it years later, "Although we grew up poor, we didn't know we were poor."

My parents had been introduced on a blind date by my mother's aunt Dot, who would live to the age of 101 and who said she had never met two people more in love. My mom, a dark-haired and attractive woman with high cheekbones, worked as a secretary in a law office at the time and had been courted by many men but had always found them wanting—until my dad came along. When he did, she was immediately, and passionately, smitten with him. A handsome man with a jaunty character, he was the first in his extended family to attend college and graduated with a degree in chemistry from Syracuse University. The two married within six months of their meeting, on June 21, 1947.

It was Dad's chemistry degree that took them to Laurel, a Deep South (and, back then, strictly segregated) city of about twenty-five thousand, surrounded by dense pine forests. He worked in research and development for Masonite Corp., a pioneer in making siding and paneling by using heat, pressure, resins, and glues to bind together wood fibers, flakes, and chips that otherwise would be thrown out as waste.

The early years in Mississippi were, in many ways, an idyllic time in their lives. Though, as olive-skinned Italian American Catholics from the North, they were considered outsiders by some in Laurel, my vivacious mom made friends easily. And my dad, an avid outdoorsman, loved the opportunities for fishing and hunting, even building a pen in the backyard where he always kept an English pointer as a bird dog. One of his dogs, named Mike, was especially good at flushing quail.

In quick succession came four children: Paul in 1950, Larry (me) in 1952, Gina in 1954, and Angela in 1956. Our parents talked about how Paul and I would fight over Gina, a cherubic infant, with each of us claiming her as "my baby." On rare occasions, our mom's parents or other relatives would make the long train or car trip from New York to visit us. And our maternal grandmother, Elizabeth Iacono, would especially smother us with affection.

For vacations, we would gleefully pile into the family station wagon and drive a couple of hours to a ramshackle beach house we rented in Biloxi, on the Gulf Coast. Those days were filled with shrimping, fishing, and collecting seashells. I got into trouble once when, halfway back home to Laurel, Dad smelled a rotten odor and stopped the car; I had sneaked a bunch of seashells into the trunk, not realizing that inside them were snails and slugs, which had died and were now stinking up the car. Another time, when we were fishing at a nearby lake, I became overly rambunctious and managed to run off the dock while Dad wasn't looking. Knowing me, he'd had the foresight to put a life preserver on me, so I was under for only a few seconds, and he pulled me out when I bobbed to the surface.

At work, Dad made a name for himself after being awarded several U.S. patents for developing formaldehyde resins that improved the fiberboard that Masonite manufactured. My parents were living the American dream, using education to rise from hardscrabble immigrant work to a more comfortable middle-class life.

But my fond memories of these good times are overshadowed by the growing realization, even in childhood, that something wasn't quite right with Mom. I recall overhearing snippets of her conversations with friends and relatives about feeling a lump in her breast but having been told by her doctor that it was nothing to worry about. Later, she would often lament, wondering why the doctor had ignored her anxiety initially, before the tumor grew bigger.

Once, after she had undergone a breast cancer operation, we were visited by one of my dad's sisters, who was a nurse. "She asked me to view her surgery site because it was so painful. The area was just dreadful-looking, and I asked her had she seen her doctor recently," my aunt Marion recalled. "Yes, she had, and all the doctor would say to her was that the pain was all in her head and needed no further attention. I asked your mom to please see another doctor because it just did not look right. As it turned out, the pain was caused by the second breast being cancerous as well."

I didn't see my mom much during the summer of 1960. We were in the process of moving from Laurel to Chicago, after my dad got a promotion. But the family didn't go there right away because mom was convalescing from one of her major surgeries at her parents' tiny two-bedroom house in Norwalk, Connecticut. There wasn't enough space for all four of us kids, so our two sisters stayed there while my brother and I spent a couple of months living with our dad's mother, Marianna Ingrassia, on the family farm. It was in some ways a blissful summer for me and Paul, a carefree extended vacation during which we scampered around the farm with our uncles and played with our many cousins. We looked forward to the occasional eighty-five-mile drive with a relative to Norwalk for weekend visits with our mother and sisters. But invariably, Mom would be exhausted and would spend much of the time resting in bed, while our grandmother Elizabeth tried to put a good face on everything and not show how worried she was.

After we settled in suburban Chicago, my mom went through hopeful cancer-free periods punctuated by battles with new tumors. Maybe it was because we were young and our parents were trying to protect us, or because cancer was a feared disease and a topic that people avoided discussing in the 1960s—but I can't recall our talking much about mom's recurrences. A few surviving letters between her and my grandmother give a glimpse of the haunting specter her cancer cast over everything.

"I felt real sad to hear you are going back to hospital," my grandmother Elizabeth wrote to my mom on September 30, 1962. "I just finished talking to Gloria, she said to me she thought it was a wise thing, because the doctor know [*sic*] what he is doing."

In another letter, written by my mom in what appears to be 1966 or 1967, she recounts being in pain, both from medication she was taking and from having contracted hepatitis—apparently, while getting a blood transfusion related to her cancer surgeries. "Last night I was miserable—I bet it's those pills for the adrenal glands. I should have let him change them—in addition to the hepatitis. The cramps & pain I couldn't take—even the cramp and pain pills didn't ease it. . . . Joie [my mom's younger sister] said a lot of hepatitis is going around. I know of no case here—mine would be from the blood transfusion in June. . . . I can't understand why the doctor didn't call; surgeons are always so busy. . . . I hope I can write & tell you I feel good—I'd do anything. Thank God I can walk and cook."

During one of the periods when she felt well, in between her cancers, she took up painting, which she had enjoyed as a girl growing up, in part as a distraction from worrying about whether another tumor would be found. "I started another picture with snow and it's coming out nice. . . . We'll be starting new art classes in February, and it will give me some outside interest," she wrote to my grandmother in January 1967. And in a letter a month later: "I've been drawing a little. I drew Gina in charcoal and my neighbor thinks it really looks like her. I feel real good." Looking back, I now realize that amid the constant suffering, her greatest pain, no doubt, was the growing fear that she might never have the joy of watching her four children grow up.

She had been in and out of the hospital so often that I didn't think anything was different when she went back for another stay in the early spring of 1968. So I was confused when a coworker of mine interrupted me on Sunday morning, March 31. I was fifteen years old, in the middle of working a four-hour brunch shift as a busboy at a nearby restaurant, Olde North Pancake House. I had just cleared a table and taken the dirty dishes to the kitchen when the chef, who knew our family, told me with a stricken look on her face that my dad was waiting for me in the parking lot out back.

When I got to the car, I saw that a friend of my parents was behind the wheel, and my dad was sitting in the backseat. He opened the door from inside and beckoned me in. We locked eyes—his were teary and red—and the next words he spoke changed my life. "Mom died," he said. I was shocked, and we wept together as he clutched me in his embrace. She was forty-two and, by then, had endured cancer and its painful treatments for about a decade. The malignancy, I later learned, had metastasized from her breasts and ravaged her liver, lungs, and abdomen.

It was heartbreaking for all of us, but especially for Gina, then thirteen, and Angela, eleven. They were so young when Mom had her first cancer that they had scarcely any memories of her before—before cancer, when she was a radiant woman in her twenties, taking joy in raising her young family, hosting parties with new friends, sharing confidences, and looking forward to a long life.

Though I recall with intense clarity the moment I learned she was gone, I somehow have mostly gauzy images of what followed in the weeks and months after she died. I remember my friends consoling me at the funeral Mass. I remember standing with my dad and siblings at the cemetery on a raw and windy April morning while Mom's casket was lowered and visiting the gravesite often, after Sunday Mass.

I remember Dad hiring an older woman to help out at home, and how we hated her bland cooking; it wasn't nearly good as the spaghetti and meatballs, braciole with tomato sauce, chicken cacciatore, or veal parmigiana our mom and her mother had made for us. I remember not doing anything for my sixteenth birthday a couple of months after Mom died, because I didn't feel like celebrating. I don't remember being angry much, though I'm sure I was, but I do remember spending a lot of time by myself and becoming fatalistic, ruminating on how life sometimes brings bad things over which you have little control.

Even in my grief, like most teenagers, I was soon engrossed in the daily activity of life—attending my high school classes, running cross-country and track, socializing with my pals, trying to get a girlfriend, and becoming transfixed with politics in that highly political year of the assassinations of Martin Luther King Jr. and Robert F. Kennedy, of Vietnam War protests and of clashes at the Democratic National Convention in downtown Chicago. The disbelief and denial over my mom's death faded eventually, though not the emptiness or the sadness. She was one of 318,500 Americans who died of cancer in 1968. It was tragic, but what was there to say?

There would be, alas, much more to say. Cancer was far from done with my family. We didn't know it then, but the legacy of our mother's illness would linger menacingly over our lives for many years to come. My mom's fear of missing what the future held for her children was indeed well placed, it turns out. But the reason was far more complicated and painful than she or any of us could have imagined, and it would take decades of research by doctors traversing the scientific unknown before there would be any answers.

2

CHRISTMAS 1966 WAS A HAPPY TIME FOR NED AND NANCY KILIUS. THE YOUNG couple, both from the Los Angeles area, had met and fallen in love while students at San Diego State University. They married in August 1965, shortly after Ned graduated with a degree in business; Nancy, a year younger, left school before getting her degree—not all that uncommon for women back in the 1960s. Ned was offered a job as a salesman for Colgate-Palmolive, and the two moved to Seattle and bought a small house for $18,200 in the suburb of Kirkland a year later. Nancy soon became pregnant and, on August 6, 1966, gave birth to a baby boy they named Darrel.

A few months later, to escape the dreary, rainy winter weather, they flew to Southern California to spend the holidays and show off their newborn baby. They stayed with Nancy's family in Downey, a southern suburb of Los Angeles, and spent time with Ned's family in Oxnard, a distant northern exurb. Ned (his given name was "Edward," the same as his father's, so he had always gone by the nickname "Ned") was feeling tired and napped a lot, but with a demanding job and a new baby, that hardly seemed surprising.

At some point during their visit, relatives remarked that Ned seemed to have lost weight. Back in Seattle, he continued to feel lethargic and started having minor nosebleeds, which prompted him to see a doctor after a few weeks. He was admitted overnight while waiting for test results. That evening, at home with their baby, Nancy came across an article in *Reader's Digest* about the comedian Red Skelton's son dying of leukemia in Los Angeles in 1958. It sent her mind racing, and the next morning at the hospital her worst fear was confirmed: Ned, only a month after turning twenty-three, had been diagnosed with acute myeloid leukemia. "It was an omen," Nancy thought of the article she had read.

Ned's prognosis—as for all leukemia patients—was grim; at the time, the chances of surviving even five years was only about 15 percent, and many patients died within a year. Nancy's mind flashed back to a conversation with Ned before they got married: at his father's urging, Ned had told her there seemed to be a lot of cancers in the Kilius family. But it didn't bother her at the time, much less affect her decision to marry him. She thought, *Well, some families have heart attacks and some have cancers.*

Ned's doctor in Seattle advised him and Nancy that they would need help, lots of help, coping with Ned's intensive chemotherapy treatment, especially with a newborn baby. Maybe they should go home to their families, he gently suggested. So they headed back to Southern California, where they could lean on their families for support during what everyone knew would be an exceedingly difficult period.

Looking for treatment options, Ned scheduled appointments with doctors at the University of California, Los Angeles. After confirming the diagnosis, the doctors there weren't any more encouraging than the physicians in Seattle. But the UCLA doctors did offer a small glimmer of hope: they had heard of a clinical trial with experimental chemotherapy for leukemia patients being conducted by the National Cancer Institute. The doctors could help Ned get into the trial, but it would mean uprooting and moving for a while to the East Coast, far away from their families. Ned and Nancy didn't hesitate. Though the clinical trial probably offered only a small chance of beating Ned's cancer, that was better than no chance.

In February, they flew with baby Darrel to the East Coast. They rented a one-bedroom apartment in Baltimore's historic Hampden neighborhood, an area lined with two-story row houses near the old U.S. Marine Hospital, which had been renamed the U.S. Public Health Service Hospital, where Ned would be treated. Because chemotherapy can deplete white blood cells, and thus increase the risk of infection, Ned basically moved into the hospital to avoid germs. He didn't want Nancy to bring Darrel with her on visits, where he would see his father and others who were sick on the hospital ward. Ned and Nancy were active in a Lutheran parish back home, so Ned called a nearby Lutheran church and found a grandmother to babysit Darrel while Nancy sat with Ned several hours every day at the hospital to keep him company and cheer him up.

Ned's treatment was going as well as expected. The chemotherapy, thankfully, wasn't making him too sick, and he didn't seem to be getting worse; despite the fear of infection, his doctors occasionally let him go home to their apartment on weekends. For all the challenges, Nancy and Ned settled into a routine that made the situation bearable.

Then, one afternoon in early June, after visiting with Ned, Nancy came home to find the babysitter in a panic. While picking Darrel up from his high chair after lunch, she had felt a small lump inside the elbow of his right arm. It was the size of a marble. Nancy wondered why she hadn't noticed it before, as she bathed Darrel every day. It had to have appeared suddenly, she thought.

Nancy had been so focused on Ned's health that Darrel didn't even have a pediatrician yet. She found one who could see her baby the next day. The doctor, alarmed after examining him, advised Nancy, "I want you to see a surgeon tomorrow." Then, he repeated it for emphasis: "Tomorrow." So she made an appointment with a surgeon at Johns Hopkins Hospital. It was several miles south, so inconvenient, but she thought Darrel might get the most attentive care there.

The surgeon did a biopsy of the lump, and tests confirmed that Darrel had a cancerous tumor—a rhabdomyosarcoma, a very rare soft-tissue malignancy that afflicts only about five hundred people a year in the United States. Darrel was barely ten months old. It was unusual for a baby to get cancer of any kind, but especially a rhabdomyosarcoma.

Not sure how to proceed, the surgeon called other physicians he knew at other children's hospitals. Radical surgery was the main weapon for fighting tumors like Darrel's. The typical treatment, the doctor advised, would be amputation of Darrel's arm all the way up to the shoulder, to keep the cancer from spreading. Nancy caught her breath. To her relief, the doctor quickly added that, given the small size of Darrel's tumor, the consensus was to try an alternative—a resection, or removal, of the biceps, taking the tumor out at the elbow but also the muscle tissue above it, where the malignancy might metastasize. It would be a major operation, but Darrel would still have his arm.

Irma Kilius, Ned's mother and Darrel's grandmother, flew to Baltimore from the West Coast to be with Nancy, and the surgery was performed on June 6. A few days later, it was time to take the bandages off. The surgeon, worried about Nancy's initial reaction to seeing Darell's disfigured arm, wanted her to wait outside his room, but she insisted on being there. When the doctor unwrapped the bandages, Darrel immediately moved his arm, as if the surgery hadn't removed a large portion of his upper arm muscles. To Nancy, it was a blessing. Maybe, just maybe, a year that had been unrelentingly horrible until now was going to get better.

Indeed, a couple of months later, Darrel's follow-up radiation and chemotherapy were completed with no sign of the tumor having spread, and Ned's doctors felt his leukemia was sufficiently in remission that they released him in early August. Though Ned wasn't feeling great, the young couple and Darrel flew home to Kirkland, happy to leave behind the constant gloom of cancer wards, chemo infusions, and appointments with doctors. They went back to "playing house," as Nancy called it, hoping—really, praying—that life had returned to normal.

But Ned's remission didn't last long. After a week or so, he started having a hard time breathing. Late one night, Nancy was so scared that she called a local doctor, who advised her to get a paper bag and have Ned breathe into it. Still worried, she called the pastor at their church, who came over and drove them straight to a hospital emergency room. Ned might have died otherwise. His leukemia had caused severe respiratory acidosis, with high levels of carbon dioxide in his bloodstream causing him to hyperventilate as he gasped for oxygen. The young couple spent their second wedding anniversary in the hospital, then flew back to Baltimore so Ned could be with the doctors who had been treating him.

Ned clearly was in a fight for his life. Though father and son had both had cancer at the same time, none of the doctors treating either of them suggested any connection. Leukemia and rhabdomyosarcoma are entirely different malignancies. No veteran cancer researcher would have suggested the two were related. Yes, it was a wildly unlikely occurrence— but it was a coincidence. In a country with tens of millions of families, tragic, statistically unlikely things can happen.

3

D R. FREDERICK PEI LI ARRIVED AT THE NATIONAL CANCER INSTITUTE IN THE summer of 1967, while Ned and Darrel Kilius were both undergoing treatment. One of the first things Li did was jot a short letter to a few other young doctors he knew in town. Just twenty-seven years old, he was fresh off a two-year internship and residency program at Bellevue Hospital in New York and had just accepted a position in the NCI's epidemiology department. A fledgling group of only about a handful of researchers with offices above a dress shop in Bethesda, Maryland, the department had as its mission to examine patterns of disease that might provide clues about susceptibility and early detection.

In truth, the epidemiology department wasn't just small; it was a backwater. The prestigious jobs at the NCI were held by doctors concocting experimental chemotherapy therapies or researchers conducting lab studies to determine the causes of cancer, especially possible viral causes that were then considered the leading suspect for most tumors.

In his letter, Li mentioned that he was looking for instances of uncommon cancers—such as Hodgkin's disease, lymphosarcomas, multiple myeloma. In particular, he noted, "I would be interested in cases, 1) associated with other unusual diseases, 2) occurring in patients with congenital anomalies, 3) having family histories of lymphoma or leuke-mia, 4) having history of unusual exposure to potential carcinogens."

Li was a bit of a whiz kid—he had graduated from high school at sixteen, college at twenty, and medical school at twenty-three. He had chosen to go into public health in part because of his family's unusual background. His father had served as a general in Chiang Kai-shek's Kuomintang, or National Revolutionary Army, and later as a provincial governor, and his mother was the niece of a mayor of Shanghai. The middle of five children, Li was seven years old when his family moved to the United States in the late 1940s as Mao Zedong's Communist forces took control of their country.

Once prominent and well-to-do, his parents were forced to start over again. They opened a Cantonese restaurant called Good Will in New York City's Washington Heights neighborhood, earning a bit of derision from some compatriots; as Li's eldest sister, Virginia Li, put it, "Tongues wagged about the fact that the former governor and his lady had sunk so low as to open a chop suey house." Li's mother was the hostess, and his father was the cashier; to help make ends meet, the children worked occasional shifts at the restaurant, where they and their parents some-times watched in frustration as U.S. immigration officials raided the business and hauled off waiters and dishwashers who had entered the country illegally from China.

The restaurant eventually thrived enough that the family sold it and moved in the mid-1950s to White Plains, where they opened a bigger, classier restaurant, China Garden. A far cry from their humble initial endeavor, it was one of the first Chinese restaurants on the East Coast to feature traditional dishes, such as lychee duck, roast squab, shark fin soup, seafood clay pot, and crêpes Mandarin.

Fred Li, with jet-black hair and a round face, had a winning person-ality even though he often had a serious demeanor. He was known at the University of Rochester Medical School for coming to gatherings with a doctor's black bag stocked with ingredients like soy sauce, black vine-gar, and Chinese wine and whipping up meals for colleagues. At medical school, Li took a year's break for a trip around the world, spending time at state-run health agencies in Europe, the Middle East, and Asia, where he saw the impact that public health service doctors could have on sick populations.

Back in the United States, at the end of his two-year internship and residency at Bellevue Hospital in New York 1967, Li fêted about a dozen of his colleagues at a banquet at the family restaurant. He selected all the dishes the group dined on—which was helpful, as for some, it was the first time they were eating at a Chinese restaurant. On such occasions, colleagues who had known him as reserved saw a different Fred Li, more jovial and comfortable and reveling in his Chinese heritage.

Li's favorite saying from the time he was a young child, his siblings recall, was "I can do it." So it was no surprise to them that he chose to focus his medical career on cancer asking himself, "What can I do that is the hardest thing?"

Less than two months after joining the NCI and sending the letter to friends asking about unusual medical cases, Li attended a dinner party where someone mentioned to him that a young father and his baby son were both being treated for cancer in Baltimore. It was the kind of off-hand, corridor chatter that physicians often share with one another and is quickly forgotten. But, recognizing that the odds of this were astronomical, Li had a hunch that it would be worth his time to learn more about the family's history.

He raced to the office the next day to tell another colleague, Dr. Joseph Fraumeni Jr., who also was intrigued. The two had met for the first time only that summer, after Li joined the NCI, but they had immediately hit it off. While both were competitive, they were also collaborative and shared an intellectual curiosity for exploring uncharted medical territory.

Fraumeni, at thirty-four, a few years older than Li, was lanky, with a receding hairline, penetrating eyes, and a quick smile. He had joined the NCI's epidemiology department five years earlier, in 1962, as only its second professional. Like Li, he was also the son of immigrants, though

Fraumeni had enjoyed a more comfortable upbringing. His father had arrived with his own parents from Italy as a child around 1910; he later became an optometrist, serving the Italian American community in Boston's North End. His practice flourished, and the family moved to a large French Norman–style house in the suburb of North Reading. Fraumeni's father belonged to a riding group called the National Lancers, and he was chosen in April 1941 to play the coveted role of Paul Revere, traveling on horseback in the annual reenactment of the "midnight ride" to Lexington.

Congenial and soft-spoken—and off the end of the bell curve with how introverted he was, according to a personality test he once took— Fraumeni was also athletic and smart, which helped him get elected class president his senior year of high school. He graduated near the top of his class and was accepted at Harvard College. There, he got good but not great grades, and he felt shunned and treated like an outsider among the many WASP classmates who were well-to-do prep school graduates and often the second or third generation of their family to attend Harvard. Fraumeni once got scolded and put on "social probation" for briefly bringing a coed into his dormitory lobby while he fetched an umbrella, a transgression he felt would have been overlooked if he had attended Groton or had influential parents. He earned money to help pay his tuition by, among other things, going to chaperoned high school socials where he was paid ten dollars for the evening to dance with students.

At Harvard, Fraumeni majored in what at the time was called social relations, a degree that involved the study of psychology, anthropology, and sociology, but he joined a student premedical society because he hoped to become a doctor. At one point, the group visited Massachusetts General Hospital to sit in an amphitheater and watch a patient being cut open for an abdominal operation. Fraumeni got queasy from the sight, and had to walk out, so he decided it would be best not to become a surgeon.

Instead, at Duke University School of Medicine, he initially planned to become a psychiatrist. But after graduation, he found himself drawn to unusual cases while making the rounds during his hospital residencies, first at Johns Hopkins Hospital and then at Memorial Sloan Kettering Cancer Center in New York. "I notice that you always steer me toward interesting patients," the senior physician with whom Fraumeni worked at Sloan Kettering told him. "Why is that? I think it's because you are like a Sherlock Holmes. You're interested in puzzles and the causes of disease." Fraumeni decided to study epidemiology. At the time, it wasn't a field that an ambitious young physician aspired to. Indeed, from his class at the Harvard School of Public Health, where he studied after his internships, only a handful of students majored in epidemiology.

Fraumeni turned down jobs that paid more money—at Harvard and the University of Miami—partly because he liked the National Cancer Institute's mission and partly because the job would satisfy his military service obligation without the prospect of his being sent to Vietnam.

At the NCI, the self-effacing Fraumeni found a kindred spirit in the man who had hired him, the head of the epidemiology department, Dr. Robert Miller. A pediatrician by training, Miller had worked for the Atomic Bomb Casualty Commission in Japan in the 1950s, studying the effects of radiation fallout on fetuses. "There are no Nobel Prizes for epidemiology, but epidemiologists can help point the way," Miller wrote in expounding on his team's primary purpose. "I'd like to think of it as the study of peculiarities in the occurrence of disease as revealed by the study of the patient, his family, or the community. . . . One of the problems in finding such clues to the origins of cancer is that there are not many good, new clue finders."

Upon arriving at the NCI in 1961, Miller had asked himself, "What can I do to make a difference nationally?" His philosophy was that it was a good idea to look where no one else was looking; as a reminder to colleagues, Miller later in his time at the NCI kept a framed copy of a 1971 cover of the *New Yorker* showing eight seagulls standing on a rooftop, with seven looking in one direction and the other staring in the opposite direction. He decided to focus on childhood cancers, both because of his training as a pediatrician and because so little was known in this area. But there was no central repository for data on such cases, so he worked with vital statistics offices to retrieve death certificates of children nationwide who had died of cancer and then scoured them, looking for patterns. In addition, after Fraumeni joined Miller at the NCI a year later, the two traveled to children's hospitals around the country. Searching for unusual case histories, they would spend a couple of days hunched over a desk reviewing records often kept in basement filing cabinets.

Early on, Miller and Fraumeni spotted possible links between childhood malignancies and other conditions, such as birth defects. They discovered that children with a rare kidney cancer called Wilms tumor, often under five years old, also had aniridia, meaning they lacked irises. Why the two were related was unclear, but the discovery of this previously unknown correlation between a cancer and another condition proved significant enough that a paper Miller and Fraumeni coauthored about the anomaly was published in the *New England Journal of Medicine* in 1964.

More important than the finding itself was how the connection was found: by mining the NCI's early database of childhood cancers. So when Li told Fraumeni in mid-1967 about a young father and baby son being simultaneously treated for cancer in Baltimore, their epidemiologic instincts—together with the records they had painstakingly gathered that indicated how rare this was—prompted them to look at what was going on.

But one challenge they faced is that cancer remained a black box, its causes still largely confounding even to the best scientific minds.

4

IN 1966, THE YEAR BEFORE LI AND FRAUMENI CAME ACROSS THE UNUSUAL CASES OF Ned and Darrel Kilius, the renowned scientist Dr. Peyton Rous was awarded a Nobel Prize for Physiology or Medicine for his cancer research.

Typically, Nobels are awarded for work done many years before the scientists are recognized for it. Even by that measure, Rous's Nobel stood out, because he was honored for research conducted more than a half century earlier, in 1911. At age eighty-seven, not only did Rous become the oldest Nobel recipient ever, but the fifty-five years between his famous experiment and his prize was the longest gap ever.

Rous had all but stumbled into studying cancer. He graduated with a medical degree from Johns Hopkins University in 1905, only to decide that because of his personality he wasn't well suited to being a "real doctor" treating patients. A couple of years later, he received a grant that the Rockefeller Institute for Medical Research was offering young scientists. While at the institute, he initially did some work on lymphocytes, a type of white blood cell. But the director of the institute, who had been overseeing its cancer research lab, decided he wanted to instead focus on studying polio, a feared disease then afflicting many children. Would you take over the cancer lab? he asked Rous.

One day, a farmer brought to Rous's laboratory a black-and-white-speckled Plymouth Rock hen with a large tumor, a soft-tissue sarcoma, growing on its right breast. Rous conducted an experiment to see if the bird's malignancy could infect another chicken, transplanting cells from the tumor into a hen from the same flock. The transplanted cells developed into a new sarcoma. Then, wondering if something infectious could account for the new tumors, Rous minced a bit of the tumor in saline solution, strained it through a filter to eliminate any contaminating bacteria or tumor cells, and injected this liquid extract into healthy birds. Lo and behold, they, too, developed sarcomas. Rous attributed the new tumors to "a minute parasitic organism," or a virus.

It was a scientific breakthrough—not that it was immediately recognized as such. A recurring theme in medicine, indeed in much of science, is that discoveries by newcomers are ignored or questioned by the experts. After all, if what was purported to have been discovered were something truly worth discovering, wouldn't a more experienced scientist have been the one to discover it? Rous must have done something wrong, the skeptics said. Despite his best efforts, the extract could have been contaminated. So certain of this were other scientists that no one even bothered trying to replicate Rous's experiment. Complicating matters was that viruses, and their role in transmitting disease, were little understood at the time.

Given the reaction, Rous moved on for a while. He solidified his renown as a distinguished scientist by doing notable research on blood, the liver, and the gallbladder before returning to study cancer in the 1930s, when his earlier work was validated by others, who discovered a tumor caused by a virus found in rabbits.

When Rous was finally awarded a Nobel, many scientists thought the honor was long overdue. His lasting influence on cancer research was underscored by the fact that many top scientists in the 1950s and '60s were sharply focused on trying to definitively establish links between viruses and human cancers, with environmental factors a distant second.

In his Nobel lecture, delivered in Stockholm on December 13, 1966,

Rous asserted his belief that viruses caused most cancers, even while acknowledging one difficulty with the theory: "No virus has as yet been found that indubitably actuates neoplasms in man." He even added that "Innumerable attempts [by researchers] have consistently drawn blanks." He went on to say that exposure to chemical agents might be a possible cause, even as he conceded that research still hadn't yielded any convincing evidence for that. However, Rous didn't mince words when it came to dismissing possible genetic causes of cancer. "Numerous facts, when taken together, decisively exclude this supposition," the new Nobel laureate pronounced.

Rous's confidence in what was known about cancer belied the fact that very little was understood at the time, even though cancer has engendered fascination and fear for millennia. What is believed to be the first historical mention of cancer dates to 3000 BC, during the reign of the early pharaohs, in an Egyptian papyrus that refers to tumors or ulcers of the breast that were cauterized and removed. Hippocrates, who died circa 370 BC, would describe lumps as *karkinos* and *karkinomas*—from the Greek word for "crab," because the tumors he observed often looked akin to tentacles, resembling crab's legs.

Several hundred years later, a Roman physician named Aulus Cornelius Celsus made key observations about the perplexing ailment. He noted that carcinomas appeared to be "a spreading disease," and that even after being cut out, "the excised carcinomas have returned and caused death."

Over the following centuries, others went on to describe further characteristics of tumors as they sought to better recognize and treat them: that they occur in every part of the body; that tumors causing illness often had a different consistency and feel than lumps that were benign; that malignant tumors often were incurable.

Hoping to improve understanding of the dread disease, the Academy of Sciences, Humanities, and Arts of Lyon, France, in 1773 offered a prize for the best report on *Qu'est-ce que le cancer?* (What is cancer?) The winner was Bernard Peyrilhe, a surgeon who wrote an essay about the nature of tumors, their growth patterns, and cancer's possible cause, suggesting that some substance in the body triggered tumors. Peyrilhe tried to test his theories by injecting fluid from a human breast cancer into a dog through an incision on its back. But the dog developed an abscess and yelped so fiercely that his assistants drowned the distressed animal.

Around the same time, in 1775 in London, a surgeon named Percivall Pott noticed that chimney sweeps—workers who started as "apprentices" when they were younger than ten—often developed tumors on the skin of their scrotums. The malignancy frequently didn't occur until years later, and Pott suggested that the long and frequent exposure to soot while climbing up and down narrow chimneys had led to the cancer. It was the first time a possible environmental carcinogen was identified, and this helped lead to Parliament's passage of the Chimney Sweepers Act in 1788, requiring suitable clothing for the workers and raising the minimum age of apprentices.

Nearly a century later, in 1866, a French surgeon named Pierre Paul Broca delved into the medical history of his wife's family after she developed breast cancer. Of twenty-five women over several generations, he found that eight others also had breast cancer. He published his research *Traité des tumeurs* (Treatise on Tumors), but so little was known about genetics that others expressed doubt about his suggestion that heredity might be a factor.

Scientists like Peyton Rous began studying cancer more systematically in the early twentieth century, as the disease was recognized as a growing public health problem, with U.S. cancer deaths rising to 115,000 in 1927, from 70,000 in 1910. Still, efforts to get increased public funding for cancer research languished. Then, in its March 1937 issue, *Fortune* magazine published an article with the provocative (and accurate) headline "Cancer—The Great Darkness." Noting how little was known about cancer, and how little was spent trying to find out, *Fortune* asserted, "Society has the power, if not to directly call forth light from those sparks, at least to finance the brains and equipment at which it might conceivably be called forth." The article added to a growing swell of public calls for more government support for scientists studying cancer. Just four months later, Congress unanimously passed a bill creating the National Cancer Institute, with money for a well-equipped laboratory at the agency's new office in Bethesda, Maryland.

If not much was known at the time about what caused cancer, the new agency was emphatic about what did not. NCI pamphlets published in the late 1930s and 1940s, while mentioning animal experimentation and heredity, carried prominent captions on the cover stating, "Did you know: That cancer is NOT hereditary or contagious?" An American Cancer Society video, *The Traitor Within*, produced in 1946 to encourage early detection and treatment, dismissed the suggestion that cancer might be genetic, intoning, "Everyone's chances of developing cancer are just about the same regardless of heredity."

Potential environmental carcinogens began to receive more attention after the intriguing publication in 1950 of the first articles suggesting a link between tobacco smoking and lung cancer. It took over a decade, but in 1964 the U.S. surgeon general published a report outlining the health hazards of smoking.

But viruses—in line with Peyton Rous's thinking—remained the primary focus of many researchers. The NCI in the early 1960s announced a "Special Virus Cancer Program" dedicated to searching for viruses that cause human cancer. Funding for the program accounted for more than 10 percent of the NCI's contract budget, exceeding half a billion dollars over the next decade, more than any other line of research.

Heredity wasn't totally ignored. But even geneticists were cautious about linking it with cancer. In *Genetics and Disease*, a primer written in 1965, Dr. Alfred G. Knudson Jr. included a chapter on cancer toward the end of the book. "Family studies revealed occasional instances of more than one case in a family, but this is little more than expected by chance; single hereditary factors play a very small role.... Although these unusual examples of cancer attributed to dominant genes are interesting, they leave unanswered the question of the role of heredity in common cancers."

5

IN THE LATE 1950S AND 1960S, WHEN FREDERICK LI AND JOSEPH FRAUMENI WERE training to be physicians, a medical book called *Eleven Blue Men and Other Narratives of Medical Detection* was popular reading at many medical schools. It was a favorite of their boss at the NCI epidemiology branch, Robert Miller.

Published in 1953, the book was a compilation of a dozen articles that originally appeared in the *New Yorker* magazine's Annals of Medicine feature. All told how forensic investigations solved puzzling medical cases—like what ailed the eleven men who showed up at Manhattan hospitals with a bluish hue to their skin, cramps, and retching. (It was not carbon monoxide poisoning, as initially suspected; instead, an extensive inquiry eventually determined that the likely culprit was in food the victims had eaten at a restaurant where the cook had accidentally mixed toxic sodium nitrite with salt.)

Presented with a case of a young father and baby son both having cancer at the same time, Li and Fraumeni were now detectives with a medical mystery to solve. But where to begin? They knew that two cancers in a family, while unusual, could be a coincidence. The two physicians would need to build a comprehensive Kilius family medical history—not just for the current generation, but for multiple generations going back as far as they could. And not just for one branch of the family, but for the extended family. How many of the relatives had developed tumors versus what would be expected for the overall population? What were the types of cancers? What might the malignancies have in common or not? At what ages were the family members diagnosed, and where were they living at the time? What would possible explanations be? The answers might provide valuable clues to assemble pieces of the puzzle.

Fraumeni, with Robert Miller, had come across a different cancer-prone family the year before, in 1966, when a boy had been admitted to the National Cancer Institute with a lymphatic system cancer. They learned that the boy's sister had a liposarcoma, a soft-tissue cancer; another brother had a bowel cancer; and their father had a bone cancer. The doctors weren't sure what was going on—perhaps it was some kind of environmental exposure, or an oncogenic (i.e., cancer-causing) virus—but they didn't study the family closely, as they were busy working on other projects.

Now that Li had joined the NCI, they had more manpower to delve into the Kilius family. One challenge was that Ned and Darrel Kilius were members of a sprawling clan dispersed around the United States. Their Kilius forebears had come to America from Germany in the mid-1800s, settling initially in Ohio. Many of the children, grandchildren, and great-grandchildren of the first generation had married, so some now had different surnames: Stansberry, Kingsley, Prine, Daugherty, Ernst, Howard, Godwin. Starting in the early 1900s, a number of family members had joined the nation's westward migration, departing in search of new opportunities in California, Arizona, Nevada, and New Mexico, and had lost touch with one another.

The first step of what would be a long journey by Li and Fraumeni—longer than they ever imagined—came on September 8, 1967, when Li wrote a letter to Johns Hopkins seeking Darrel Kilius's medical records. (He and Fraumeni already had access to Ned Kilius's records because the Public Service Hospital where he was being treated was connected with the National Institutes of Health, the U.S. government medical research agency that oversees the NCI and other specialized health care institutes.) Li then traveled from Washington to visit Darrel's doctors at Johns Hopkins, in Baltimore, where he met Nancy Kilius. When it came to the family history, however, she couldn't offer much help. Nancy had been a member of the Kilius family for just two years, having married Ned in 1965. Besides, she was consumed with looking after her ailing husband and baby son.

But on that visit to the hospital, Li had a stroke of luck in also encountering Irma Kilius, the mother of Ned and a grandmother of Darrel. Irma had flown to Baltimore from her home in Oxnard, California, in early June, as soon as she heard Darrel had cancer, and had made several subsequent visits. A graduate of UCLA with a business degree, Irma was a strong-willed woman with a take-charge personality who had helped start and run a successful company selling office machines, Ed's Typewriter Service, with her husband, Edward. Though Ned's and Darrel's doctors at times felt she could be overly intrusive, Irma was determined to do everything possible to help the doctors save her son and grandson.

Irma wasted no time in trying to assist Li after meeting him. The very evening that she returned to California after a long flight, she assembled a partial family tree for him and Fraumeni and mailed a one-page letter to Li the following day, September 21. The genealogy she outlined showed several generations of two branches of the family, including her husband Ed's. It indicated that Ed's younger brother Charles had died of lung cancer, though her letter didn't indicate at what age. And one of Charles's three daughters, Joyce Kilius Ciafardone (a first cousin of Ned's), had died of lung cancer in her twenties.

But it was another name in the family tree provided by Irma that stood out most of all: Michael Howard, the first child of another of Charles's daughters, Joan. Michael had had a rhabdomyosarcoma soft-tissue cancer as an infant—just like Darrel, his second cousin. The letter didn't say—perhaps because Irma had mentioned it to Li when they met—but Michael's tumor was in the muscle in his right shoulder.

When doctors diagnosed Michael with cancer at age two in May 1962, they noted that he had the deceiving appearance of a "healthy, husky boy." But the tumor had progressed so far that surgeons removed most of his upper arm muscles—his entire deltoid around his shoulder as well as part of his biceps. The surgeon observed in the post-op report: "Prognosis of course is very poor, but good for immediate operation." A month later, doctors again operated on Michael to remove tumors they found in his lymph nodes, and they described his outlook as "very grave." He died on August 18, several months after his tumor was detected. Irma concluded in her letter, "We hope we have helped in some small way, and perhaps one day some common denominator will give you the answers."

Li and Fraumeni were astonished. Not only did there seem to be a lot of cancers in the family, but two second cousins had been diagnosed as babies with the same rare soft-tissue cancer. That was virtually unheard of. There are only five cases of rhabdomyosarcoma reported annually for every one million children in the United States.

Another intriguing (and important) fact: the two young cousins didn't live near each other. Michael lived in San Bernardino, California, east of Los Angeles, while Darrel lived outside Seattle and, then, a few months in Baltimore before his cancer diagnosis. Though it was far too early to rule out, this and the fact that Michael had died in 1962 reduced the likelihood that the cousins had caught a similar cancer-causing virus or been exposed to the same environmental risk.

It was an aha moment for the two epidemiologists.

If there were many things that researchers didn't know about cancer at the time, on one thing they agreed: cancer is a disease of the aging. Four out of ten Americans get cancer during their lifetime, a figure that sounds staggeringly high. Yet the number masks the fact that the odds of getting cancer in childhood are infinitesimally small. Before age ten, only 0.17 percent of children will develop any type of cancer—or, fewer than two out of one thousand children. And the risk factor doesn't increase much for many years. By age twenty, only one in three hundred Americans will develop cancer. Even by age thirty-five, the chance of getting cancer is still less than 2 percent, and that rises to only about 5 percent by age fifty. It's only in the later stages of life that the odds of getting cancer rise dramatically. Over age seventy, one in three men and one in four women will develop cancer.

The reason, scientists came to understand, is in the very nature of what cancer is. Although there are myriad types of malignancies—soft-tissue cancers, bone cancers, blood cancer (leukemia), skin cancers, and many more—they have one thing in common: bad cells growing out of control. It turns out that there are trillions of cells in the human body, and many are constantly mutating. But very few of those mutated cells become cancerous. Why? Because some cells are specifically programmed to regulate cell division and mutation, so the body is equipped to stop most potentially cancerous cells from multiplying out of control and becoming malignant.

As the body ages, this constant battle inside us between good and evil—the superior forces of cancer-fighting cells and the inferior but relentless forces of bad cells—eventually tips the odds in favor of cancer. It is simple math: with each passing year, the more mutations you have over time, the greater the chance that one of those mutations will grow uncontrollably and become malignant after evading the cells meant to regulate growth. By the time a person turns sixty, he or she will cumulatively have had to survive countless more mutations than at age five or ten or twenty.

Understanding this, Li and Fraumeni were determined to find what might possibly explain two young second cousins like Darrel Kilius and Michael Howard both developing rhabdomyosarcomas. But there still was a lot of work ahead to build a more extensive family tree with detailed medical histories. A handful of cases, and family members' memories of other cancers, are one thing. Records including pathology reports and medical case histories that could confirm the diagnoses and causes of death are another thing altogether—and would be essential for a rigorous scientific inquiry.

6

LI AND FRAUMENI PONDERED HOW THEY COULD TRACK DOWN ENOUGH generations of the scattered family to create an extensive genealogy. Fortunately, Irma Kilius's letter offered a clue. It mentioned that her husband, Edward Kilius, had a cousin who lived in Georgetown, Ohio, a rural community southeast of Cincinnati—though the two men hadn't been in touch for twenty years.

Starting with the limited list of names in the letter, Li began composing a batch of letters to anyone he thought might have the detailed information he and Fraumeni needed. The letters typically began, "The National Cancer Institute of the National Institutes of Health is conducting an epidemiologic study of a family surnamed Kilius which has an unusual family aggregation of cancer." In the days before computers and digitized data, this was slow and time-consuming work. But it was also easier in one way: laws hadn't yet been passed restricting the disclosure of sensitive patient health information or the release of vital documents like death certificates.

For starters, Li sent letters to two doctors of Edward Kilius, the father of Ned and grandfather of Darrel, because Edward's wife, Irma, had mentioned that he had had malignant skin lesions from his back removed a few years earlier, though he now was in good health. Li also had learned from Irma that Edward's mother, Cora Stansberry Kilius, had died around 1930 at around the age of forty-five, possibly of cancer—so he wrote to a hospital in Norwalk, California, where she had been treated.

Other letters went to hospitals in Phoenix, Arizona, that provided records showing that Edward Kilius's brother Charles, another son of Cora's, had gone to see doctors in late 1962 complaining of a dull soreness in his chest after several years of wheezing with a cough. Surgeons removed a malignant tumor in his right lung, but it was too late to be of much help. Just forty-eight years old, he died in June 1963. Li contacted hospitals in Reno, Nevada, and Cleveland, to get the medical history of Charles's daughter Joyce, confirming that she was first diagnosed with lung cancer at age twenty-three and died in June 1967 at age twenty-five.

The more they learned, the more pieces of the puzzle they still had to fill in. As they came across names of other family members from different branches—Florence Johnson, a sister of Edward Kilius's mother, Cora; Edward's married sister, Iola Kilius Kingsley; Henry Daugherty, a son of Edward's mother's other sister, Sena Stansberry Daugherty—Li would reach out to Irma Kilius for help in tracking them down. "I realize that it is somewhat unpleasant for you to have to dig into family history at a time when both Ned and Darrell are both [sic] ill," he wrote to her in early November 1967. But he offered up some encouraging news, too. Though her son Ned was back in the hospital in Baltimore, his doctors advised Li that his leukemia "is responding to treatment and we have achieved results in his case which would not have been possible a few short years ago." Even so, Irma and her husband, Edward, were bracing themselves for the worst. "We realize [Ned's] condition is terminal, and yet we hope," she responded in a letter to Li, while offering to continue to help him.

Getting detailed medical records of family members who had died recently—Michael Howard, Charles Kilius, Joyce Kilius—turned out to be relatively easy. However, others whom Li contacted for information about earlier generations often didn't have, or couldn't find, documents he was seeking. "Our records only go back 25 years and then we destroy them," Li was informed by Bethesda Oak Hospital in Cincinnati, where he had been told two siblings from an earlier generation of the family had been treated for cancer.

But with lots of forensic legwork, Li and Fraumeni managed to piece together a genealogy going back to the early part of the century and found evidence of more cancers. Again, Irma Kilius provided some key information. She dug out a handwritten letter from 1937 from a cousin of her husband's. It had the name of a law firm in Springfield, Ohio, that had handled estate work for some family members. When Li contacted the firm, he was told that a 1953 fire had destroyed the files he wanted. But he managed to track down family members in Ohio anyway, by locating a sale of property in county records.

While Li and Fraumeni couldn't locate all the documents they would have liked, what they found confirmed that not only had Edward Kilius's mother, Cora Stansberry Kilius, had cancer, dying at age forty-four in 1930, but both her sisters probably had as well—one of whom, Florence Johnson, born Lily Mae Stansberry, had died at forty in 1936, and the other, Sena Stansberry Daugherty, at twenty-seven in 1916. The 1937 handwritten letter also said that Edward's grandmother Minnie Mefford Stansberry, born in 1867, "wasn't so old" when she died of cancer as well, though the details couldn't be determined.

By November 1967, Li was able to advise a physician colleague in Baltimore treating Ned Kilius that "We have been able to trace [the family] back for nearly 200 years. However, since records of vital statistics have been available only in the last 80 years, I have included all the members of the family tree who died in the present century. As you can see, there are a large number of cancers on the male side of the Kilius family."

Still, even with what seemed to be an unusually high number of cancers, Li and Fraumeni felt it was too early to draw conclusions. As Li wrote to one family member while seeking information, "Malignant diseases are not generally considered to be hereditary." For one thing, some branches of the family seemed cancer free. The only son of Walter Kilius, an older brother of Edward's dad, wrote back after Li contacted him to say he had always enjoyed excellent health and that "My father died in early 1954 of a coronary while on a European vacation. He was 69 years of age at the time of his death. He had an unusually healthy life with no surgery or any serious illnesses." And what would explain why Robert and Raymond Kilius, the two older sons of Irma and Edward, didn't have cancer, while their younger brother Ned and his son, Darrel, did?

In addition, the complicated medical histories of some family members raised the possibility of other causes for the seemingly high rate of cancers. Li scoured the medical records of Joyce Kilius Ciafardone, who was just four feet, seven inches tall and weighed eighty-four pounds and had died of lung cancer shortly before Li and Fraumeni began studying the family. He noticed that she had had Turner syndrome, a rare chromosomal disorder affecting only females. It causes short stature, delayed sexual development, and, it was suspected at the time, an increased likelihood of cancer.

He wrote to Joyce's mother, Jeanne, that this "may help to explain the cause of her malignancy." Then Li added, "It is comforting that we are so far unable to identify any familial conditions in the Kilius family known to predispose toward malignancies. It is possible that the unusual aggregation of malignancies in the Kilius family was unfortunate chance occurrence. A family study such as the one we are conducting is often very difficult to do." In part, Li and Fraumeni felt it would be helpful to provide this reassurance to avoid causing undue alarm. But it was also because they still really weren't sure of what was going on.

As Li and Fraumeni continued digging, tragedies in the Kilius family mounted. Though Ned had seemed to be improving, his condition deteriorated in early 1968. He died on February 10 at age twenty-four. His mother, Irma, sent a letter a couple of weeks later to Li with details she had dug up about members of the Midwest branch of the family, adding, "We can't help our son Ned as he passed away Feb. 10th, but it would give us great satisfaction if we can help in any way." Li responded with a letter of condolence, writing, "Even though Ned is gone, we will carry on with our work."

Nancy Kilius, numb and distraught over her husband's death, returned home to Seattle and went back to college to complete her teaching degree. Though Darrel's cancer was in remission, she worried every time he coughed that he might be developing lung cancer.

The rest of Darrel's childhood would, perhaps remarkably, be cancer free. But it didn't take long for yet another cancer to appear in the extended family. In August 1968, Joan Kilius Howard Vance, just twenty-eight years old, noticed a lump in her left breast. She had already suffered the sadness of her first child, Michael Howard, dying of the rhabdomyosarcoma in his arm in 1962, with the stress in the family contributing to the breakup of her marriage. Her father, Charles, died of cancer the next year, and her younger sister, Joyce, had died of cancer in 1967. Joan's other two children from her first marriage, Gerald and Tamera (whom everyone called Jerry and Tammy), were healthy, and Joan had since remarried and, only months earlier, given birth to a new baby, in March 1968. "Patient has a miserable family history," the doctor who examined Joan for her breast cancer at St. Mary's Hospital in Reno, Nevada, noted in his report.

Though vaguely aware of the Kilius cancer history before the study began, some family members were alarmed by the mounting numbers. "Last night was the first time we actually charted the family and marked those with cancer, and it amazed us . . . one does not realize the high percentage until he sees it on paper," Irma Kilius wrote to Li.

Joan underwent a radical mastectomy on September 3, 1968, but would die in April 1969.

These explosive cases of cancer in the family surely meant that something other than random occurrence had to be at work, Li and Fraumeni agreed. But in line with the current thinking of cancer experts at the time, they wondered if it could be an unidentified and undetected virus that had somehow been transmitted among family members, only to surface sporadically over the years, even though some of them lived far apart.

On the off chance that lab tests on family members that had been collected over the decades by doctors might yield clues, Li started requesting slides with tissue samples from hospitals where deceased family members had been treated. To supplement this, he and Fraumeni also decided to collect tissue samples from living family members. After conferring with colleagues at the NCI, they dispatched a small team to Southern California, home to the biggest concentration of the extended Kilius clan. In a letter to Irma Kilius, Li explained, "Our colleagues in the laboratory suggest that a virus may have a role, since both of these tumors can be occasionally produced in selected animals by infection with specific viruses." Still, he added in a note of caution to temper expectations of the tests yielding a quick answer: "The significance of these findings with regard to human tumors is unknown. Despite intense effort, we have been unable to show that viruses cause human tumors."

On several occasions, Li asked family members if mothers in the Kilius family breastfed their babies. It seemed an odd query, but some lab studies had found that female mice transmitted cancer viruses directly to their offspring from their mammary glands. Though similar human cancer viruses still hadn't been found, Li and Fraumeni didn't want to rule out the possibility of an unknown virus causing tumors in children of the families. However, the Kilius women told Li they either hadn't breastfed their children or that they had done so only briefly, so this was dropped as a possible cause.

In mid-1969, about thirty members of various branches of the Kilius family traveled to the home of John and Janette Godwin, on a cul-de-sac in Orange, California. The family had moved there in the 1960s, at a time when the population of Los Angeles was growing rapidly and sprawling suburban subdivisions were replacing the once-vast orange groves that gave the city its name. Janette was the oldest daughter of Charles Kilius and sister of the now-deceased Joan and Joyce. She and John, a former football player at the University of Southern California, had two young daughters and a son, thankfully all of them healthy and cancer free.

To avoid alarming the children about the real purpose of the get-together, their parents billed the day as another family reunion. Some of the children thought it odd that they didn't recognize a few of the adults. The real purpose of the gathering dawned on them when the visitors started drawing blood samples and snipping tiny bits of skin from everyone's forearms. Some of the children scattered around the neighborhood, hiding until their parents managed to find them.

Back at the NCI in Washington, the samples were tested, but nothing unusual was detected.

Though the search for a definitive answer for the cause of the cancers was elusive, the number of cancers Li and Fraumeni counted in the family was stunning: all told, fourteen of thirty-five family members in the branches they tracked over five generations had developed cancers (in the lung, ear, pancreas, nose, and breast), and ten had died in their forties or earlier. Their sleuthing also indicated that the high cancer lineage may not have started with the original Kilius ancestors, but with Thomas Stansberry and his wife, Minnie Mefford Stansberry, who were born in the 1860s and had three daughters. All three daughters had died of cancer at early ages, and there was a high cancer rate among the children and grandchildren of the two sisters who married. But there was no unusual cancer history in the Kilius branch, not until a Kilius son married one of the Stansberry daughters in the early 1900s.

This indicated that any cancer predisposition, if there was one, appeared to have originated in all the branches of the family, including the Kilius branch, through the Stansberry line. This squared with what Irma Kilius had written to Li early on, in November 1967: "I can recall my father-in-law telling us that there were many cases of cancer in the Stansberry family."

As unusual as the extended Kilius family was, Li and Fraumeni knew they couldn't build a scientific paper around one family; it was far too small a sample. But thanks to the research that Fraumeni and the head of the epidemiology department, Robert Miller, had conducted earlier into childhood cancers, they didn't have to look far to find other cancer-prone families. Li and Fraumeni began sifting through the records already collected from seventeen hospitals around the nation; they also reviewed death certificates of all children under fifteen who had died of cancer between 1960 and 1964. They found 698 cases of children who had succumbed to soft-tissue cancers.

From this data, they identified a couple of other instances of two siblings in other families who had developed malignancies at between one and eleven years old. Delving into their histories, they found that other members of those families also had cancer. In a fourth family, which they came across while searching a national childhood cancer mortality registry, they found yet another set of young siblings with cancer; further inspection of those siblings' hospital charts also revealed a family history of malignant tumors.

Collectively, the rate of cancers among siblings in these four families was fifty times higher than in the overall population. And as with "Family A"—as Li and Fraumeni had come to refer to the extended Kilius family to protect their privacy—the cancers in the other three families (which they called B, C, and D) were varied; this set them apart from families in which multiple members had experienced the same "site-specific" cancers, such as breast cancer, which was among the few cancers at the time suspected of possibly having some kind of unknown hereditary connection.

As they began drafting a paper for submission to an academic journal, Li and Fraumeni agreed they needed to list potential explanations for the seemingly unrelated tumors in these families. It could be nothing more than chance, a statistical oddity; out of tens of millions of families in the United States, it would hardly be surprising for a handful of families to have multiple members with different types of cancer. Or it could be what scientists call referral bias: if you start by focusing on unusual cases of families with cancer, there is a higher probability of finding more cases than in a random sample of families. Or, even though Li and Fraumeni's tests for viruses on tissue samples from the Kiliuses were negative, maybe it was a virus they couldn't detect despite examining tissue samples.

Finally, though they felt confident in ruling out an environmental factor with Family A because some branches lived apart, maybe there were unknown carcinogens that led to tumors. Indeed, some of the family members themselves wondered if the heavy smog in Southern California might be causing the cancers, though this wouldn't have explained Darrel Kilius's tumor, as he had been born in Kirkland, Washington, and had never lived in California.

While putting the final touches on their medical journal article, Li and Fraumeni debated how strongly they could word their paper. When it was published by the *Annals of Internal Medicine* in October 1969, the title they gave it—ending with a question mark—reflected their hesitation: "Soft-Tissue Sarcomas, Breast Cancer and Other Neoplasms: A Familial Syndrome?" Fraumeni and Li had sweated and argued over the question mark. Li was the more conservative of the two. He insisted they simply didn't know for sure, and in the end, Fraumeni had reluctantly agreed.

Taking care to include caveats, their article still pointed toward a novel concept: "These findings suggest a new 'familial' syndrome of neoplastic [tumorous] diseases in which hereditary or oncogenic agents, or both, may have a causal role.... An inherited predisposition for these tumors appears likely, although it is premature to assign a precise genetic mechanism."

The paper drew scant attention when it was published, but it did intrigue a few researchers, like Louise Strong. Then twenty-five years old, with a background in mathematics and statistics and a keen interest in genetics, she was in her last year at the University of Texas Medical School. "I never paid much attention to epidemiology.... I was very surprised to see a department or branch, I should say, of epidemiology reporting on families that had these unique aggregations of cancer," Strong would later recall. "After the paper came out, and people saw it, there was the question of what is this clustering, what does it mean, what is it about, how do we look for it at our institution? It was a pretty vague description, unusual familial cancer aggregation, unusual cancer types, the 'unusual' word kept repeating itself. Multiple primary tumors in multiple generations."

But, for the most part, the hypothesis that heredity might be involved was greeted largely with deep skepticism. When Fraumeni and Li presented their findings, other researchers challenged them. Relatively little was known about genetics, and to have a genetic susceptibility to cancer was almost unheard of. The prevailing notion was that familial cancer was exceedingly rare and that when it occurred it was sort of a fluke. And in the few cases in the medical literature describing possible hereditary causes of cancers, they involved the same type of cancer, like breast or colon tumors. Some of the cancer research luminaries openly scoffed at Fraumeni and Li, telling them, "Why are you studying genetics? It's not important, genetics is not a major factor."

But Li and Fraumeni were undeterred—especially after learning, within weeks of the publication of their paper, of yet another childhood cancer in Family A. In November 1969, John Godwin, who had just turned three years old, was diagnosed with Wilms tumor, a rare kidney cancer. He was now the third young cousin in the same generation—along with Michael Howard, who had died of cancer as an infant, and Darrel Kilius, whose cancer was in remission—to develop a malignancy.

Initially, John's physicians had told his mother, Janette—whose two sisters, Joyce and Joan, had died of cancer before age thirty—that he had the flu. But John, once a chubby child, failed to get better and rapidly began to lose weight; tests determined he had cancer. He began chemotherapy and radiation treatment, with his two older sisters trying to assuage his fears by telling him he was going into a spaceship on days when he had radiation.

John, constantly sick from his treatments, survived less than six months, finally succumbing to cancer on April 27, 1970. His death devastated his parents. For more than a year, they insisted on leaving everything in his bedroom undisturbed. "If you do go in there, don't touch anything," they would tell his two sisters, then nine and five years old.

Despite doubts that these seemingly unrelated tumors might have a hereditary connection, the latest tragedy in Family A convinced Li and Fraumeni that they should keep following the families in their study.

7

I T IS HARDLY SURPRISING THAT A 1964 ACADEMIC PAPER ON "MEDICAL GENETICS IN Nebraska" got little notice in the medical world. The article was published in the *Nebraska State Medical Journal* in Lincoln, an obscure title edited far from top research centers on the East and West Coasts.

The paper didn't offer news about a groundbreaking lab discovery or new medical hypothesis. It mostly discussed a variety of diseases in some families observed by the University of Nebraska College of Medicine's "medical genetics research team"—a somewhat lofty description for a staff of just two people, a physician geneticist, Dr. Henry T. Lynch, and his assistant, a medical social worker, who were occasionally aided by medical students and consultants. The article listed more than a dozen cases in several families of a variety of possibly hereditary conditions, such as myotonia dystrophica, a progressive muscle wasting; atrial septal defect, a hole in the wall separating the heart's upper chambers; and a brittle bone disorder called osteogenesis imperfecta.

Seventh on the list was a brief mention of cancer: "Carcinoma of varying types has been shown to be present in an unusually high frequency in four families. Patients with two and three primary cancers have been encountered in some of these families. This work is in its early phase, and while a genetic etiology is possible, more studies will be necessary in order to further the role of hereditary factors."

The article, with Lynch as the lead author, offered help to referring physicians on cases of any illnesses that might involve inheritance. It noted, "Nebraska, with its predominantly rural population, is ideally suited for genetic investigations. Rural families often keep careful records of their kindred[,] which makes for rapid and accurate collection of data. In addition, several generations of the family are frequently available for study in the immediate area."

Conducting research in the relative obscurity of Middle America, Lynch—like Li and Fraumeni—was an outsider with an inkling that heredity had a far more important role in diseases, including cancer, than many in the medical establishment believed at the time. Then thirty-six years old, he was at the beginning of an improbable and circuitous journey that would make him a renowned pioneer in cancer genetics research.

Lynch had grown up in a working-class family in New York City during the Great Depression and dropped out of school at fourteen. Two years later, in 1944, he used an older cousin's ID card to enlist in the navy. He served in the European and Pacific theaters as a gunner, suffering permanent hearing loss from the concussive pounding when the artillery was fired. A towering figure at six feet, five inches tall and tipping the scales at 250 pounds and sometimes even 300, Lynch became a boxer—nicknamed "Hammerin' Hank"—after his discharge from service at the end of World War II and earned a high school equivalency degree.

Despite—or perhaps because of—his early lack of education, Lynch poured himself into academics, getting a bachelor's degree from the University of Oklahoma and a master's in clinical psychology from the University of Denver. He then began pursuing a PhD in genetics, intrigued about a possible hereditary basis for psychiatric disorders, before deciding to get a medical degree at the University of Texas at Galveston and doing his residency at the University of Nebraska College of Medicine in Omaha in the early 1960s. After Lynch started teaching, his medical school students gave him the sobriquet "dancing bear," because of his imposing bulk and animated lectures.

Lynch's interest in the role of heredity in cancer became a single-minded passion after a doctor at the Omaha Veterans Administration Hospital asked for his thoughts on a patient with a strong family history of colorectal cancer. The patient, who was being treated for alcoholism, explained that he drank heavily because he believed he would one day die of cancer, like most of his relatives. With the help of Anne Krush, a medical social worker who would become a longtime research partner, Lynch put together a family history, finding that many members of the patient's family had developed colorectal cancer along with, in some cases, other malignancies.

After making a presentation about the family at a conference of the American Society of Human Genetics in 1964 in Boulder, Colorado, Lynch was approached by a medical geneticist from the University of Michigan who happened to be there. She knew of another family with a history of similar malignancies. Together, she and Lynch worked with a team that reviewed medical records showing that the two families—dubbed Family N (for "Nebraska") and Family M (for "Michigan")—both had a staggering number of tumors over several generations, especially colorectal cancer but also a variety of other malignancies.

Lynch was the lead author in a paper published in the *Archives of Internal Medicine* in February 1966 titled "Hereditary Factors in Cancer: Study of Two Large Midwestern Kindreds." In passing, the article mentioned another cancer-prone family discovered in 1895 and followed for thirty years by Dr. Aldred Warthin, a pathologist at the University of Michigan. Warthin was one of the first to speculate that there might be "cancerous fraternities" in which "some influence of heredity" could be a factor. But with no way to prove his conjecture, his suggestion never gained traction in the scientific community.

Though Lynch's paper was published many decades after Warthin's, it couldn't point to definitive scientific proof of a genetic cause, either, as the field of molecular biology still wasn't advanced enough. While suggesting that heredity appeared to be a possible factor, the paper observed that "the mode of inheritance is not clear." And Lynch acknowledged—as Li and Fraumeni would in their 1969 paper—that the large numbers of cancers in the two families could simply be a chance occurrence or could have been caused by environmental factors. Or it could be a viral agent, Lynch's paper noted, as "The high incidence of multiple primary tumors in the N and M kindreds is not unlike that found in several animal strains which have been infected with the polyoma virus." Despite noting this uncertainty, the paper concluded on a hopeful note: "Intensive studies of 'cancer families' such as these may lead to new clues to the etiology of cancer."

Lynch was confident that he and his colleagues were onto something, but the article got little attention. Not only did it suggest the contrarian notion that heredity was more important than cancer experts believed, but Lynch was working for a medical school in Omaha, Nebraska. Surely, if he were a first-rate scientist, he would have a position at a more prominent medical school or research institution.

Indeed, to Lynch's consternation, word filtered back that some researchers were questioning his methodology. Though his article had been peer reviewed, and he had studied genetics at MD Anderson, the renowned medical center in Houston, critics intoned that his work was a bit too descriptive; that while there were many confirmed cases of cancer in the two families, a fair number were unconfirmed; and that, to put it bluntly, Lynch had been inclined to find what he was hoping to find, rather than using scientific rigor to seriously examine other explanations.

Despite the general skepticism, Lynch's article did catch the eye of the director of the pathology department at the University of Michigan. Would Lynch, he asked, like to take custody of the documents and specimens from the cancer-prone family gathered by Aldred Warthin decades earlier? Lynch quickly agreed and began taking frequent trips to Michigan to update those earlier findings, at times gathering at family reunions with members of what he called Family G—he said the G stood for "Germany," a nod to the family's origins, though it really was for the family's last name—who were still being afflicted with an unusually high number of cancers three-quarters of a century later.

Among the few others to show serious interest in Lynch's work at the time was a student at the Yale School of Medicine named C. Richard

Boland, who was writing a thesis on the high incidence of cancer in his own family. Boland's father, a physician, was one of thirteen children, and at the time an astounding eight of them, including him, had developed malignancies (mostly colorectal tumors), all before age forty-five, and two others eventually would as well. In addition, his grandfather and great-grandfather had died of colon cancer, as had other male relatives. He wasn't sure where to start, as so little had been written in academic journals about familial cancer clusters. One faculty member told him the cancers were probably due to bad luck or chance. But when Boland came across Lynch's papers, he sent him a letter seeking his insight. "This disease is running in my family," he wrote. "Would you help me?"

To Boland's surprise, a large envelope soon arrived from Omaha; it was stuffed with big diagrams of family trees Lynch had assembled. The cases Lynch had collected confirmed for Boland that he had picked a good topic for his thesis, as there were other cancer-ridden families like his—meaning the incidences of cancer might be more than simply chance occurrence. The experience, along with his own family history, inspired Boland to devote his career to searching for causes of colon cancer. Boland later surmised that it was because of Lynch's irritation and disappointment over the snubbing of his work in the broader cancer research world that Lynch had eagerly helped a lowly medical student.

Lynch's studies also slowly began to draw attention in the rural Midwest. Doctors in small and medium-size towns far from prominent medical centers often felt ignored and were keen, even desperate, to get advice for treating patients. Lynch soon began fielding telephone calls: "Gee, you know I've got a family here that I think may be the kind of family that you're talking about."

Encouraged by their interest, Lynch tapped this growing network of family doctors to build on his research. If a doctor alerted him to an intriguing case, Lynch's colleagues would mail envelopes with a thick questionnaire to extended family members to get their medical history and records. Then Lynch, along with his research colleague Anne Krush—and occasionally with Lynch's wife, Jane, a nurse, and their son, Patrick, who had joined the team while pondering a medical career—

would pile into a Winnebago camper and travel to towns in Nebraska and other nearby states to meet in person with and gather more data from cancer-prone families. The town's family practitioner—often, there was just one doctor and no specialists—would make his office available for the weekend. Ahead of the visit, Krush typically arranged with a family matriarch to reach out to several generations to make sure they would cooperate and show up, much like the role Irma Kilius played in getting relatives to assist Li and Fraumeni. With the family members assembled, Lynch and his team conducted free physical exams and counseled patients and the doctors on treatments. Like Li and Fraumeni, he always made sure to take skin and blood samples, creating a vast collection over time—with the thought that, someday, the samples might be the key to unlocking the cause of the cancers. At the end of the session, Lynch occasionally posed for a photograph sitting at a table surrounded by a dozen or more relatives.

As he found more families with extensive cancer histories, Lynch—like Li and Fraumeni—became more convinced that something genetic had to be going on, though he didn't know what. At one point, he applied for a research grant from the National Institutes of Health, hoping to delve more into the causes of what he was calling a "cancer family syndrome."

The NIH team reviewing Lynch's grant request visited Nebraska but turned him down, indicating that it had doubts that his findings showed heredity was behind the cancer clusters. Given that many of the family members in Lynch's studies were farmers who worked with fertilizers and pesticides, the NIH doctors suggested he examine environmental factors more closely.

Frustrated, but accustomed to rejection, Lynch scurried to get funding for his family studies from other sources, such as the Damon Runyon Cancer Research Foundation, named after the newspaperman and short story writer who died of throat cancer. Lynch wasn't going to be dissuaded simply because some self-appointed experts at the NIH and big-name medical schools scoffed at his ideas.

8

A T ITS PEAK, THE ANN LANDERS ADVICE COLUMN WAS SYNDICATED TO MORE than twelve hundred newspapers and read by tens of millions of people. The column typically would advise (and sometimes lecture) readers on how to deal with a difficult mother-in-law, philandering spouse, irritating coworker, or nosy neighbor; on other days, the columnist might weigh in on long-running household debates, such as the correct way to hang a roll of toilet paper.

But Eppie Lederer, who wrote the column under the "Ann Landers" pen name, skipped her standard agony aunt fare on April 20, 1971. Instead, she urged readers to write or call their representatives in Congress to support the proposed National Cancer Act: "Today you have the opportunity to be part of the mightiest offensive against a single disease in the history of our country." More than one million of them dutifully followed her instructions.

Lederer didn't mention that she had been encouraged to write the column as part of a relentless and skillful campaign orchestrated by a rich socialite and philanthropist, Mary Lasker, to get the law passed. Long an advocate for cancer research, Lasker had made it her life's mission after her husband, Albert, a successful advertising executive, was diagnosed with colon cancer in 1951 and died a year later. Mary Lasker strategically cultivated allies in the medical world, most prominently Dr. Sidney Farber, who had pioneered the use of chemotherapy to treat young leukemia patients (and helped found what would become the Dana-Farber Cancer Institute in Boston). Like Lasker, Farber had a keen sense for public relations, putting a face on the tragedy of childhood cancer by creating a charity he called the Jimmy Fund, supposedly named after one of his patients. (The patient was Einar Gustafson in real life, but Farber wanted to protect his privacy, and the name "Jimmy" had a better ring to it.)

Lasker and Farber were both frustrated that, despite decades of growing efforts by scientists to understand what caused tumors and how to treat them, cancer stubbornly remained the second leading cause of death in the United States after heart disease. Something had to be done. If America could land a man on the moon, as it had in the summer of 1969, surely it could solve cancer, they insisted. So, on December 9, 1969, the Citizens' Committee for the Conquest of Cancer that Lasker founded took out full-page ads in newspapers calling for President Richard Nixon to declare a "war on cancer." To pressure the president into action, the ad began with the challenge "Mr. Nixon: You can cure cancer."

A blue-ribbon National Panel of Consultants on the Conquest of Cancer was authorized by Congress, and Lasker used her connections to guide the selection of some of the group's members. The panel, carefully picked to impress Washington politicians, included luminaries such as Benno Schmidt Sr., the prominent financier who was the panel's chairman; Laurance Rockefeller, a scion of the fabulously wealthy oil family; Lewis Wasserman, a powerful Hollywood movie mogul; Mary Wells Lawrence, a Madison Avenue advertising executive; labor union leader I. W. Abel; and a number of doctors (including Sidney Farber, as cochairman) to enhance the group's medical bona fides.

The panel issued a report in November 1970 with a clarion call for a substantial increase in cancer research funding. "Cancer is a disease which can be conquered. Our advances in the field of cancer research have brought us to the verge of important and exciting developments in the early detection and control of this dread disease, but as a nation we have not put forth the effort necessary to exploit the full potential of these gains," the report asserted. It noted the comparatively paltry sum spent on finding a cure for cancer: "For every man, woman, and child in the United States, we spent in 1969: $410 on national defense; $125 on the war in Vietnam; $19 on the space program; $19 on foreign aid and only $0.89 on cancer research." While the report acknowledged that "the nature of cancer is not yet fully known," it proffered that there is "strong suggestive evidence" that viruses cause some human cancers, as well as certain chemicals and some types of radiation. Genetics didn't merit a single mention.

The U.S. senator from New York Jacob Javits, citing the report approvingly, announced, "We can do for cancer what the Salk vaccine did for polio," later going even further in claiming, "we believe we are close enough to a final breakthrough."

More than a few scientists felt the endeavor was not just unrealistic, but also recklessly misguided. Cancer was still barely understood. Rejecting the moonshot analogy, a distinguished Columbia University cancer researcher, Sol Spiegelman, argued, "An all-out effort at this time would be like trying to land a man on the moon without knowing Newton's laws of gravity."

Still, even in a year of deep divisions between Democrats and Republicans and fierce protests over Vietnam and race relations, the PR campaign was so effective that Congress approved the National Cancer Act with near unanimity, by a vote of 79–1 in the Senate and 350–5 in the House of Representatives. Nixon signed it into law in December 1971 at a ceremony in the White House with 250 guests in attendance—including Mary Lasker, who received a ceremonial signing pen from the president for her role in advocating for the legislation. With hundreds of millions of dollars a year in additional funding for cancer research, optimists blithely predicted a cure for cancer soon could be found, perhaps even in time for America's bicentennial celebration in 1976.

But Spiegelman's skepticism about the daunting challenges ahead proved prescient. Not long after the bill's passage, Nixon appointed a new director to the National Cancer Institute, Frank Rauscher. A renowned virologist, he had discovered a tumor-causing mouse virus in 1962 that was named for him, the Rauscher leukemia virus. That finding had provided impetus to the NCI's Special Virus Cancer Program, begun in the mid-1960s.

By the time of Rauscher's appointment, upward of $500 million had already been poured into the program, though it had not yielded any significant evidence of viruses that caused human cancers. But Rauscher still firmly believed the answer to the cause of most human cancers would be found in viruses, if only scientists kept looking—which the new funding would help them do.

As in any war, the top general determines the strategy—how many troops to deploy and where to aim the artillery. Rauscher, the new top general in the war on cancer, directed the NCI's increased firepower at viruses. Under his guidance, a pie chart was drawn up and distributed to the agency's scientists to illustrate the main targets for the NCI's research efforts: viruses filled much of the space, environmental carcinogens got a much smaller share, and possible genetic factors were given a tiny wedge, almost like an afterthought. When research money was doled out, projects aimed at identifying cancer-causing viruses got priority over other lines of inquiry.

Robert Miller, who oversaw Li and Fraumeni at the NCI's epidemiology branch, was none too pleased with Rauscher's dictate. Even though he reported to Rauscher, Miller made sure that Li and Fraumeni could continue pursuing their research on the role of heredity in cancer-prone families. True to Miller's contrarian nature—which he proudly displayed, with the framed cover of the *New Yorker* of a lone seagull on a rooftop looking in the opposite direction of the rest of its flock—Miller declared to his team, "No, no, family cancer could be genetic as well as viral or environmental."

9

EVEN AS GENETICS CONTINUED TO GET SHORT SHRIFT AT THE NCI, A PAPER PUB-
lished in April 1971 in the *Proceedings of the National Academy of Sciences* was creating a stir among researchers studying hereditary causes of cancer. Unlike Peyton Rous's discovery of a tumor-causing virus in chickens, its findings were based not on a laboratory experiment but, rather, on a theoretical concept from an inquisitive scientist.

The article, using statistics and complex probability equations, put forward an explanation for why children in families with a history of developing a rare eye cancer tended to get more tumors, and at an earlier age, than children with the same malignancy but no family history of the cancer. In doing so, the paper offered a new and compelling hypothesis about the role of genetics in cancer, or at least some cancers.

The paper was authored by Alfred G. Knudson Jr., a forty-nine-year-old geneticist trained as a pediatrician who, in 1965, had written the medical textbook *Genetics and Disease*. Knudson had attended college at the California Institute of Technology, just fifteen minutes away from where he grew up in Pasadena, California, to study physics or mathematics. While at Caltech, he had stumbled across a course on genetics and, immediately intrigued, decided he would study medicine instead.

It was in the 1940s, a time when genetics was so much an emerging science that he found almost no mention of it in textbooks, when he went to Columbia Medical School after graduating from Caltech. While doing his medical residency in New York, Knudson was assigned to a rotation at Memorial Hospital, where he spent time in a children's cancer ward. "How can these little kids—one, two, five and six-year olds—get cancer?" he wondered.

After getting a PhD in biochemistry and genetics, Knudson worked for a while as a pediatrician, treating patients, but in his heart he was increasingly interested in research. His 1965 book on genetics had mostly highlighted other conditions—mutations associated with sickle-cell anemia, immune system disorders like lupus, congenital defects that cause dwarfism—but it prompted him to leave the hospital for the lab to study cancer. Initially, he focused his efforts on leukemia, the most common childhood cancer. In keeping with the prevailing wisdom, he briefly sought to determine if a virus might be the cause.

But this didn't lead anywhere, so he shifted his attention to trying to understand the cause of solid tumors that develop in body organs and tissues. That's when his early training in physics proved valuable. "If an explanation is complicated, it is wrong" was a saying Knudson had learned from his physics professors. He kept their words in mind as he pondered what triggered cancer. It was known that mutations in cells were connected to tumors, but that a single mutation wasn't enough. Many experts estimated that it could take five, six, or seven different mutations, or "events," before cells became cancerous. But no one was sure.

It struck Knudson, who was then working at MD Anderson Cancer Center in Houston, that a good way to resolve the riddle would be to look at a form of cancer that would enable him to narrow down and even rule out extraneous factors—like a childhood cancer. "A hereditary tumor that could be found even in a newborn child must be as simple as cancer can be," he told himself, because the odds were very low that an environmental carcinogen or a virus might have caused mutations in a baby and led to a tumor.

Knudson zeroed in on retinoblastoma. A rare eye cancer found mostly in young children, the malignancy was especially intriguing to him, as in some cases a parent would develop the tumor as a child, and then his or her child would develop one, often at a very early age—and sometimes these young patients would develop tumors in each eye or multiple tumors in one eye. With this parent-and-child pattern known, it was widely assumed (though not proven) that retinoblastoma was one of the "single-site" cancers that might occur in a specific body organ in a hereditary form. But there was another tantalizing piece of the puzzle to ponder. In other cases, children develop a malignancy in just one eye and, generally, when they are a bit older. In most of these cases, neither of the child's parents has been afflicted with retinoblastoma, so these were believed to be a nonhereditary form.

Knudson asked himself, *What might determine the differences in children who developed multiple tumors and children who had only one? How might a hereditary form of retinoblastoma work genetically, versus a nonhereditary form? Could this help explain how cancer is triggered?*

For clues, Knudson determined that he needed records of enough patients to discern patterns between the two different groups of children with retinoblastoma—data such as the number of malignancies; the ages at which they occurred; and the time elapsed between the child's first, second, or even third tumor. One challenge, given how rare retinoblastoma is, was to find enough cases to do a statistically valid comparison. Often, medical records of "bilaterals" (children with a tumor in each eye) didn't include detailed family histories. Knudson scoured the medical literature and eventually found papers published in Holland and Britain in the 1960s that convinced him that, as widely assumed, retinoblastoma almost certainly occurred in both hereditary and nonhereditary forms.

But to understand what might account for the differences between the two forms, he still needed extensive records of many more patient cases to analyze. Luckily, he didn't have to look far. Sifting through archives at MD Anderson, where he worked, Knudson came across files kept by painstakingly detail-oriented ophthalmologists who had meticulously tabulated data on patients they had treated dating back to 1944—everything he needed, from the age of the children when they were first afflicted, to the number of tumors each had, to whether the tumors were in one eye or both, to their family histories. This gave him forty-eight cases of children with retinoblastoma, some of them babies as young as two months and many less than one year old. The cases were almost evenly divided between those with multiple cancers (thus, likely hereditary cancers) and those with just one cancer (almost certainly nonhereditary). Then, using a mathematical model known as the Poisson distribution (which can predict the likelihood of a given event happening over a period of time), Knudson calculated the statistical probability of how many tumors would occur, and at what ages. The computation was based in part, as well, on an estimate of the number of cells in the area of the retina where the tumor occurs, along with the estimated rate of mutations occurring constantly in human cells. When he compared what the model predicted with the actual data on tumors in the forty-eight children, they matched—including the fact that a small number of children with the hereditary form get only one tumor and 5 percent of children whose parents had eye cancer didn't develop any tumors.

From this, Knudson deduced the likely explanation for why children with the inherited form of retinoblastoma get multiple tumors and at earlier ages. Everyone inherits two copies of each gene, one from the mother and one from the father. He theorized that if a baby is born with a mutated gene on one of the copies, it would take only one other spontaneous mutation on the other copy of the same gene for something to go awry—that is, for cells to start growing out of control and become malignant. But if a child is born without a mutation in the critical gene, it would take two things to go wrong for retinoblastoma to occur. This would explain the higher frequency of tumors and at earlier ages in children with the presumed inherited form of retinoblastoma compared with the noninherited form. And his mathematical model showed that as few as two mutations in a gene—not a half dozen—were needed to trigger cancer.

What became known as Knudson's "two-hit" hypothesis was published in a paper titled "Mutation and Cancer: Statistical Study of Retinoblastoma." Like many breakthroughs, it was greeted with some skepticism, because it was based on a mathematical calculation rather than scientific evidence gathered in a lab experiment. Knudson hadn't proven—and couldn't prove conclusively—what specific genetic mutation was connected with an inherited form of retinoblastoma in a patient. And even if his hypothesis was correct, determining which gene or genes might be involved wasn't yet possible, given the limitations of laboratory technology at the time.

Still, Knudson's paper marked a milestone. He had set out to see if he could explain how one rare cancer, retinoblastoma, worked and had ended up providing a broader intellectual framework for understanding how inherited cancers might develop and why hereditary cancers can occur earlier and more often in affected family members who might be born with a genetic mutation.

Fraumeni and Li at the National Cancer Institute hadn't yet met Knudson, but they read his article with excitement and discussed it with their boss, Robert Miller. While the complex mathematical calculations in the paper were difficult to understand, even for researchers like them, the logic behind the hypothesis was simple and brilliant, all three agreed. They immediately recognized that Knudson's two-hit theory could help explain the high rate of cancers (including early childhood cancers) in the Kilius family and others they were studying.

Genetics might still be outside the mainstream of cancer research, but Knudson's paper validated their belief that in looking for genetic causes, they were onto something, maybe something big.

10

AT FAMILY GATHERINGS OF THE EXTENDED KILIUS CLAN, WORD OF NEW CANCERS was shared in hushed tones to avoid worrying the children or over-shadowing the festivities too much. But it was impossible to avoid the belief among them that the family was cursed.

Not long after the first paper by Li and Fraumeni was published, three-year-old John Godwin developed cancer and died months later. Around the same time as John's diagnosis, Edward Kilius visited a dermatologist to check out small growths on his back. He and his wife, Irma, were understandably unnerved by the lesions, as their son Ned had died of leukemia a year earlier, and their baby grandson, Darrel, had been stricken with a rare soft-tissue cancer in his arm. Edward's doctor removed five malignancies, all of them basal cell carcinomas, a fairly common, slow-growing skin cancer that is easy to treat when detected early. Fortunately, that was the case with Edward, and he was fine, but the skin cancers were just the beginning.

Just over a year later, in January 1971, Edward was having difficulty urinating and decided to see a urologist. After examining him, doctors initially diagnosed the cause as prostatic enlargement, not unusual for a man of sixty-two, Edward's age. Irma Kilius, who continued to send updates about the family to Dr. Li and to ask about any new research findings, tried to be upbeat when she wrote a letter later that year, telling him that "Our family seems to be getting along o.k."

But Edward's prostate problem got worse, and in early October 1971, a medical procedure by a new doctor found evidence of early stage prostate cancer—not long after another physician had told Edward his prostate was "entirely within normal limits" and revealed no malignancy. "The patient has a very, very strong familial history of carcinoma and in fact is in a study group through the National Institutes of Health," his new doctor indicated while writing up Edward's case history. Edward immediately underwent cobalt radiation treatment, five days a week for seven weeks. It worked. The good news was that there was no evidence that any malignant cells had metastasized.

Still, Irma was worried about what the latest cancer in the family might mean, and she wrote to Dr. Li expressing concern about their grandson Darrel, even though he had not developed any new tumors. "We have been told by doctors that no one has lived more than 12 years with rhabdomyosarcoma and, of course, we hope that our only grandchild will be the exception."

Irma's fears for her husband were realized a few years later, in August 1975, when Edward was diagnosed with yet another malignancy—a leiomyosarcoma, a rare soft-tissue tumor in the small intestine, just below the stomach. Surgeons removed an abdominal mass, and Edward underwent chemotherapy.

He wouldn't survive this cancer, dying on April 11, 1976, at age sixty-six, though, to Irma's relief, the end was less painful than it could have been. "He suffered just two days, which was a blessing," she told Li. But Irma, still distraught, added, "I have been in a state of shock since Ed's passing. So our family history goes on and on. Meanwhile, I am alone, feeling sorry for myself, but realize I have to go on somehow. It is difficult after 40 good years with a wonderful husband. Yet, I realize, too, that he lived longer than anyone else in the family and can be thankful for that."

Yet it wasn't just the Kilius branch of the extended Family A being studied by Li and Fraumeni that was being afflicted with new cancers. With Irma Kilius's help, Li and Fraumeni had tracked down and continued to follow members of the Daugherty branch, which had stayed in Ohio as many of their relatives moved west in the early part of the century. In late 1969, a younger cousin of Edward Kilius's named James Daugherty was diagnosed at age thirty-five with larynx cancer after complaining of hoarseness. James was the latest member of the Daughertys to develop cancer at an early age. His father, Henry, a first cousin of Edward's, had died of pancreatic cancer in 1941, when he was thirty-two years old. Henry's only sibling, his younger sister Berneda Daugherty Ernst, had her first breast cancer at age thirty-three and died of her second breast cancer at forty-six in 1958; and Berneda's only child, Phyllis Ernst Prine, had died of uterine cancer just six years later, when she was thirty-four. (Henry and Berneda's mother, Sena Stansberry Daugherty, had died at an early age of breast cancer, as had both her sisters, Cora Stansberry Kilius, Edward's mother; and Florence Johnson, whose name at birth was Lily Mae Stansberry.)

James Daugherty, a hospital maintenance worker, survived his first cancer in 1969. Then, in February 1973, he had what his doctor thought was a chest cold, but it didn't go away. In April, a doctor told James he had pneumonia, but he started to rapidly lose weight, more than thirty pounds. Soon, he developed a persistent cough and had difficulty swallowing food; he was diagnosed with an inoperable tumor in his right lung.

James told his doctors that he wasn't aware of any family diseases, puzzling his doctors, who figured he must be in denial. "The patient's father's side of the family has been investigated by the NIH for evaluation of a possible immunological defect resulting in multiple carcinomas and sarcomas. The patient himself denied in discussion any predilection to such problems," according to a write-up of his medical history. James began radiation treatment in May, but his cancer was too far along to help; just thirty-nine years old, he died of lung cancer on August 31, 1973.

Less than two years later, James's only child, Debra, began having trouble walking. A member of her high school's marching band flag team in Georgetown, Ohio, she would occasionally stumble and fall. Doctors initially said she had phlebitis in her legs. But in the summer of 1975, not long after she graduated, she was diagnosed with a spinal cord tumor. She was eighteen years old. The operation to remove the tumor lasted ten hours, and Debra then began intensive radiation therapy, spending months lying flat in a body cast while her spinal cord healed.

With so much focus on treating her cancer, no one realized for a while that she was pregnant, and her uterus was exposed to X-rays dozens of times. When her due date arrived, her body cast had to be temporarily removed so Debra could have a caesarean section, and then it was replaced. Remarkably, she had a healthy baby girl, and over time Debra recovered and was able to walk again.

When news of Debra's malignancy, in the wake of her father's death, came to the attention of Li, he wrote to her oncologist seeking details for his research: "You may be interested to know that recently several additional members of the family residing in California have also developed cancer.... We are convinced that the neoplasms represent expressions of some genetic defect."

The seemingly endless cancer cases were taking not just a physical toll on Family A, but a psychological one as well. Few things are as wrenching in life for a parent than losing a child. The death of John Godwin at age three in January 1970 caused tension in his grief-stricken family. His father, also named John, began flying into rages, distressing his wife, Janette, and their two young daughters, Jill and Jennifer. The trauma inside the family caused Jennifer, who was six and had been a good student, to have to repeat the first grade.

A couple of years later, the Godwin family moved from Orange, California, to La Jolla, near San Diego, to be closer to John's side of the family, in an effort to get more emotional support and to distance themselves from the tragedy. But it didn't help much. John, having seen his wife Janette's two sisters, Joyce and Joan, die as well as his son, was still having a difficult time coping with the idea that Janette and his daughters might develop cancer at some point, too.

With research by Li and Fraumeni still having no definitive answer for the cause of the family cancers, members vacillated between thinking it was just bad luck and worrying if the thick smog that often engulfed Southern California at the time might be causing the malignancies. Some in the family grasped for anything that might help ward off tumors. When Jill and Jennifer Godwin visited their grandmother Jeanne—whose first husband, Charles, and two of their three daughters had died of cancer—in Carson City, Nevada, she would pull out a "juicer" at breakfast. She insisted they drink a concoction of carrot, celery, and spinach juice because she believed a healthy diet might protect them from cancer.

The two girls hated the vegetable mixture. But they forced it down anyway, as they feared upsetting their grandmother and getting cancer.

11

ARE SOME PEOPLE PREDISPOSED TO CANCER? AND IF SO, WHY? Though occasional cases like the extended Kilius clan intrigued researchers, answers to these seemingly simple questions were still elusive several years after the war on cancer had been launched. On December 10–12, 1974, some of the best and brightest minds in cancer research gathered in Key Biscayne, Florida, in the hope of shedding light on the topic.

There was Ernst Wynder, who as a young scientist in 1950 had authored the first paper linking lung cancer to smoking. There were Alfred Knudson Jr., now a rising star in cancer circles thanks to his "two-hit theory" of cancer causation; Henry Lynch from Nebraska, still an outsider but no longer so easily dismissed; Anna Meadows, a pediatric oncologist from Philadelphia who was doing research on children who survived cancer; and, of course, Joseph Fraumeni and Frederick Li, along with a contingent of colleagues from the National Cancer Institute.

The conference was titled Persons at High Risk of Cancer, with the goal of focusing the discussion of what could be a sprawling topic. Over two and a half days, with few breaks amid dozens of presentations to enjoy the seventy-degree weather, speakers described their research and theories. But the scholarly discussions on cancer-prone populations were punctuated with intense debate and disagreement.

Some attendees pointed to growing evidence of genetic factors. "The question is no longer whether cancer susceptibility in man can be inherited, rather, how do susceptibility genes act and interact with environmental influences and how may gene carriers be identified?" asserted David E. Anderson, a colleague of Knudson's at MD Anderson in Houston. An epidemiologist at the Mayo Clinic, Bruce S. Schoenberg, echoed this, giving belated recognition to Henry Lynch for his studies of families with high cancer rates. "Other investigators reported similar families that point to genetic determinants, although environmental factors cannot be excluded with certainty," Schoenberg noted.

Still, while viruses were starting to share the limelight as the main cancer research, with environmental factors beginning to gain ascendance, some continued to express doubt about hereditary causes. A microbiologist called "for studies to assess the possibility that oncogenic viruses are responsible for certain combinations of multiple primary cancers." This prompted a riposte by Alfred Knudson: "Despite intense investigation, we still do not have one proven case of a human malignant tumor caused by a virus." Knudson hastened to add that he remained puzzled by the accumulating information about what triggered malignancies. "Viewing all these genetic and environmental factors brings us to the questions: who are the people at risk and what are the risks? Many of you will do as I did and personalize the consideration. I, for example, for the fact that I have one first-degree relative and seven second-degree relatives who died of cancer; that I have Scandinavian ancestry; but I have lived in Los Angeles, New York, and Texas; and that I have worked with radioactivity, with tumor viruses, and with children with cancer. I don't know what all this adds up to."

More than anything, a recurring topic was how little was still known for certain about the causes of cancer. In a summary of the discussions after the conference, Fraumeni wrote, "At present, epidemiologic studies of high-risk groups are often high-risk ventures: slow, complicated, tedious, expensive." Unstated by Fraumeni was that this description could apply to his research with Li, which had begun seven years earlier, when they happened upon the Kilius family—and that still had no end in sight.

Far from being deterred by the lack of consensus, however, Fraumeni came out of the meeting energized. Though many in the cancer research world still downplayed heredity, the gathering showed that it was finally starting to become part of the conversation, albeit slowly.

He and his NCI confederates wasted little time in planning a second gathering, one that would be a bit of a coming-out event for proponents of the hereditary causes of cancer. The conference, on the Genetics of Human Cancer, was held just a year later, in early December 1975, at a recently opened hotel in a then largely undeveloped part of Orlando, Florida. Disney World had opened four years earlier, but the conference was distanced from there—so far that one organizer likened the location to being in the middle of the Gobi Desert, surrounded by large tracts of empty wasteland.

But no one minded, because a who's who of cancer genetics stars would be speaking—Alfred Knudson, again; along with Anna Meadows (whom he would marry the next year) and Louise Strong, one of Knudson's young protégées at MD Anderson, who in 1969 had been one of the few cancer researchers intrigued by Li and Fraumeni's original paper; Henry Lynch and his wife and son; Mary-Claire King, a twenty-nine-year-old researcher at the University of California, Berkeley, who was starting to study women from families with high rates of breast cancer for possible hereditary causes; Mark Skolnick, also twenty-nine, an assistant research professor at the University of Utah, who spoke about how extensive genealogies of Mormon families could further the study familial predisposition to cancer; Fraumeni and Li; and cancer genetics experts from Japan and Russia.

As word about the conference spread that fall, researchers not initially invited clambered to get a spot on the agenda. "I've got to come to this meeting," many pleaded in calls to Dr. John Mulvihill, chief of the

NCI's Clinical Genetics program, who was lining up speakers for the conference. To accommodate as many as possible, he agreed to add a "poster" session, where scientists who couldn't be squeezed into the schedule for a presentation were allowed to erect a poster display describing their research.

As the conference unfolded, some researchers openly questioned the prevailing theories about the role of viruses. On the first day of the conference, after a presentation by Robert C. Gallo of the National Cancer Institute on viruses and cancer, Gallo was challenged by another prominent virologist and immunologist, Hilary Koprowski: "I am not so enthusiastic as you about the role of viruses in human cancer. . . . We still need much more evidence even to postulate they are viral etiology," he said, forcing Gallo to concede, "I do not dare to say that we have proven that any viruses cause human cancer."

As at the 1974 conference, a few discussions became heated, even contentious. At one point, Henry Lynch floated the idea of a national cancer registry to identify, and help treat, families with unusually high rates of cancer. This prompted one attendee to respond, "As a geneticist I have great enthusiasm for looking at the genetic background in cancer, but Dr. Lynch's proposal is a little bit frightening if I understand correctly. The idea of having centers all over the country keeping track of cancer-prone families, given our current state of knowledge, really concerns me."

Dr. Lynch, accustomed to (but tired of) having his ideas dismissed, testily shot back, "I find the lack of such a registry system frightening, particularly when you realize the work that goes into family studies and the good that can be accomplished through early cancer detection. The present cancer registries throughout the country have a paucity of information that is functionally useful to the clinical oncologist." Growing more passionate, he added, "In these families many of the members are extremely fatalistic, particularly the older people who have been saddened by the loss of so many relatives. In some families . . . the fatality rate has been virtually 100% among affected persons. Death from this disease should be preventable." Then, in a condescending comment, a Harvard pediatrician and geneticist named Park S. Gerald said to Lynch,

"What is acceptable in Nebraska may not be as acceptable in other parts of the country."

One presentation that got some of the veteran cancer researchers buzzing was by Mary-Claire King, of the University of California at Berkeley. A onetime political activist in her early twenties, King had been considering dropping out of science when a professor told her he had a project that might be worthy of her interest. On January 1, 1974, she had begun studying why women in some families had a far higher rate of breast cancer than the population as a whole. Families with high levels of breast cancer had first been described in medical literature in 1866 by French doctor Pierre Paul Broca. But a century later, scientists had made little progress in understanding what might be the cause of breast-cancer concentrations in families.

King, in a talk titled "Genetic Markers and Cancer," discussed how her lab was conducting studies to find possible genetic markers in the chromosomes of cancer-prone families that might help explain susceptibility. Like virtually every speaker, King cautioned against a breakthrough anytime soon. Progress had been slow, as some of the data were contradictory, she acknowledged: "Critics correctly point out that spurious associations may arise from inappropriately lumping together different diagnostic conditions. . . . It is evident that, although statistically significant associations between individual genetic markers and cancer do exist, they are for the most part relatively slight. They are not yet useful for the detection of individuals at high risk for cancer nor in the differential diagnosis of cancer." Still, she added, if any markers could be pinpointed, "The presence of the genetic marker could, of course, be detected long before the process of carcinogenesis is clinically apparent. If, in addition, the chromosomal site of the genetic marker is known, the location of closely linked cancer-related genes could also be estimated." In these two succinct, carefully worded sentences, King had conveyed the hope, the goal, of cancer genetics researchers: that, someday, their work could further the understanding of hereditary causes of tumors and help more patients survive and live longer.

Fraumeni and Li took turns onstage as well, both speaking about "familial cancer," asserting that cancer-prone clans could offer clues to understanding all kinds of cancer. Fraumeni noted that statistical studies had shown that "a small but increasing percentage of cancers are being recognized which exhibit patterns of inheritance. . . . In general, the risk of the same neoplasm developing in a close relative of a cancer patient is about three times greater than would be expected in the general population."

He conceded that this wasn't the same as identifying a specific genetic cause and—in a nod to the growing body of evidence on chemical carcinogens, including some studies he himself had done—noted that subtle and complex "interactions with environmental influences" might work in combination with inherited conditions. But there was growing evidence, he concluded, that "familial occurrences of cancer usually suggest genetic susceptibility."

Li's presentation described the medical detective work he and Fraumeni had been doing on cancer-prone families. After publishing their first paper on the Kilius family and others in 1969, he explained, the two had decided to continue tracking them. Would the family members keep developing tumors at a high rate? they wondered. Six years later—just in time for the opening of the conference—Li and Fraumeni published a new study after accumulating enough data for an initial answer: yes. Emphatically so.

They had lost contact with one of the original four families, but the number of new cancers was striking, not just in the extended Kilius clan but in the other two families, too. In the intervening years, "eight of approximately fifty surviving members of the three families have been diagnosed with new malignancies," Li and Fraumeni reported in their brief follow-up paper published in the December 1975 issue of the *Annals of Internal Medicine*. Overall, five of the patients with new malignancies were in their thirties or younger, and some had developed multiple cancers. Just as before, there was a variety of malignancies: breast cancer, thyroid, brain, larynx, lung, prostate, bowel. While still acknowledging that the causes "remain obscure," Li and Fraumeni added that "These findings provide additional evidence for increased susceptibility to breast and other cancers."

After he spoke, Li faced lingering skepticism over their hypothesis. Dr. Kurt Hirschhorn, a prominent geneticist at New York University, quizzed him, asking, "I wonder if this has been analyzed as to the possibility of chance." Li responded, "Your point is well taken, and you may be right. On the other hand, we identified those families for the study because there were so many affected cases.... But we really do not know what the mode of inheritance is, or whether, in fact, inheritance is a factor."

Still, at the conclusion of the conference, it was clear that the attitude inside the cancer establishment toward heredity was starting to change. A renowned scientist wrote about the proceedings, "The study of cancer genetics has come of age. At a time when major programs are underway to determine the environmental causes of cancer, it is important to review the genetic factors that interact with the environment to produce cancer." The scientist was none other than Frank Rauscher, the head of the NCI who had long downplayed the role of hereditary causes of cancer and had instead championed the belief that viruses were the cause of many, if not most, malignancies.

Not that it mattered to Li and Fraumeni what any remaining skeptics were saying. They were already working on the next stage of their research into families that appeared to have a predisposition for cancer.

12

FOR ANY SCIENTIFIC STUDY, THE MORE DATA YOU COLLECT, THE MORE PERSUASIVE
your conclusions. Li and Fraumeni knew their 1969 and 1975 papers,
based on just a handful of families, had too small a sample to counter
doubts about their hypothesis that the source of these seemingly uncon-
nected malignancies could be in genes passed from generation to generation. That might change, the two agreed, if they found enough other
cancer-prone families to expand their study.

After their 1969 paper was published, Li and Fraumeni had occasionally received calls or letters from oncologists around the nation about
families they were treating with multiple cancer cases. And colleagues
also alerted them to unusual patients from cancer-prone families being
treated at the National Institutes of Health Clinical Center in Bethesda,
Maryland, which often got referrals from regional cancer centers.

In the early 1970s, Fraumeni was helping treat a teenage boy from
Miami with an osteosarcoma in his leg. The boy's two brothers, Fraumeni learned, also had cancer; one had survived a spinal tumor and the
other had died of leukemia at age four in 1967. Fraumeni didn't know
what caused the brothers' malignancies, but he figured it could well be
hereditary, even though neither of their parents ever had cancer. Then, a

couple of years later, the father began suffering frequent seizures. NCI doctors ran some tests and determined he had a brain tumor. They then traced a long history of cancer in several generations of the father's family.

In other cases of young patients whom Fraumeni helped treat, he found that parents were in denial, having a hard time accepting that something inherited from them could be a factor in the cancers causing their children such pain. In one family Fraumeni saw, several children and one of the children's paternal grandparents had tumors. This meant it had to be the father, and not the mother, transmitting whatever was causing the children's malignancies, Fraumeni concluded. He asked the dad to donate a blood specimen for testing, in the hope of detecting a clue as to what was going on. The man responded, "Absolutely not. I'm healthy. Leave me alone." Then, six months later, the man contacted Fraumeni. He was now willing to communicate, but he couldn't speak because he had cancer of the larynx. Before they could get together, the man's wife called back and said her husband had died of lung cancer, a second malignancy he had developed within a short period.

Cases like these reinforced Li and Fraumeni's belief that some families might carry a hereditary predisposition for cancers. But chance encounters don't make a good basis for rigorous scientific research. For a valid broader study, they knew they would need a thorough review of new families to include. Finding subjects who fit the parameters of the original four families would require a systematic approach. They needed families with an array of cancers, starting at early ages and occurring over several generations—but with no obvious potential environmental or viral causes and no preexisting health conditions that could have made them more susceptible to tumors. Simply including any families they came across who had multiple cancers could inaccurately skew the results. Rather than erasing doubts, it could potentially negate years of research when it came time for other scientists to conduct a peer review of their methodology and conclusions.

How could they find families like these? For starters, they worked with colleagues at the NCI to put together a detailed five-page questionnaire for cancer-prone families, which they offered to share with other cancer researchers to enlist their help. The questionnaire was designed not just to identify families worthy of further study but, just as important, to winnow out families with extraneous cancer risks that might taint the results. It asked about everything: occupations, personal medical problems (liver, lymph node, thyroid, and lung and heart diseases were among a couple of dozen listed), medication, congenital defects, any family cancer history (including grandparents, parents, siblings, children, and "any other family members with cancer"), and possible environmental exposure ("to any poisons, chemicals or toxic materials").

Fraumeni had become especially well versed in environmental carcinogens and, thus, felt the need to avoid including families exposed to them in the hereditary cancer studies. In addition to teaming up with Li to study possible hereditary cancers, in the late 1960s he had helped conduct pioneering research that identified high rates of cancer associated with men employed at copper smelting plants in Montana. Then, in the 1970s, Fraumeni used early computer databases to spot unusual cancer rates by counties throughout the United States—finding, for example, that men working in areas with chemical factories had high rates of bladder, lung, and liver cancers, and that women in the rural South who used smokeless tobacco had a propensity to develop oral cancer.

Li, who had moved to Boston in the early 1970s to set up an office of the NCI's epidemiology branch at the Dana-Farber Cancer Institute, began recruiting medical students to help search for families, often starting with referrals from the pediatric oncologists treating those families. "We've got a family that has a child with leukemia and their sibling has an osteosarcoma," a doctor would tell him. Or, "We had a child with a soft-tissue sarcoma, and a brother who was a few years older developed an osteosarcoma. And then their mother had breast cancer." The doctors didn't know what was going on, but they thought perhaps the NCI doctors could help.

Not having time himself to sift through family histories, Li took out an advertisement for a research assistant. It caught the eye of a first-year student at Harvard Medical School, Margaret Tucker. She was looking for part-time work she might find interesting. When she arrived at Li's office for the interview, she thought he looked familiar. Tucker couldn't place his face until she saw a photograph on his desk of him and his wife, Elaine Shiang. Tucker and Shiang had lived in the same dorm as undergraduate students at Wellesley College, where Li would occasionally stop by to pick up Shiang for dates. Adding to the coincidence, Tucker and Shiang were now medical school classmates at Harvard.

Tucker remarked on the unlikely personal connection and immediately hit it off with Li. He hired her and assigned her to send out questionnaires. After reviewing the responses in the time between her classes and hospital rotations, she would call and interview families where at least two children had had cancer and at least one parent. It was an unenviable task because, in many cases, one and often two children had already died, and the parents were distraught. The conversations were often painful, but Tucker quickly found that most families welcomed the opportunity to talk with someone.

In their grief, the families were looking for clues to detect or, even better, avoid tumors in their remaining children. At that time, there still was little evidence that most childhood cancers had anything to do with genetics. So parents would ask Tucker if the cancers were caused because they lived too close to a highway, or maybe because they had been exposed to radiation. Many would say plaintively, *Why is this happening?* It pained Tucker that it was a question she couldn't answer. As gently as possible, she would tell them, "We really don't know what is going on. That's why we're doing these studies."

Tucker found the project so compelling that she occasionally skipped classes to call family members from Li's office at the Dana-Farber Cancer Institute, which was only a block away from Harvard Medical School in Boston. Often, getting the full picture required her interviewing twenty to thirty family members and cross-referencing their answers to make sure their memories were consistent. Someone would tell her,

"My first cousin had some kind of surgery. I don't know what it was, but I think it was some kind of tumor." To confirm the accuracy of the family medical history, Tucker would then request that person's permission to allow hospitals to release family medical records. In predigital days, getting the records meant writing letters to hospitals and then waiting for photocopies to be made and sent to her. Small hospitals in small towns at times often didn't keep the detailed records Tucker needed, which required her to go back to the family and find out if a different doctor was perhaps involved in the treatment, and at another hospital, which might have the documents.

Getting the full picture on each family could take a month or more—at which point, in some cases, Li concluded that the family didn't fit after all. It was slow going, but after a year or so, Tucker had helped identify an additional twenty or so families who fit the precise parameters Li and Fraumeni had drawn.

Now they had to wait. It wasn't enough that these families in the past had lots of malignancies. The question was: Would they continue developing a high rate of cancers? If they did, this would help Li and Fraumeni make more persuasive the case that heredity was a key factor in the cancers, and that it was not just a matter of "selection bias" (that is, the result of picking study subjects likely to prove one's hypothesis). And if the families didn't keep developing tumors at unusually high rates? Well, then perhaps their theory was wrong.

They knew this stage of the study would last for a protracted period. Even in cancer-prone families, tumors occur sporadically, often at long intervals. For a definitive study, it could take many years to gather enough data on the number and types of new cancers. The only thing Li and Fraumeni could be sure of was that science couldn't be rushed. They would just have to be patient.

13

THE 1970S WERE BLISSFULLY CANCER FREE FOR MY FAMILY. MORE THAN A DECADE after our mom died, she remained the only member of my proximate family who had had cancer. Her own mother and father were both in their seventies and going strong; her only sister, in her fifties, was healthy, as were that sister's two children, our cousins.

My siblings and I had graduated from college and were all employed doing things we enjoyed—Paul and I as journalists. I imagine a psychologist would have a great time analyzing us—or me, anyway. I followed Paul to college (the University of Illinois), then to the student newspaper (the *Daily Illini*), and, a few years later, to the *Wall Street Journal*.

When Paul was hired in the *Journal*'s Chicago bureau, I was working as a reporter for the *Chicago Sun-Times*. But encouraged by him—seeing how much he enjoyed the *Journal*—I applied there, too. Before hiring me, the editor in charge of the Chicago bureau, Richard Martin, first asked Paul, a rising star among the *WSJ*'s young reporters, if he would be okay with me working at the *Journal*. How would he feel, to put it bluntly, if I didn't do well and had to be fired? Paul didn't hesitate. "Of course you should hire Larry," he said. "He'll do fine." We both worked in the Chicago bureau for a while—causing confusion at times when people called to speak to Mr. Ingrassia, only to be asked, "Which one?"—before Paul moved to Cleveland as the *WSJ*'s bureau chief and I moved to Minneapolis for the *Journal*. Paul never told me about this conversation until years later. Like most siblings close in age, he and I had had our scraps growing up. But he was always looking after me, though I didn't always recognize or acknowledge it; as the little brother trying to keep up with a successful big brother, I was way too competitive.

To the extent that there was a bit of sibling rivalry, it was overshadowed by our sibling bond. At our weddings, Paul and I were each other's best man. Paul married Susan Rougeau, whom he had met at graduate school, and I married Vicki Johnson, my college sweetheart, whom I had met in a journalism class, and the two of them quickly became close friends. Vicki and I always got together with Susan and Paul to celebrate Thanksgiving and Christmas, and we both started families. Paul and Sue had a son, Adam, in 1976. A few years later, our son Nicholas and their twins, Charlie and Dan, were born just a month apart—Nick in August and the twins in September 1979.

As our journalism careers were taking off, our sister Gina had graduated from college in 1977 and taken a job as a special education teacher with a class of hearing-impaired children in Dubuque, Iowa, as she had learned sign language. Angela, the youngest, who had graduated in 1978, became a technician at an agricultural chemical company in Chicago; she quickly impressed her boss and was promoted to a demanding job in charge of state registration filings for the firm's regulatory department. In late 1979, Gina got engaged, choosing Angela as her maid of honor for the planned wedding the following August.

Life was good. Cancer, to the extent we thought about it, seemed behind us.

Then, in the spring of 1980, Angela felt something in her abdomen, a small lump, though initially she didn't mention it to anyone. But when it was still there a month or two later, she confided to her closest friend, Anita Borsdorf, who had been a college roommate and lived a floor below her in an apartment building in Chicago. Borsdorf expressed alarm that

Angela hadn't mentioned the lump before and insisted she see a doctor right away. Angela, who had always been healthy, replied, "I don't have a doctor," so Borsdorf referred her to her own doctor.

At the appointment in late May, the doctor examined Angela and did a biopsy, and Angela then headed to Wisconsin with some other friends for a long holiday weekend getaway. The next day, the doctor called Borsdorf, knowing she was a good friend of Angela's, saying she urgently had been trying to reach Angela and had left several messages, but hadn't heard back. It was in the era before mobile phones, and Angela hadn't told her friend where she would be staying that weekend, so Borsdorf didn't know how to contact her.

"Tell Angela as soon as she comes back to town that she has to come into the office Monday morning," the doctor said insistently. Sensing the urgency, Borsdorf asked if the doctor could tell her why. Hesitating, the doctor did something she normally wouldn't have done. She strongly suspected the tumor was cancerous, she told Borsdorf, and Angela would need surgery as soon as possible.

That Sunday evening, Borsdorf waited anxiously, watching for Angela to get home. When she arrived—having to walk past her friend's apartment on the way to her own—Borsdorf greeted her so they could walk up to Angela's place together.

"You're going to have a lot of phone messages from Dr. Ann," Borsdorf said; "maybe five or six, saying that it's important that you call."

Angela stared at her friend, then asked, "Do you know what she wants to tell me? Can you tell me?"

"I can if you want," Borsdorf responded. Angela nodded, and Borsdorf told her the doctor believed that what had been bothering her was a malignant tumor. Angela was shaken, but she tried to lighten the conversation by adding, "We need to name this something. What about Hortense?" Henceforth, she would refer to the tumor as Hortense.

The next day, a couple of months shy of her twenty-fourth birthday, Angela was told the diagnosis. She had a "disseminated liposarcoma in the abdomen," a rare cancer that begins in fat cells and, even then, typically occurs in older adults. All of us were stunned. The baby of the family, Angela had been only eleven when our mother died, and her age and sweet disposition made our mom's death especially painful for her.

How could this be happening again? And why her? Angela was single and just starting to spread her wings. She was a couple of years out of the University of Illinois, where she had majored in biology and was known by her friends for lugging around campus a backpack loaded with as much as twenty pounds of textbooks. Despite her demanding class load, she was an honors student, even while working part-time at a fast-food restaurant on campus and at a natural food co-op to earn spending money.

Angela's warm personality had won her many friends. She often reached out to ask how they were doing and arranged get-togethers during the summer or when school resumed. She chattered with them about her family (Gina's breaking up with one longtime boyfriend before finding the right guy; Angela's visit with my brother, Paul, and his wife, Susan, and their new baby, Adam; the news that my wife, Vicki, was pregnant and expecting to give birth any day to our first child). And she pondered the mundane (not meeting dateable guys, or having to spend ten dollars to fill her car with gas: "When do you think the spiraling price of gas will stop?").

Occasionally, Angela would confess to her friends about having a bit of angst about her future. She spent the summer between her junior and senior years of college working as a "field scout" in the small central Illinois farm town of Casey, population three thousand. The job entailed walking the cornfields and making observations about any problems she spotted in the rows of stalks. Angela said she enjoyed the friendliness of a small town and liked working in agriculture more than she had expected, but she wasn't sure it was for her. "I feel so undecided about my future that I want to have made some decisions before making commitments—and besides I've got a lifetime!"

Before the summer of 1980, there had been no reason for her to think otherwise.

Liposarcomas can be fast or slow growing, and Angela's best chance was that her tumor was slow growing, which she might be able to live with for a number of years. Perhaps because she didn't want to know the answer, Angela didn't ask her oncologist, Dr. Gershon Locker, what her odds of survival were. But he told her what he told most patients, to give them a glimmer of hope: "My goal is to enable you to live as well as possible as long as possible."

A week after being diagnosed, Angela was wheeled into surgery for an operation, with the hope that some of the malignancy could be removed. Our father sat nervously in the waiting room with Borsdorf, her friend. When the surgeon came out, the news was foreboding. Rather than being concentrated in one spot, the tumor was diffuse; the cancerous tissue was like marbling in a steak, spread throughout Angela's abdomen. "It's more massive than anticipated, so we weren't able to get out all of the tumor," the doctors explained. "It's a rapid-growing cancer." Dad started crying. First, his beloved wife, at forty-two. And now his youngest daughter—at only twenty-three? "Why didn't Angela go to the doctor sooner?" he asked wistfully.

Angela told her oncologists about our mother having had breast cancer starting in her thirties, but they didn't see an obvious connection. If Angela had breast cancer, an alarm bell might have gone off. But her liposarcoma and our mom's breast cancer, while both soft-tissue tumors, were different cancers, so they didn't seem linked. It was statistically unusual, the doctors acknowledged, for a mother and daughter to have malignancies at such young ages. But otherwise, we knew of no history of cancer on either side of our family. *Maybe it is just incredibly bad luck*, we thought.

Unable to surgically remove Angela's tumor, her doctors hoped to shrink the malignancy with chemotherapy. The cancer was advanced and had been spreading rapidly before they discovered it, but Angela remained hopeful. Though she was doing well at her job at the agricultural chemical company, she began thinking of changing careers. Concerned that our mother's cancer, and hers, might somehow have been caused by an unknown exposure to toxic chemicals—perhaps something our dad unknowingly carried home on his clothes from his research lab—she talked about applying to a master's degree program in social work at the University of Chicago.

Angela's friends had been shocked when they learned she was sick and not only because they didn't know anyone else their age with cancer. She enjoyed partying and going to bars, but she had a healthier lifestyle than most of her friends. *What the heck?* thought Susan Bonner, one of her former college roommates. *She's been trying to do everything right.*

Early on, Angela felt surprisingly good, despite the chemotherapy, and was her typically upbeat self. When Bonner unexpectedly visited her one day, Angela opened the door with a big smile.

"You look awesome," Bonner said.

"Yes," Angela responded without pausing, "except for this"—and she reached up to her head and took off her wig. She was completely bald, having lost all her hair from her chemo treatments.

Before Gina's wedding in August, Angela took a respite from her treatment for an impromptu weekend reunion with some of her college pals at the University of Illinois, where they enjoyed dinners and hit their favorite campus bar, Murphy's Pub. Angela didn't talk much about her cancer. While her face was a bit gaunt from her chemo treatments, with her wig on she otherwise looked like the Angela they knew. But early one morning, when she was still in bed, a friend got a glimpse of the toll the cancer was taking. Angela had taken her wig off at bedtime and was still sleeping. Her friend was shocked at how different and frail Angela looked, realizing for the first time how sick she was. "She looks like a little old man," her friend later told the others.

As Gina's wedding date approached, she worried about Angela. *How sick would she be on the big day? Would she have enough stamina to walk up the church's center aisle and stand for long periods as maid of honor along-side Gina during the ceremony? Would this,* she wondered to her fiancé, Michael Nystuen, *be the last happy time our family would gather?*

Though Angela's illness hovered over the weekend, the wedding was a joyous family celebration. At the reception, our dad, who once had been a heavy smoker and was having heart problems, raced around with a whistle in his mouth, which he blew whenever he needed to get everyone's attention. Angela didn't just hold up, but she even danced with our mom's father, Salvatore, who had come with our grandmother Elizabeth from Norwalk, Connecticut, along with other relatives.

But then it was quickly back to reality. Angela's longtime friend Anita Borsdorf, who had been accompanying her to chemo treatments and doctors' appointments, was interviewing for a job in Minneapolis that fall. Ever the loyal friend, she told Angela that she didn't know if she would accept if the position were offered to her.

"Why not?" Angela wondered.

Borsdorf told her she wanted to see Angela through her illness.

Angela drew a breath and replied, "I can't make any promises. I don't think I'm going to live." It was the first time she had expressed what no cancer patient ever wants to acknowledge and that some never do.

Angela did have one request of her friend, the kind of request that only the best of friends won't turn down. Angela had never had a serious boyfriend. "I don't want to die a virgin," she told Borsdorf. "Would you please help me find someone?" Borsdorf began calling guys among the large group of college friends they shared. Each, somewhat pained, responded that it didn't feel right. "I can't do that. Angela has been my friend," they would say.

Finally, Borsdorf called Angela's boss, whom Angela had a crush on. He was fond of Angela as a colleague but, understandably, he declined as well.

It wasn't to be.

Angela's last couple of months were excruciating, as it became obvious the treatment wasn't working. In the midst of her illness, our dad unexpectedly died, on October 4. He had been hospitalized because of a bad heart, but the condition wasn't considered life-threatening. Days earlier, Gina had called Dad saying she wanted to fly down from Minneapolis, where she and Michael lived, to visit him, but he insisted, "Don't come now. Come later. I'll be fine." Dad's funeral was all the harder because Paul, Gina, and I knew that Angela was getting worse. Even though she hadn't openly confided to us her fears that she might not live, we had a palpable sense that there was more heartbreak to come.

With my father's death, both our parents were now gone, so Angela needed the love of family more than ever. Unlike with our mom, we suspected the end could be near. We just didn't know when.

As the holidays approached, Angela jotted a note to herself confessing her deepest feelings: "Tears alone do not express the totalness of the pain. I have heard so many cries from my mouth that I never knew existed and wish I did not know now. My heart is shredded, I am terrified. . . . I find so much fear and all my hope is so strongly being diminished. Now at Christmas time, I dare anyone to force a smile from my lips or a gleam from my eyes. . . . Will life continue to be so horrible or does 1981 include a shred of happiness so desperately needed and achingly absent?"

By then, the tumor in her abdomen had grown so large that she looked eight months pregnant. In early January, she went back to the hospital, and in her final weeks, we gave her baths, delicately lowering her naked and swollen body into the tub. It was the only thing besides morphine that temporarily relieved her pain. Angela had one request of everyone visiting her: if you needed to cry, you couldn't do it in front of her; you had to leave the room. She had dealt with physical pain for many months, but that was one thing she couldn't bear.

Angela died at 5 a.m. on January 15, 1981. My brother, who had stayed the night at the hospital, called me at his house, where my family and I were staying, with the news. I was numb. I had thought there would be time for one last visit. Gina, then twenty-six, was especially unnerved and heartbroken. She was now the only surviving woman in the immediate family after having lost her mother and sister.

Angela was buried on a cold January morning next to our mom and dad. Before she died, she had summoned enough energy to do one final thing from her hospital bed—and on the day of the funeral, a handful of people received a note and a plant from her. Along with the plant, Angela thanked Anita Borsdorf for everything she had done, for being her best friend, for being on the journey with her. She sent Paul, Gina, and me, and some friends and her oncologist, a flowering plant with a one-word message: "Forward!"

14

WITH THREE YOUNG BOYS—A FIVE-YEAR-OLD AND TWO-YEAR-OLD TWINS—MY brother, Paul, and his wife, Susan, quickly came to accept that somebody was getting a bruise somewhere constantly. So when they noticed on Thanksgiving in 1981 that Charlie, one of the twins, had a bump in his left cheek, they figured he had knocked it while playing with his brothers.

When the bump didn't go away after a week or two, they wondered if something was wrong, and Susan took Charlie to their pediatrician in the Chicago suburb of Glen Ellyn. He and his twin brother, Dan, were laughing while the doctor examined him. "He's fine," the doctor reassured her. "That's just a hematoma"—a harmless sac of clotted blood that can be caused by internal bleeding from a minor injury—"and it will go down." But after they moved in early January to Cleveland, where Paul had been named head of the *Wall Street Journal* bureau, the bump didn't seem to be shrinking and even appeared a little bigger. Susan took Charlie to a pediatrician her new neighbors recommended.

By this time, the bump was the size of a grape. As soon as he looked at Charlie, the new pediatrician suggested they see a specialist at Rainbow Babies and Children's Hospital. On the first visit there, a pediatric surgeon told Susan, "Let's watch it for three weeks." Before long, the bump was the size of a walnut and kept getting bigger. On a Saturday night, a couple of weeks after that appointment, Susan noticed a little bit of blood oozing from the gums around Charlie's bottom teeth and drove him to the hospital.

The doctors drained some fluid from the muscle tissue in his jaw, and a few days later, they delivered the news: what other doctors initially had misdiagnosed as a hematoma was cancer, a rhabdomyosarcoma; in early stages, the two can be similar in appearance until symptoms, like bleeding, occur. Charlie had the same type of rare cancer that two cousins from Li and Fraumeni's Family A, Michael Howard and Darrel Kilius, had developed as infants—not that we or most oncologists, for that matter, knew about their research at the time.

Amid the shock and disbelief, Vicki and I, expecting our daughter Lisa at the time, immediately packed the car and drove from Minneapolis, where we were living, to Cleveland to stay with Paul and Susan and help them through this latest cancer crisis. Even as we all wondered how this could be happening yet again, just a year after our sister Angela's death, Paul and Susan focused on the most pressing questions: How bad is this? What is the treatment? What are Charlie's chances of survival?

Not good, his doctors said: perhaps 20 percent.

There are few things more tragic or dispiriting than visiting the children's cancer ward. Parents walk around in desperation, trying to smile and remain upbeat despite the palpable fear and dread. Bewildered children sit in wheelchairs or lie on beds in hospital gowns, bald from chemo and with IV needles sticking out of their forearms. Many will die despite their suffering, and the lucky ones who survive will be robbed of the carefree time of childhood. Given what Charlie's oncologist had told us about his odds, we could only pray that he would be one of the lucky ones.

About a week after he was diagnosed, Charlie went in for surgery. It didn't take long. As cancer tumors go, his was easy to operate on, and doctors were able to remove most of it by cutting into my nephew's cheek from the inside. But rhabdomyosarcoma is a particularly nasty cancer, as it can quickly metastasize to other parts of the body, most commonly to the lungs, lymph nodes, and bones. So the surgery, while successful, was only the first skirmish in Charlie's long and drawn-out battle with his cancer.

He immediately began getting heavy doses of radiation, directed at the bone and muscle tissue in his left jaw, to target any cancer cells in the vicinity of the malignancy. The goal, as Paul put it, was "to kill the tumor before it killed him."

Because Charlie was an infant, he was put under anesthesia for each dosage, so that he wouldn't move and so that the precisely targeted radiation hit the right spot on his face. Susan, covered with a lead apron to protect her from the radiation, sat next to Charlie to comfort him. After seven weeks of this radiation bombardment, whatever remained of the tumor had shrunken further, and Charlie underwent another operation to excise the remnants. Then he began what would eventually be three and a half years of chemotherapy, with toxic chemicals being dispatched on a search-and-destroy mission for any stray malignant cells that may have spread and established a clandestine cancerous beachhead elsewhere in the body.

Chemo regimens are nasty for any patient, but especially for a young child. The plan was for a week of chemo followed by three weeks of recovery. But it often didn't work out that way. The chemo meant to vanquish cancer cells also killed many of Charlie's white blood cells, which protect the body against infection. So he frequently had to spend another week to ten days in isolation in the hospital, receiving an intravenous antibiotic solution, with Susan at his side. Then, when his white blood cell count built up, he might get ten days at home before the cycle was begun all over again.

The chemo wreaked havoc on Charlie's body. He threw up often after getting the infusions and was soon gaunt and bald. But, to our surprise, it didn't seem to sap his spirit for long. At home between treatments, whenever he could muster the energy, he was determined to play with his two brothers and our son, Nick. Whatever comfort that might have given my brother and Sue, it also must have agonized them to see our healthy toddler and their other two boys next to their possibly terminally ill son.

Amazingly, Charlie beat the odds. But the heavy doses of radiation that helped save him also killed bone and muscle tissue in his left jaw. The cells lost their ability to grow, which meant the left side of his face would become lopsided over time, and he likely would need a series of reconstructive surgeries as he grew older. But it was a small price to pay for his life, Paul said, even though Charlie's appearance would increasingly bother him.

Only after Charlie was out of immediate danger and his treatment had begun did we focus again on why he had developed a rare cancer. Is there something in our family causing these cancers? If so, what? As best as his doctors could tell, it was probably, once again, a tragic, against-all-odds coincidence.

But the oncologists suggested that my brother, his two other sons, and Susan, and my son and I undergo skin biopsies. One day, we all drove to Rainbow Babies hospital and held out our forearms. The doctor pinched the skin together and then took a tiny snip; the surgical scissors were sharp, but the cut caused a painful sting. Then they cultured the tissue to see how fast the skin cells were dividing, looking for evidence of unusual growth. Nothing came of it. To this day, many decades later, a faint outline of the biopsy remains on my arm, where the skin tissue that grew back is slightly whiter than the skin around it.

We didn't have any answers for the cancers in our family, but we had something far more important. After losing our mom and our sister, we had won one battle. Charlie had beaten cancer, for now.

15

CHARLIE'S DOCTORS MAY HAVE BEEN PERPLEXED, EVEN CLUELESS. BUT UNBE-knownst to them—oncologists treating patients often don't have time to read the latest scientific literature—Drs. Li and Fraumeni were accumulating more data to prove their hypothesis that an underlying genetic factor could be at work in families like ours.

In May 1982, while Charlie was still undergoing treatment, the two doctors published another paper on the original four families in their initial study, having reconnected with the family they lost track of in the 1970s. Again, they found a stunning increase in the number of new tumors. "Between 1969 and 1981, in ten of 31 surviving family members, there developed 16 additional cancers," or thirty-two times the 0.5 cases that would have occurred among any random group of the same number of Americans over a twelve-year period.

Adding the new cancers to the ones Li and Fraumeni had recorded in the past, forty of the fifty-seven family members tracked over several generations had a total of fifty-two cancers; and a dozen of the cancers had occurred between birth and the age of fourteen, a startling number given how rare cancer is at early ages. Of the seventeen women in the four families with breast cancer, nine had been diagnosed before age thirty-five—or

53 percent. By comparison, in the overall population, only 3 percent of women with breast cancer are afflicted that young.

Debra Daugherty Armour, from the Ohio branch of the family, who had survived spinal cancer in 1975, had a recurrence, with a glioma tumor that had regrown from her spinal cord and into her brain. Just twenty-three years old, she died in March 1981, leaving behind her husband and two infant daughters, having given birth to a second baby about a year earlier. Debra had a life insurance policy, but the company refused to pay, saying the cancer was a preexisting condition. At one point after Debra died, cancer researchers tried to contact her husband, George Robert Armour, to gather more information. But overwhelmed with working full-time and looking after two little ones, he didn't get back to them.

Another young cousin from the Daugherty branch, named Thomas Prine, had died of a brain tumor at age twenty-four in 1973 (but he wasn't included in Li and Fraumeni's 1975 paper because they hadn't yet tracked him down, as he had left Ohio and was living in New Mexico). The young man's death continued the tragic early fatalities from a variety of cancers in his branch of the family, following his mother's death at thirty-three, his grandmother's at forty-six, and his great-grandmother's at twenty-seven.

Janette Kilius Godwin, a member of Family A, was also among those included on the list of new cancer patients. Her father, Charles Kilius, had died of cancer, as had both her younger sisters, Joan and Joyce, and her toddler son, John. Janette had managed to escape the family curse until 1980, when, at age forty-two, she was diagnosed with breast cancer and had a mastectomy. "For a while I thought the bad news was all over, but it seems to go on. . . . You will remember that her two sisters died of cancer at very early ages," Irma Kilius Swan, who remarried after her husband Edward Kilius died, wrote in a letter to alert Dr. Li to the latest cancer in the family.

Janette's husband, John, had become angrier in the years after their son died, and even more abusive toward Janette and their daughters. Jill, the oldest, had left home at eighteen to get away from it all and began doing drugs to deal with the family trauma. Though Janette, unlike her sisters, would survive her first cancer scare, she and John divorced after years of an increasingly tense and unhappy marriage.

With their mom getting cancer, Jill, now nineteen, and her younger sister, Jennifer, now sixteen, who as young children had watched their little brother die years earlier, were terrified. *Who would be next?* they and their cousins wondered whenever they got together. At times, they broached an especially sensitive subject: maybe they shouldn't have children.

Many in the extended family, including Janette and her daughters, were getting weary of being involved in the ongoing research project with Li and Fraumeni. It had been more than a decade, yet family members kept getting tumors and dying. Lab tests of the skin tissues and blood samples taken from Family A didn't detect anything, as the technology wasn't advanced enough to identify any anomalies. Being in a seemingly never-ending study was a constant reminder that little could be done about the tragedy that had befallen the family. Was it ever going to amount to something? Why keep participating if there wasn't going to be a cure? Despite their discouragement, they decided to continue cooperating. Someday, perhaps, the research might produce results that would help them.

Li and Fraumeni's 1982 study hadn't provided any conclusive answers, but it did underscore earlier indications that the cancers occurred among blood relatives. The tumors had started and been passed on initially only in the paternal line of two of the families in their study, and initially only in the maternal line of the other two families (including Family A); spouses who married into the families didn't suffer cancer. They felt confident in drawing two conclusions: the high rates of cancer meant it couldn't be a statistical fluke, or "chance events," as they put it; and the fact that spouses didn't get tumors all but ruled out an environmental factor, so their propensity to develop cancer likely was inherited, albeit still in some unknown way.

Though there weren't any cures for the cancers these family members were suffering, Li and Fraumeni did offer one shred of hope: with the knowledge of a possible hereditary predisposition for cancer, early detection and treatment could increase longevity. "Cancer surveillance should begin in childhood and continue even after successful treatment of one neoplasm. . . . Awareness of the family history probably resulted in earlier detection of four new cancers among the study patients," they reported. But this potential early warning didn't always help. A woman in one of the four families who had cancer in her right breast at age thirty-two was advised that she should consider having her other breast removed as a precaution, even though it was cancer free; she made a fatal decision not to. "She declined the procedure," they wrote, "and died of a second cancer in the opposite breast six years later."

The research by Li and Fraumeni finally was starting to garner more respect and attention, though many questions remained unanswered about the role of heredity in cancer. In a chapter titled "Genetic Factors" that Fraumeni contributed to the 1982 edition of *Cancer Medicine*, a reference book by leading experts on the evolving scientific knowledge of cancer, he was careful not to state more than what was known. While asserting there was evidence for "susceptibility genes" that might cause cancer, he wrote, "In experimental animals there is considerable evidence that genetic factors influence the incidence of cancer. . . . In human cancers, the contribution of genetic determinants is less evident, and often difficult to distinguish from environmental influences." He added, "Evidence for genetic mediation may be too subtle for detection by ordinary clinical and epidemiological means."

That same year, English cancer researchers who also were studying families with high levels of cancer published a paper that credited Li and Fraumeni for their groundbreaking work by naming the suspected syndrome after them for the first time. The article they wrote for the *Journal of Medical Genetics* was titled, "Two Families with the Li-Fraumeni Cancer Family Syndrome." Before then, it had been referred to simply as either a "cancer family syndrome" or SBLA syndrome, the initials for "sarcoma, breast, leukemia, and adrenal gland tumors," four of the main cancers associated with the puzzling syndrome at the time. For most scientists, this would have been an honor. And it was for Fraumeni, who was touched upon being greeted at a cancer conference in Manchester, England, by other researchers wearing sweaters and T-shirts emblazoned with the words "Li-Fraumeni Syndrome."

Li, while proud of the recognition, was less enamored. "In Chinese culture," he confided to another cancer researcher, "it isn't good to have a disease named after you."

16

L IKE MANY AMBITIOUS YOUNG CANCER RESEARCHERS IN THE EARLY 1970S, J. Michael Bishop and Harold E. Varmus at the University of California at San Francisco chose to study the role of viruses in causing malignancies. Each had ended up in a research lab only after taking a bit of a meandering journey.

Bishop went to Gettysburg College with the plan to be a physician, but he was tempted along the way to become a historian, philosopher, or novelist, not a scientific researcher. Preference tests he took suggested he would make a good journalist, musician, or forest ranger. In the end, he decided to stick with his chemistry major, though, by his own admission, he graduated "with diffidence and the bare minimum of credits." While attending medical school at Harvard University, Bishop found himself drawn to the "glamour and intrigue of molecular biology." After getting his medical degree, he joined the National Institutes of Health, but soon was lured away by the University of California, San Francisco. Though it wasn't recognized as a top research institution at the time, he figured a young scientist would have more opportunity to make his mark there.

Varmus, like Bishop, had entered college, at Amherst, initially thinking he wanted to become a doctor, following in his father's footsteps. But as an undergraduate, he switched to studying English literature, though he did take a class in organic chemistry, which his faculty adviser counseled he should leave, because he was doing poorly, a suggestion Varmus ignored. After getting his undergraduate degree, he next got a master's degree in English at Harvard. Only then did he again change his mind and decide to become a doctor after all. After being rejected twice by Harvard Medical School—one interviewer told him he should join the army because of a lack of "focus"—he managed to get into Columbia Medical School.

In 1969, not long after completing his hospital residency and toward the end of a stint at the NIH in Bethesda, Varmus went on a backpacking trip to California; while there, he visited the UCSF lab where Bishop had begun working the year before and said he would like to join Bishop to conduct postdoctoral research. Bishop agreed, later recounting that "Judging from the length of his beard, I figured he was the kind of free spirit who would do well."

For one of their projects, Bishop and Varmus decided to conduct an experiment on viral cells that were believed to have a role in causing cancer. The hypothesis was that viral genes inserted themselves into normal cells and, in so doing, carried cancer-causing material. The virus they studied was the Rous sarcoma virus—the same virus that Peyton Rous, in 1911, had found caused cancer in chickens, work for which he subsequently won his Nobel Prize. Using the latest molecular biology laboratory techniques, Bishop and Varmus expected their experiment to prove that the viral cells had left their genetic trace in normal cells that then became cancerous.

To their surprise, they found something altogether different. The oncogene (or cancer-causing gene) in the Rous sarcoma virus actually was a normal cellular gene gone awry, and not a viral gene. The study Bishop and Varmus published in 1976 showed that the seeds of cancer were embedded in our normal genetic makeup. The viral gene, rather than causing cancer, simply carried the oncogene that was responsible for controlling cell growth and division, resulting in cancer when a mutation enabled cells to grow unrestrained—though why such mutations occurred still wasn't clear.

The startling finding (which would win Bishop and Varmus a Nobel Prize in 1989) helped change the direction of cancer research by challenging the long-held belief that most cancers are caused by viruses. While some are, it turned out that the vast majority of tumors had nothing to do with viruses. Scientists over a couple of decades had spent hundreds of millions of dollars trying to prove something that wasn't true. But, ironically, the money hadn't been totally wasted, as Bishop and Varmus were using research dollars from the NIH virology project for the experiment that would undercut the prevailing theory about viruses and cancer.

With that, more attention started to focus on other causes of cancer, such as environmental carcinogens and diet, and slowly, on the hypotheses promoted by pioneers such as Li, Fraumeni, Knudson, and Lynch on possible hereditary causes of cancer. In the wake of the groundbreaking research by Bishop and Varmus, other scientists began racing to look for potentially cancer-causing suspects lurking among our normal cells. In particular, researchers wondered if there were any genes that could be identified as oncogenes—specific genes that were often found in malignant tumors.

Remarkably, two researchers working independently, one in the United States and one in Great Britain, in the late 1970s zeroed in at the same time on the same gene that seemed to appear often in cancer cells. It was named *TP53*, for a protein (p53) produced by a gene that had a molecular weight of 53,000 hydrogen atoms, hence its name. One of the studies, from the laboratory of Arnold Levine at Princeton University, was reported in the May 1979 issue of *Cell*; the other came from a group led by David Lane at the Imperial Cancer Research Fund in London and was reported in the March 15, 1979, issue of *Nature*.

The p53 gene (technically *TP53*, though commonly called the p53 gene) was notably present when normal cells in hamsters and mice were transformed into cancer cells, the researchers found. "The role of this protein in transformation is unclear at present," noted the paper by Levine, whose work—like that of Bishop and Varmus—was an outgrowth of previous research begun on viruses and cancer.

The finding, while intriguing, posed more questions that scientists couldn't yet answer and sparked a spirited debate over p53's importance. What was the purpose of the p53 gene? Did it, as some researchers suspected, play a central role in causing cancer, perhaps by propagating rapidly growing cancer cells? Or was it, as others believed, just a bystander, a benign gene whose presence was merely incidental? Only a deeper understanding would determine who was right. Though it would take more lab work—much more—to find the answer, the discovery added to the growing excitement among scientists that further research could provide important clues about what causes cancer.

Perhaps more important than any individual finding, the growing lab work by Varmus, Bishop, Levine, Lane, and others was starting to bring the role of genetics in cancer to the forefront—a sea change from the late 1960s and early '70s, when skepticism about heredity was widespread. After decades of flailing about, scientists were starting to have a greater understanding of the human genome, aided by improved lab technology, as they sought to shine a light on the "black box" that cancer long had been.

The next challenge was determining if a specific inherited genetic mutation could be connected to a specific type of malignancy. Whoever got there first would be guaranteed a prominent place in the annals of cancer research. There were several potential targets, particularly cancers that came in presumed hereditary forms, including breast cancer and colon cancer, which statistically had been shown to occur at much higher rates in certain families. But one team of scientists turned their attention to retinoblastoma, the eye cancer in children that Alfred Knudson had used to develop his "two-hit" hypothesis in 1971, a concept that was finally validated by other scientists in the early 1980s.

Scientists had come to understand that there are two types of genetic mutations that can occur in cells: inherited, germline mutations carried in all the cells of a person born with the defect (and that can be passed on from parents to children) and sporadic, spontaneous somatic mutations that are constantly occurring in cells and often are harmless and aren't passed on. New experiments had proven Knudson's hypothesis that when there was just one mutation in a specific area of a chromosome (the structure inside cells that contains genes), a person would not get retinoblastoma cancer. But a second abnormality on a second, complementary chromosome fragment led to a malignancy. So if a person is born with an inherited mutation, that means only one more event, or mutation, can trigger cancer; in the noninherited form of retinoblastoma or other cancers, two random, somatic mutations in a gene must occur.

This knowledge added support to Knudson's idea that the affected, or mutated, retinoblastoma gene was paired with a normal or good copy of the same gene called an anti-oncogene, or a "cancer suppressor" gene, that somehow blocked cancer from occurring in its normal condition. When the good copy of the gene also developed a defect, however, the combination of mutations in both genes contributed to cancer formation.

But every chromosome contains hundreds to several thousand genes, and researchers had not determined precisely what gene within the chromosome contained the flaw that led to retinoblastoma. And finding the one gene that was the culprit would be a daunting task.

The effort to identify it began in 1985, when a thirty-one-year-old research oncologist, Dr. Stephen H. Friend, showed up at the Whitehead Institute for Biomedical Research, a laboratory headed by Robert Weinberg, a prominent researcher at the Massachusetts Institute of Technology known for his work on cancer-causing genes. Friend had majored in philosophy at Indiana University, with the idea of pursuing a career in medical ethics, but he decided he needed to become a doctor to fully understand the complicated issues they face in treating patients. He got a medical degree and a PhD in biochemistry and then became a pediatric oncology resident at Children's Hospital in Philadelphia, where he met Alfred Knudson and Knudson's wife, Anna Meadows, also a prominent cancer researcher. One day, while Friend was on duty, a father walked in with his year-and-a-half-old son. The dad was missing an eye from retinoblastoma, and the child had retinoblastoma, so it was clearly a hereditary form of the cancer. "I know I gave this to my son," the anguished father said. From that moment, Friend vowed he would work to find the cause of retinoblastoma.

Friend informed Weinberg that he would like to work on identifying the gene for retinoblastoma. Key to making this possible was a lab technique called Southern blot analysis, named after Edwin Southern, the Scottish molecular biologist who developed it in the mid-1970s. The method was at the time rudimentary and laborious, and tricky to master; an article published in an academic journal in 1987 contained ten pages of detailed instructions to describe the multiple steps for lab workers to follow. But it was a revolutionary advance in molecular biology because it allowed scientists to examine specific fragments of DNA, the molecular structure inside our cells that carries detailed genetic information governing how our bodies develop and function.

Scientists start by using an enzyme to "cut" the targeted DNA fragment they want to analyze. Then an electrical charge moves the fragments through a gel (a sheet of Jell-O-like material), separating them by length and into strands. Blotting paper (giving the process its name) is then applied to lift these fragments off the gel, and they are treated with a radioactive probe so segments of the DNA fragments can be exposed on X-ray film.

Completing all the steps took a day or so, and scientists had to be careful to avoid contamination. When the procedure was performed correctly, the end result was a series of columns on a sheet of film with what appeared to the untrained eye to be an indecipherable jumble of short lines or even smudges. But for trained scientists, the image enabled them to peer inside a specific gene in a person's body—and compare a gene from one person to the same gene from another person. So, for example, they could use snippets of DNA from patients with retinoblastoma and juxtapose them to snippets of the same DNA fragments of cells from people who were cancer free, and see any differences—and thus look for a mutation in a gene from the cancer patients that might have caused their tumors. This method is called gene sequencing because it involves looking at the sequences, or the position, in which those fragments occur within a DNA snippet.

Weinberg was impressed with Friend's determination and intrigued by his ambition. But he also was skeptical that Friend could achieve his goal. "That's all very good, but you don't know how to clone genes," he replied, referring to the gene sequencing process. Assuming they could find someone who was proficient in cloning individual genes, there was another obstacle. Where would they start looking among the thousands of genes?

Serendipitously, another young researcher, named Thaddeus Dryja, was working at the Massachusetts Eye and Ear infirmary, a short one-mile walk across the Longfellow Bridge over the Charles River from Weinberg's lab. Dryja, who had treated some patients suffering from retinoblastoma tumors, had kept samples of their tissues. The two decided to collaborate, and they recruited a colleague from Weinberg's lab who knew how to use molecular biology methods to isolate specific genes. They focused their search on a particular chromosome that had been identified by other scientists as a likely place for the defective gene. But the chromosome was large, containing upward of a thousand genes, which would make it difficult to home in on the one with an inherited mutation they could link to retinoblastoma.

Building on existing research by Dryja and others, and with a bit of luck, they made an informed choice to focus their search on the area of the chromosome where the mutated gene was indeed located. After months of laboratory work, comparing genes from normal retinal cells with those from patients with retinoblastoma, they managed to isolate the mutated gene—the first time a single gene predisposing someone to cancer had been identified.

Just as important as locating the *Rb* gene (short for "retinoblastoma"), they determined that it actually wasn't an oncogene, or cancer-causing gene. Rather, it was a mutation in what they called an antioncogene—the first identified tumor suppressor gene that had the power to prevent potentially cancerous cells from forming malignant tumors. A normal, functioning tumor suppressor gene detects potential cancer cells and either repairs or causes the death of these bad cells before a malignancy can develop. But the mutation they discovered prevented the *Rb* tumor suppressor gene from doing its usual job.

In the October 16, 1986, issue of *Nature*, the Weinberg-Friend-Dryja team reported their groundbreaking finding, which the *New York Times* covered with a front-page story. The news ricocheted around the cancer research world. If a mutated gene predisposed a person to the inherited form of retinoblastoma, there must be similar mutations linked to other types of malignancies. And perhaps there were other tumor suppressor genes linked to other cancers that, when mutated, couldn't perform their task properly. Sure enough, in 1987, a team of researchers identified a defect on a chromosome (though not the exact gene) believed to be connected with many colon cancers; the finding confirmed what Henry Lynch in Nebraska had suggested two decades earlier, in the 1960s, only to be dismissed at the time by many others in the cancer research world.

Even up to that point, Lynch at times would be greeted with polite condescension when he went to medical conferences and described his research of families riddled with colon cancer. "These are interesting families, but you must be just finding black swans every once in a while," he would be told, a reference to very rare occurrences in nature. Now, however, there was overwhelming evidence that the skeptics had been wrong. Inspired by the discoveries, and armed with more sophisticated laboratory equipment and techniques, scientists began racing to find other genetic defects linked to cancer.

Li and Fraumeni had keenly followed these developments. Nearly two decades after their original 1969 paper, their pioneering work on the genetics of cancer was starting to be widely lauded—and their goals were becoming more ambitious. In 1987, Li was invited to give the keynote lecture at an international symposium on cancer research in Tokyo. In addition to the twenty-four cancer-prone families in their latest study that wasn't yet completed, he noted, only twenty-one other families had been reported in academic literature with what seemed like a similar syndrome. "Why have we pursued studies of this rare syndrome for nearly two decades? The disorder affects only a few families and has almost no public health impact," he said. "The reason is that several major forms of childhood cancer are involved and that another component, breast cancer, is the commonest neoplasm among women in many parts of the world. . . . Our approach is to study the rare, but hopefully informative, families with this cancer syndrome to gain new insights into genetic mechanisms involved in breast cancer and childhood neoplasms in general." What began as a study of four unusual family histories was beginning to provide a deeper understanding of cancer and its causes.

Li and Fraumeni's original premise was strengthened even more in September 1988, when they published "A Cancer Family Syndrome in Twenty-four Kindreds" on their findings on the expanded group of families they had been tracking for more than a decade. By every statistical measure, the rates of cancers in these families continued to be far higher and the tumors occurred much earlier in life than in the overall population. By age seventy, 90 percent of these high-risk family members had developed cancer—many different kinds of tumors among them, with some members experiencing multiple malignancies—more than double the 40 percent lifetime rate of cancer in the United States. Even more, a staggering 79 percent of the cancers in these families occurred before a person was forty-five, versus less than 10 percent in the population overall.

Despite these overwhelming numbers, Li lamented in his lecture in Tokyo, his and Fraumeni's efforts over the years to find genetic proof of a hereditary link had been futile: "We have conducted laboratory studies to seek the gene(s) involved in this cancer syndrome. The initial studies . . . [have] yielded little definitive data."

Now, with advances in identifying mutations in individual genes, Li and Fraumeni recognized it might finally be possible to find the cause of the high rate of cancers in the families they were following. But neither of them had the specialized lab skills to perform the gene sequencing tests. They needed to find someone who did.

17

CANCER, SADLY, DOESN'T WAIT FOR HALTING ADVANCES IN MEDICAL TECHNOL-ogy or for scientific breakthroughs. In January 1987, I got a call from my sister Gina.

I had seen her just a few months earlier, when she and her husband, Michael, had visited me and my family in Boston in the fall. The two had met in the late 1970s in Dubuque, Iowa, soon after Gina ended a long relationship with her previous boyfriend. Michael, a psychiatric social worker, was counseling a family with deaf parents who had hearing children, and he suspected the children—who translated Michael's comments for their mom and dad by using sign language—weren't accurately conveying to their parents what he was saying. He needed a professional to interpret for him.

Gina was teaching a class with deaf students at a middle school, and using sign language had become second nature to her—so much so that, without her thinking about it, her hands often would shape the words even when she was chatting with us and her friends. After interviewing several interpreter candidates, Michael chose Gina. The two of them hit it off, and so began a whirlwind romance. Though Gina moved to attend graduate school in New York City a few months after they began dating, they stayed together, writing multiple love letters to each other every week and traveling back and forth every couple of months. After Gina graduated with a master's degree in counseling psychology, she and Michael moved to Minneapolis, where Vicki and I were living.

Gina was happier than ever. Her grief over our sister Angela's death, just months after Gina's wedding, had slowly receded. She and Michael had bought and fixed up a duplex, sanding and painting on evenings and weekends, and were thinking of having children. Her adventurous spirit and zest for new experiences helped them quickly build a strong network of friends. Gina's career was taking off. She had become enamored with personal computers while using them in classrooms, even buying a "portable" (the size of a small suitcase) before powerful laptop PCs became common. After a couple of years, she left teaching and used her computer proficiency and instructional skills to get training jobs in the corporate world, and she began selling software from their basement as a side business.

After the death of our mother and then of our sister, Gina had embraced a healthier lifestyle. She read the latest books on wellness, took yoga classes, and began seeing a homeopath and a masseuse. She became a bit obsessed with fitness and ate a more nutritious diet. "I've always liked salads, but I don't eat salads quite the way Gina does," Michael would quip. But he gamely went along, as she felt it would contribute to a longer life—and reduce her risk of getting cancer. She and Michael would head out to the country for long biking trips with friends, and run road races together. In the summer of 1986, she began training for her first Twin Cities marathon, running fifty to sixty miles a week, often around picturesque Lake Harriet, near where they lived.

As late summer turned to fall, Gina was bothered by an irritating cough. She was hypervigilant about her body; any unusual ache or pain would spark anxiety. Once, while on a business trip, she called Michael worrying about a pain in her bottom, thinking that something might be seriously wrong. In his soft-spoken and soothing way, he reassured her that it sounded like she had developed a hemorrhoid (which it was).

When her cough persisted, Gina decided to consult a doctor. He advised her that it was probably caused by something she had breathed in. Each fall, Lake Harriet is invaded by legions of Canada geese heading south, leaving mounds of droppings everywhere; perhaps she had breathed in spores floating in the air. Perhaps it was an unusual bacterial infection, or maybe she had inhaled a fungus, or fine dust from the window frames she and Michael were sanding while not wearing masks, the doctor suggested. Or it might have even been something she inhaled in the air from our children's pet parakeet while visiting us, or while she was playing with cats at a bed-and-breakfast where they had spent a few nights. It might be a previously unknown allergy.

Could it be cancer? she asked. Her physician dismissed the notion, saying she was far too young and healthy. Besides, none of the other cancers in our family were lung cancer. Still, to be safe, she underwent a couple of chest X-rays, but they didn't spot anything that looked suspicious.

Then she went from coughing up mucus to coughing up blood. Her doctors decided to admit her to the hospital between Christmas and New Year's Eve and perform a bronchoscopy, an uncomfortable procedure in which a scope is put down the throat and windpipe and into the airways. A screen displays the visual so the doctor can view the images being captured by the scope's camera. Michael joined Gina in the room to watch the procedure. Before starting, the doctor, expecting to see a fungal infection or some kind of mold, told Gina and Michael that she'd be able to tell them right away what she had found.

Toward the end of the procedure, Michael saw the doctor's face turn a shade of white, and the doctor shifted the monitor out of their sight and quickly pulled the scope out. She said, "Oh, it's not working, something's wrong," and abruptly left the room.

What just happened? Michael wondered silently.

It wasn't until the next morning, after Gina's overnight stay, that the doctor returned. The news was what Gina had long feared: she had lung cancer.

"It's a serious cancer. We're not sure what to do," the doctor told them, adding that she was referring Gina for a follow-up appointment with cancer specialists at the University of Minnesota. It was then that Michael realized that, the day before, the doctor—who had developed a warm relationship with Gina—probably was so surprised and worried by what she saw on the scope she couldn't bring herself to say how problematic it looked.

After returning home from the hospital that day, Gina and Michael got together in the evening with two of their closest friends, Mike and Leslie, a married couple. Gina told them she was worried, but she was confident she could beat the cancer. "A lot of people get cured from cancer," Michael added, remembering a statistic he had seen that there were nine million cancer survivors in the United States. "You know, cancer for a lot of people is a treatable disease." Even more, they believed it was in their power, Gina's power, to determine the outcome; if she truly believed she could overcome her illness, and refused to accept the possibility it might be terminal, that would increase the likelihood of survival.

Their friend Leslie, who was finishing her medical residency, was more alarmed. She thought to herself, *This is bad, bad, bad.* But knowing Gina and Michael needed encouragement and support at this point, she kept that to herself.

The following week, Gina and Michael met with oncologists at the University of Minnesota, who told them Gina had a large-cell carcinoma that was more aggressive than many types of lung cancer. More typical of men than women, it is a type of malignancy that occurs most often around sixty years of age, with 95 percent of cases associated with smoking. Gina was none of these; she was a woman, had only recently turned thirty-two, and was a nonsmoker in excellent physical condition.

When Gina phoned me after learning the detailed diagnosis, I could hear the anxiety in her voice even before she delivered the bad news. In earlier conversations, she had expressed concern that her nagging cough wasn't going away and frustration that her doctors were puzzled over its cause. But she hadn't told us about her hospital stay or the bronchoscopy. The news that she had cancer came as a shock, and I scheduled a trip to Minneapolis to spend time with her as she began a combination of radiation and chemotherapy treatment because her tumor was inoperable.

In a diary she began writing on January 12, shortly after her diagnosis, Gina admitted she was frightened. "I'm searching for the whys, the randomness," she wrote. To steel herself for the nastiness to come, she added, "The battle has begun—A MIRACLE IN PROGRESS. I will overcome this with the love of Michael, my family and relatives and friends."

The combined radiation and chemotherapy treatments were harsh, causing her to vomit, often violently. "I want *my mom*," she wrote in her diary on February 10, underscoring the words. "Am I the same age as when my mother first got ill? Is this grief for my mom I'm trying to release?" To ease the nausea, Gina tried taking Marinol, a synthetic marijuana, but it didn't help. So her friends Mike and Leslie drove to a farm in southern Minnesota, where they had been connected to a young farmer who not only raised sheep and goats but also cultivated and sold marijuana. Worried about being caught, they bought a stash and stuffed it into a large Tupperware container and raced back to Michael and Gina's. They baked the bud into a batch of brownies—and eating them indeed eased Gina's nausea from chemotherapy and reduced her vomiting. She began bringing some of the "magic" brownies to her hospital treatments, sharing them with other patients in her "chemo club."

Early on, Gina's treatment, while draining, seemed to be going well. For a break, she and Michael went to the Florida Keys for a week's vacation near the end of March. They went swimming, boating, and deep-sea fishing and lazed on the beach. "I am almost back to normal strength," Gina wrote in her diary on March 27, though adding that "I still tire & need to be aware of resting before the aches and pains begin."

Gina sent us an upbeat postcard, with photos of her looking happy and relaxed on the beach. "Thanks for all your support, calls, flowers, cards and drawings! You've really touched my heart & soul—I'm going to lick this with support from you, friends and MD's care." But she was putting a brave face on for us and herself. She broke into tears during the three-and-a-half-hour flight home to Minneapolis, bracing herself for more treatment.

In early April, though she still felt miserable at times, she wrote optimistically in her diary, "I feel the cancer is in remission—really gone . . . I believe my pain will subside—I need to let go of it and my fears" and "Diagnosed on Jan. 9 and done on April 9th."

But the pain wasn't gone, and the treatment wasn't done—and the tumor wasn't disappearing. Her early confidence wavered. "Was I too cocky before, too sure?" she asked herself in a diary entry on April 24.

Grasping for something, anything, she increasingly turned to alternative medicine. Although she had gone along with the chemo and radiation treatment, Gina firmly believed in mind over matter—that enough inner strength could defeat a disease like cancer. It was a period when theories abounded that tumors in some cases could be a manifestation of unresolved emotional issues and that healing the spirit could heal the body. She began taking homeopathic remedies, using healing crystals, seeing a psychologist, meditating with a spiritual counselor, and combing Asian markets for recommended foods. She and Michael went on a macrobiotic diet—organic vegetables, seaweed, root veggies, and soups—that they jokingly called the "macro-neurotic" diet. It lasted about a month, before they went back to enjoying cheeseburgers and ice cream.

"I am worthy of being healed. I am beginning to realize all I need is inside me. . . . My cells, listen up, we/you are carrying pain that is not yours. I command you now to release it," Gina wrote in her diary. And in another entry, she described a "breakthrough" with Echo, her spiritual counselor: "She saw my body split in two—one half my new beliefs and consciousness changing, the other half holding on for the past, i.e., my old beliefs. . . . My task, to confront my fears, is to write all my fears and visualize giving the list to God and saying I have no more use for these."

But the New Age methods weren't shrinking her tumor, either. Gina resumed chemotherapy in May, writing that "I'm finally seeing it as an ally—a needed ally to keep me whole." Alas, by the end of May, the tumor was growing, and Gina began to realize that her valiant but desperate battle might be nearing its end. She decided to stop the treatment, as it was only making her feel miserable.

I was at work in the *Wall Street Journal*'s Boston office one day in early June, chatting with a colleague at his desk, when a phone call was transferred to me. "It's terminal," Gina said simply. We cried, and I had a hard time catching my breath. My wife, Vicki, and I and our two children flew to Minneapolis to be with her. Gina's rapid decline was so unexpected that our brother, Paul, and his family had gone to Europe for vacation, but they came back early so we could be together one last time. Paul tried to persuade Gina to resume the chemo regimen and keep fighting, but she had made up her mind. In whatever time she had left, she wanted to see friends and family at home, free as much as possible from IV tubes and doctors' appointments.

Even decades later, it is painful for me to read the alternating professions of confidence and expressions of anguish in Gina's diary entries. I realize now that because she felt that staying positive was critical to helping her defeat cancer, she was telling us that things were going well, that she was winning the battle, while concealing her growing worry. Or maybe it was what I chose to hear, not wanting or being able to hear anything else.

Gina wanted to die at home, not in a hospital room. But as the cancer spread inside and outside her lungs, she was gasping for air and felt like she was suffocating, even when hooked up to an oxygen tank in her bedroom. It became too uncomfortable to sleep flat in a bed, so she spent most of her time in a chair. Even worse, in the last few months she had begun experiencing excruciating pain as fluid built up in the pleural cavity around her lungs; it had to be drained by a tube inserted in her side, a procedure that itself was so agonizing, she occasionally passed out.

On the Fourth of July, she told Michael she needed to go to the hospital. From inside the ambulance, they watched revelers bicycling, hiking, swimming, and having picnics—the simple pleasures of everyday life they had enjoyed together not that long before. Michael's mind wandered back to a six-mile race in Minneapolis he and Gina had run on a sweltering day the previous July. At the end of the race, Gina had an uncharacteristic look of panic on her face. "I can't breathe," she had told him. "Something's wrong." He had reassured her that most of the other runners felt terrible, too. "Give yourself an hour, and you'll feel okay." And she had. Thinking back, he wondered to himself, *Was that the start? Was she aware of something at that point?*

When they arrived at the hospital, Gina's breathing was so distressed that the doctors and nurses thought she was dying right then. But she rallied. A doctor took Michael aside and told him, "It's too bad she's having this experience." Michael nodded in agreement, but the doctor could see he'd misunderstood. He wasn't talking about the cancer, as such, but Gina's general level of health—because she had led such a healthy life and was so fit and had such a strong heart when her cancer began, the doctor explained, "her suffering is going to last longer." Michael tried to process the message, thinking, *She's being punished because she's taken such good care of herself? Why would a doctor choose this moment to tell me that?*

Given her healthy lifestyle and her body's resilience, her doctors said she might hold on for another two weeks or even two months. Gina's friends had always known her as vibrant, with a sparkle in her eyes, always wanting to go and do—to party, to run, to cycle, to travel. Now anyone who hadn't seen her for a while but was visiting her hospital room to say goodbye was shocked at how thin and shrunken she had become.

It was just a matter of time. On July 22, Gina died. Only years later would I learn that doctors at the University of Minnesota had told her and Michael when she was diagnosed in early January that her cancer was terminal. "You should get your affairs in order," one had said bluntly, noting that there were signs the malignancy was already starting to spread outside her lungs. "You probably won't last more than six months." Gina had decided not to tell me, Paul, or even most of her close friends, as it would have been acknowledging the inevitable fact that she would soon die. Until she had exhausted all medical and spiritual remedies, she wouldn't, couldn't, accept the prognosis, believing she could win the battle if only she summoned enough willpower.

The doctor, sadly, had been right: she died six months and a couple of weeks after her diagnosis.

Her doctors didn't offer any possible reasons for Gina's having developed a rare cancer that usually strikes people much older, though her autopsy noted, "Family history is remarkable in that her mother died of breast cancer at age 42. Her sister died of liposarcoma of the abdomen at age 24. . . . She has a nephew who has rhabdomyosarcoma presently in remission." Despite the growing research into the genetic causes of cancer, Gina's doctors hadn't considered heredity as a possible factor. Even though Gina died nearly two decades after the first paper by Li and Fraumeni, their work wasn't widely known among clinical oncologists—who, after all, were more focused on treating patients and staying abreast of the growing array of chemotherapy cocktails and radiation therapy techniques than following the latest academic articles on the causes of cancer.

Paul and I didn't push Gina's doctors for an explanation, either, because we thought we already knew the answer. In the 1970s and '80s, the number of known or suspected work-related carcinogens had exploded—silica dust, diesel exhaust, sulfuric acid, formaldehyde, dioxin, ethylene, asbestos, beryllium, vinyl chloride, benzene, chloroform, arsenic, and the pesticide DDT, to name only a small percentage. That had reinforced our belief that the cause was environmental—likely some ingredient our dad had used while working as a research chemist, or possibly pesticides that were sprayed frequently to kill bugs in the woods near our house in Laurel, Mississippi, in the 1950s. Not long after Gina died, her husband, Michael, wrote a letter to a forest products research scientist, asking about a possible environmental link. The response he received began, "Your recent letter to me concerning your in-laws' family history of terminal cancers was chilling." However, the researcher said, while some chemicals involved in the production of wood products were known carcinogens, like formaldehyde, "the likelihood of carrying sufficient quantities on clothing to contaminate the household is unlikely." The researcher concluded, "I wish I could provide you with more useful information, but the field of epidemiology, though fascinating to the latent detective, is fraught with many uncertainties and dead-end searches." Still, absent a better explanation, the carefully worded response didn't dissuade our thinking.

In one of her last diary entries, Gina had mused, "Why did it start? So many questions, so few answers. . . . There is more to this illness than meets the human eye. Someday I'd like to understand but after six months I'm tired of analyzing or maybe I'm just realizing that analyzing it doesn't get me anywhere except frustration."

It would be too late for Gina, but as she wrote these words, teams of cancer researchers—after years of frustration themselves—were using the newest laboratory tools to finally get closer to answering why.

18

THE TEN-STORY BRICK-AND-CONCRETE BUILDING AT 149 THIRTEENTH STREET IN Boston's Charlestown neighborhood stands just minutes away from some of the oldest and most storied sites in American history. It's a short walk to Bunker Hill, where the British and rebel colonists fought one of the first battles of the revolution in 1775, and to the mooring place of the USS *Constitution*, the three-masted wooden-hulled frigate nicknamed "Old Ironsides" that was launched in 1797 and defeated four British warships in the War of 1812.

Nearly two centuries later, in 1989, the ramshackle area was in need of urban renewal, making it an ideal spot to establish a new medical research laboratory affiliated with Harvard's Massachusetts General Hospital. The much-coveted lab space was created in part to lure young scientists to conduct research—including Stephen Friend. It was unusual for someone in his mid-thirties to be given carte blanche to pursue whatever projects interested him. But Friend had been catapulted to rock star status in cancer research circles after his success in helping to identify the *Rb* cancer suppressor gene. Now Friend was keen on making medical history here, by finding new projects to build on that groundbreaking discovery.

In early 1989, he visited Dr. Li at Dana-Farber with what he described as a wild idea. If Li and Fraumeni let him use tissues they had collected from some cancer families, his lab would search for the genetic mutation behind the cancers. Li didn't hesitate, as he and Fraumeni had been seeking someone to study the tumor and blood samples they had collected from members of cancer-prone families since the late 1960s. "That's a wonderful wild idea," he replied. "If you're wanting to work on that wild idea that may have a completely uncertain chance of working, we'd be delighted to help."

Friend then began recruiting research fellows to help with what he knew would be a challenging and arduous project. One of the first researchers he interviewed was David Malkin, a postdoctoral student from Toronto. The son of two physicians and the brother of a third, Malkin had planned to become a physicist before being told by a professor that he liked to talk too much to be a good one, so he decided instead to pursue his second dream, of becoming a doctor. While doing a residency in pediatric oncology at the Hospital for Sick Children in Toronto after graduating from medical school, he had spent two months on an elective training stint in Boston in 1987.

While there, Malkin had consulted on an unusual case of a family with three children who all had cancer—one with leukemia, another with a Wilms tumor, and the third with a brain tumor. By chance, a colleague of Malkin's had asked Frederick Li to review the family's history with them. The experience of working with the family and with Li stimulated Malkin's interest in pursuing hereditary cancer research and had brought him back to Boston in the spring of 1989 to further study molecular genetics after completing his residency.

Over lunch at the Legal Sea Foods restaurant in Cambridge, Friend explained to Malkin that he wanted to find the genetic mutation behind Li-Fraumeni syndrome. Though the syndrome was unknown even by many doctors, Malkin of course had heard of it and was intrigued, given his contact with Li a couple of years earlier. Friend told Malkin that Li had agreed to let his lab test tissue and blood samples that Li and Fraumeni had collected from the cancer-prone families. "They don't know what its cause is," Friend said, so it likely would be difficult to figure out. Malkin jumped at the idea, immediately responding, "If that's what the project is, I'm game."

When Malkin arrived at Friend's seventh-floor lab in the summer of 1989, the space was still fairly spartan. There were a few other technicians trying to familiarize themselves with a new model of a machine to help with gene sequencing, a Perkin Elmer 480, which was still wrapped in plastic shipping material. Their first task was to learn how to use it.

A far bigger challenge was where to start their search for a mutation linked to Li-Fraumeni syndrome. The plan—as with the discovery of the defective *Rb* gene by Friend and his team at the Weinberg lab a few years earlier—was to look for any differences between the genes of Li-Fraumeni syndrome family members with cancer and those without. With skill, and luck, they might find a genetic mutation that was common to those with cancer but that those without cancer did not have. Initially, with tissue samples provided by Li, they decided to focus on determining if these family members had mutations in the *Rb* tumor suppressor gene that Friend had helped discover in patients with retinoblastoma. Perhaps, they conjectured, the cause of the eye cancer and the malignancies in some LFS patients might be related, as both involved tumors that occurred at very young ages, even in babies and toddlers. In addition, some patients with retinoblastoma occasionally developed osteosarcoma, a bone cancer that is a frequent malignancy in LFS families, along with breast, brain, and lung cancers; leukemia; and soft-tissue sarcomas.

Li also suspected that a mutation in the *Rb* gene played a crucial role. In March 1989, after learning of another cancer in a member of the Kilius family, Dr. Li had reached out to the patient's oncologist: "Thank you for calling me regarding the unfortunate new finding. . . . Currently, we are trying to map and clone this 'cancer gene.' We believe the gene is within or near the locus of the retinoblastoma gene. . . . Essential to the analysis is any fresh tumor tissue from members of the family."

After the search for the miscreant gene was underway, Li and his colleagues at Dana-Farber began meeting with Friend, Malkin, and others on their team every week or so to brainstorm and review the lab work. The gene sequencing procedure was so technical that the discussions were, at first, difficult for Li to follow. So he started taking classes on molecular biology and genetics, explaining to other members of his staff, "I want to understand what they're doing. I want to be able to really be on top of this."

It was slow going, even with the latest, state-of-the-art equipment that automated some steps of the gene sequencing process. Months into their efforts to spot mutations in the *Rb* gene in the blood samples of the Li-Fraumeni families, they hadn't found anything. The lack of progress was frustrating, but they weren't the only lab scientists having a difficult time deciphering the genetic mysteries of families with Li-Fraumeni syndrome.

19

I N THE SUMMER OF 1986, A RECENT BIOCHEMISTRY GRADUATE FROM THE STATE UNI-
versity of New York at Stony Brook piled her belongings into her Toy-
ota Corolla and drove 1,700 miles from Long Island to Texas. Farideh
Zamaniyan was the daughter of Iranian immigrants who had left their
country in 1979, shortly before the hostage crisis. To the disappointment
of her parents, Zamaniyan had decided to become a research scientist
rather than a practicing physician. Her academic passion was genetics,
and she was heading to the only place in the world where she wanted to
pursue her graduate studies, the MD Anderson Cancer Center at the University of Texas in Houston, a leader in cancer treatment and research.

Shortly after Zamaniyan arrived, her faculty adviser told her that a
geneticist with expertise in childhood tumors, Dr. Louise Strong, had
long been collecting tissue samples from cancer-prone families. The
patients had been diagnosed with something called Li-Fraumeni syndrome, which Zamaniyan had never heard of. Early in her career, Strong
had been a protégée of Dr. Alfred Knudson's when he was at MD Anderson, and she had been so intrigued by his work that she began focusing
her research and clinical work on children with cancer and their families.

Strong and Dr. Michael Tainsky, Zamaniyan's faculty adviser, had been growing cultures of cells from the skin tissues, called fibroblasts, when something odd happened. Normal skin fibroblasts die after being cultured for a while. But some of these cells had continued growing and growing. Rather than die, the cells seemed to have become "immortalized," in the parlance of microbiologists. Strong and Tainsky had never observed this before. They initially suspected that the cultures had been contaminated, which could explain why the cells didn't die. But they performed a number of tests and couldn't find any evidence that they were tainted. Also, they noticed another thing that struck them as unusual: over time, the cells started to change their appearance, and when examined under a microscope, they looked similar to cancer cells. The researchers didn't know exactly what was going on, or why.

Tainsky asked Zamaniyan if she would be interested in working with the cells and looking for answers. Zamaniyan could hardly contain her excitement. This was exactly the type of challenging and important work she had envisioned doing when she left her close-knit immigrant family and moved to a city where she didn't know a soul.

The assignment for what became her thesis project was to start all over and see if she could replicate the results by growing new cultures using the fibroblasts from Strong's catalogue of Li-Fraumeni family tissues. If she could grow the cells, and if they also became immortalized, she would then seek to perform a transformation with them—that is, inject them into mice and see if the mice developed cancer tumors. That way, she and Tainsky might be able to determine if something was going on genetically with the tissues that could be related to the tumors.

Step one—culturing cells from the tissue to see if they became immortalized—itself took more than a year. Typically, fibroblast skin tissue culture cells can be grown in a petri dish and divided for up to thirty "passages" (or generations), at which point they die. Each generation takes a week or two to grow before the cells divide, and needs constant observation. It is a repetitive task that can't be speeded up. Culture, grow, divide. Culture, grow, divide. Culture, grow, divide. Thirty times.

Zamaniyan would arrive in the lab at eight o'clock every morning and often work until seven or eight in the evening, usually spending five hours a day or more in the culture room observing and recording what was going on with the cells from multiple families and taking care to ensure they weren't contaminated. The work could be tedious, but Zamaniyan found it intellectually stimulating, as she sensed that she was on a journey that could end up someplace important. After more than a year, her experiment confirmed that the cells she cultured had become "immortalized" and that it wasn't the result of contamination.

But she and Tainsky still were perplexed: *Why was something happening that they had never before observed? Typical human cells don't spontaneously immortalize.*

For the second stage of the study, the cells were injected into nude mice, a strain widely used in biomedical research. (Nude mice are bred so they lack a thymus, resulting in an inhibited immune system that makes it easy for their bodies to accept and grow foreign tissues, such as human cancer cells or viruses, without rejecting them. Another characteristic is that they are hairless, hence the name "nude mice.") Zamaniyan would then extract the cells and use a laboratory technique that enabled her to look at them through a high-powered microscope and examine images of pairs of chromosomes from the mice to see if they had been altered. What she saw was startling: many had been. They looked like tumor cells. The chromosomes were riddled with abnormalities; they had changed into malignancies. Under Tainsky's guidance, Zamaniyan conducted multiple tests to confirm the switch from normal to tumor cells, with uncontrolled growth and potential for developing malignancies. It meant, the two were certain, that some genetic mutation in the cells was causing the malignancies in LFS families.

Which gene, though? The MD Anderson labs at the time didn't have much expertise in the gene sequencing techniques needed to locate the specific gene. But Louise Strong had a long relationship with Li and Fraumeni, having first met them in the mid-1970s, at one of the cancer genetics conferences in Florida they had helped organize; Fraumeni had even developed a bit of a personal bond with Strong, having driven her to the airport so she could fly home after her father died during one of the conferences.

Strong reached out to Li and offered to let him use the skin-derived cell lines from Li-Fraumeni patients that had been painstakingly cultured and transfected into mice by Zamaniyan. Li was happy to accept them. The more tissue samples from families to work with, he figured, the better the chance that Friend's lab might find the mutation that was proving so elusive.

20

STEPHEN FRIEND AND FREDERICK LI HAD KNOWN THEIR SEARCH WOULDN'T BE easy. But as the weeks of failure turned into months, the question of whether they were looking in the right place loomed ever larger. Then came clues that perhaps they were not.

As Friend's lab was focusing on finding an *Rb* genetic mutation in Li-Fraumeni families, the p53 gene, discovered a decade earlier by Arnold Levine and David Lane, was being increasingly studied by other researchers trying to divine its role in cancer. And for good reason. After realizing that p53 was found in more than half of all malignancies, cancer experts believed it probably was an oncogene—a gene that triggered cancer by enabling cells to grow out of control.

Then, in late 1989, two studies published by other scientists would catch the attention of Friend and his team. The first inkling came with the publication of a paper in September 1989. A team of researchers in Toronto had injected mice with cells containing a mutated p53 gene, and many of the mice had quickly developed a number of different cancers—an array of malignancies strikingly similar to that of families with Li-Fraumeni syndrome. "These animals have an increased tumor susceptibility, exhibiting a particularly high incidence of lung adenocarcinomas, osteosarcomas, and lymphoid tumors," the article noted. Some mice developed rhabdomyosarcomas. Overall, 22 of 112 mice in the experiment developed a total of twenty-seven tumors, while only a single mouse out of 62 mice in a control group of littermates developed cancer.

The paper's conclusion, which added credence to observations about the nature of p53 in some earlier studies, was maybe more important than the data: the p53 gene was not an oncogene that caused cancer but, rather, an anti-oncogene "whose expression interferes with the neoplastic process." That is, like the *Rb* gene, p53 was a cancer suppressor gene—the opposite of what researchers had assumed in the years after it was identified. Rather than causing cancer, p53's normal function was both to prevent cells from becoming malignant and even to kill cancerous cells. The Toronto team postulated that a mutation in p53 somehow turned off the gene's cancer-fighting powers, thus increasing the likelihood of tumors developing.

David Malkin learned about the article from a colleague in another cancer lab in the building in Charlestown. Reviewing the paper, he thought to himself, *Hmm, these mice developed a wide variety of tumors. Well, that's interesting, because it sort of resembles the Li-Fraumeni humans.*

A few months later, *Nature* published the results of a study of p53 gene mutations in human tumors. The authors, including renowned cancer researcher Bert Vogelstein at Johns Hopkins Medical School in Baltimore, declared that "p53 mutations play a role in the development of many common human malignancies." This built on another article, published by Vogelstein and his colleagues earlier in 1989, linking a p53 mutation to colorectal cancer.

Taken together, the papers buttressed the new consensus that p53 was a cancer suppressor gene whose powers were inactivated by a mutation. None of the papers identified the precise location of the suspect mutation on the p53 gene, but one of the Vogelstein team's papers provided a pointer: it noted that the mutations were clustered in four "hot spots" on the p53 gene—in effect, suggesting a rudimentary map for where on the gene to look.

The p53 papers prompted Friend and Li, along with Malkin, to confer. "It looks like we have a better candidate gene to work with," Malkin posited. In early 1990, they decided to stop looking for an *Rb* genetic mutation in Li-Fraumeni cancer patients, instead turning their attention to testing the tissue samples for p53 mutations.

Making an educated guess about the general area to look for a defect, even with a rough road map based on the Vogelstein paper, wasn't easy. Before the pivot, it was as if they had been looking for a road in Canada when the road was actually in the United States. Now their task was more akin to finding a road in Illinois—but there still were hundreds of possible roads to check.

As spring turned to summer, Malkin began delegating some of the more tedious Southern blot gene sequencing tasks to a Stanford University undergraduate, David Kim, who had nabbed a coveted summer fellowship from the American Cancer Society between his junior and senior years. Summer fellows had to find their own lab position, however. Kim, whose family lived in Lexington, Massachusetts, wanted to find a position in Boston, so he could live at home and commute. He called various facilities before finding that the relatively new lab headed by Friend needed an assistant. Explaining the project to Kim at the outset, Malkin said, "It's kind of a shot in the dark."

Malkin and Kim usually arrived at the lab around 7:30 a.m. or earlier, and they often stayed late into the evening, when the magnified images of the gene segments from the DNA samples were finally ready to be examined. For their last task before heading home, they would put the films on a big screen and look at them, comparing the sequences of the fragments from a cancer patient with those of a family member who was cancer free.

For weeks after Kim started his fellowship, the result was the same: nothing, with basically no differences seen between the DNA sequences of cancer patients and their healthy relatives. They would then start over on a new set of gels, using a snippet from a slightly different spot on the p53 gene. The work was repetitive and monotonous, as much lab work can be, but each time, they had to be painstakingly careful to avoid mistakes that might result in wasted work. This was crucial, because they had a limited number of tissue and blood specimens to work with, and careless miscues might cause them to run short. *Don't screw up*, Kim kept reminding himself.

Then, at around 8 p.m. one day in early August, Malkin and Kim spotted a difference in the sequence—a mutation on the p53 gene of a Li-Fraumeni patient that happened to be in one of the four p53 "hot spots" that Vogelstein's team had suggested. Accustomed to not finding anything, they wondered if they were wrong. "Are you sure?" Malkin asked, and they looked at the image again. Yes, it clearly was a mutation they were seeing on a p53 fragment from a family member who had cancer.

The next morning, when Friend arrived at the lab, Malkin raced to tell him the news. Friend agreed that what they had spotted looked promising. Though he was excited as well, he also knew that in labs mistakes can happen—and that the worst mistake is not recognizing a mistake. So he promptly told Malkin and Kim, "Okay, do it again." They needed to repeat the sequencing to make sure they had gotten it right, that there weren't any errors, and that the gel hadn't been contaminated. Several days later, after repeating the test on the same tissues, a review of the new images confirmed their findings.

But they weren't finished. They needed to perform sequencing on DNA derived from blood cells from other individuals, to make sure there wasn't an anomaly in the first person's samples. This step would be easier, because they knew exactly what fragment of the p53 gene to sequence and where to look for a mutation. All told, they examined tissues from five different cancer-prone families, collected by Li and Fraumeni and by Louise Strong, and found that all had p53 mutations clustered in the same small region of the gene—at codons 245, 252, and 258 and two at codon 248 in the five families. (The p53 gene has 393 codons: that is, snippets, or sequences, with genetic coding that regulates cell function.)

In the middle of repeating the gene sequencing, Malkin had some news for Friend. He was planning a weeklong vacation in Maine, with his girlfriend, a law school student in Toronto.

Friend was taken aback. "What the hell?" he responded. "What do you mean a week holiday? You can't take a week holiday now."

Malkin held his ground, assuring Friend, "It will be good. It will clear my mind, and I'll come back gung ho." He didn't tell Friend that he was planning to propose to his girlfriend, so canceling the vacation or even cutting it short was a nonstarter. There was still more work to do—double- and triple-checking the data, writing up the paper, and getting it reviewed by a prestigious academic journal. After such a long time slogging in the lab, what would another week matter, anyway?

But he and Friend didn't realize they were in a race. Unbeknownst to them, a rival team in another lab had been conducting the same research—doing gene sequencing to look for a p53 mutation on DNA samples from a different cancer-ridden family with Li-Fraumeni syndrome. And, remarkably, more than a year into its work, the other lab was also on the cusp of success at precisely the same time, in early August 1990. Identifying the specific p53 mutation causing a variety of hereditary cancers in families was going to be electrifying news, one of the biggest findings in oncology in years.

Who was going to be first?

21

DR. ESTHER HWEI-PING CHANG, A DIMINUTIVE FIVE-FOOT-TALL BALL OF ENERGY, came to the United States from Taiwan in 1968. Like Frederick Li, she came from a well-connected Chinese family. Her father had worked with Nationalist leader Sun Yat-sen and later as an air force commander, leaving for Taiwan in the late 1940s in the wake of the Communist take-over when she was a toddler.

Chang, who was planning on a career in medical research, knew it would help to get an advanced degree in the States, and she chose Southern Illinois University because an older sister was already studying there. After earning a PhD in microbiology, she decided to stay in the United States and joined the National Cancer Institute. Her interest in viruses had led her to participate in groundbreaking work on the *ras* gene in humans—cancer-causing viruses first discovered in rat sarcoma (hence *ras*) tumor cells.

In the early 1980s, Chang decided to leave a comfortable position at the NCI. Though well regarded there, she wanted more independence to pursue her own projects. She took a teaching and research position at the Uniformed Services University of the Health Sciences in Bethesda, Maryland, which trains its graduates for government (especially military) service. If Friend's lab at Harvard's Massachusetts General Hospital was the medical world's equivalent of the New York Yankees, well funded and stocked with top-tier talent, then Chang's lab at Uniformed Services was a low-budget Minor League team brimming with skilled strivers seeking their chance to shine.

While pondering where to focus the efforts of her lab's small team, Chang came across a 1979 academic paper, "Genealogy of Cancer in a Family," in the *Journal of the American Medical Association.* The family described in the article, the Southerland family, had a tragic history, its members afflicted with a variety of cancers over a half dozen generations, with many getting cancer as children—much like "Family A," the Kilius-Stansberry family, in the original 1969 paper by Li and Fraumeni. In the latest generation of one branch of the Southerland family, two brothers had died of cancer before age ten, a third had his cancerous leg amputated when he was a teenager, and a couple of years later their father developed a brain tumor. The family's medical history was so unusual that they had been referred for treatment to the NIH hospital in Bethesda and came under the care of Dr. William Blattner, the lead author of the 1979 paper. One of the article's coauthors was Blattner's boss at the National Cancer Institute, Joseph Fraumeni, who had been consulted on their case and had guided Blattner in researching and writing the paper.

Blattner had documented cancers in the family going back to 1865. Like Li and Fraumeni, he couldn't be certain of the cause, but it had to be heredity, he would tell colleagues: "Whatever this defect is, it is happening in that primordial, cellular level that is functioning at the earliest phases of embryonic development." He considered possible viral and environmental causes, but found no evidence to support either, especially given the different types of tumors over many generations. As Li and Fraumeni had done with members of the cancer-prone families in their research, Blattner collected tissues from the Southerlands. "What I'm doing right now isn't going to help you," Blattner told them when he sought permission to gather blood, skin, and tumor samples, "but it could help a lot of people in the long run."

When Chang contacted Blattner in the mid-1980s and asked if she could have tissues and cell lines from the Southerlands so her lab could study them, he readily agreed. The science behind gene sequencing was so new that Blattner confessed he didn't fully understand what Chang was planning. But he helped her select which family members' cell lines should be tested, so she could look at the genes of relatives with different types of tumors as well as some who were cancer free.

Chang likens genetic research to fishing in the ocean: first, you need fishing poles, and then you need to figure out where to drop your line. Having cell lines from a cancer-prone family gave her a few fishing poles. Not knowing where to drop the line, she initially wanted to determine if there was something different about the skin fibroblasts, or tissues, of these families.

In 1987, the prestigious medical journal *Science* published an article by Chang and her team describing a "unique characteristic" found in the skin cells of certain family members. Typically, a certain level of radiation kills normal cells. But cells from this family were far more resistant to radiation, requiring higher doses to be killed. The researchers identified a cancer-causing oncogene, *raf,* in these radiation-resistant cells, the paper noted, which "may provide insight into the heritable defect underlying the familial disposition to a variety of cancers." (Underscoring the tight-knit world of cancer gene research, the nine coauthors on the paper included Joseph Fraumeni and Blattner, because of their earlier work with the Southerland family.)

While the results of this initial study didn't provide clues about any inherited genetic mutation linked to the Southerlands' cancers, the stories Chang heard of the family's suffering, together with the unusual finding, made her want to continue studying their cells in the hope of learning more. *If I could find the fundamental cause*, she thought to herself, *maybe we can develop a treatment for these kids.* Working on a limited budget at a government institution, she needed to find a grant to fund more research on the Southerlands' genes.

Writing a research grant application is like making a sales pitch. To persuade the National Institutes of Health to give her a pot of money—she reckoned the work could take up to three years and cost several hundred thousand dollars—Chang had to explain what her lab would do and why she thought it could produce valuable results. She and her colleagues pondered what might impress the key reviewers among the two dozen scientists on the panel assigned to review her proposal. Dr. Shiv Srivastava, a member of her team who was helping to write the grant application, had recently read the latest literature on the p53 gene. The team had an idea—to look at the possible role of p53.

Chang's grant application, submitted to the NIH in June 1989, was titled "The Status of Suppressor Genes in a Cancer-Prone Family." It noted that their goal would be "to define the inherited genetic defect in a cancer-prone family" and that "particular emphasis has been placed on a possible role of suppressor genes in the development of the tumors in this family." She proposed an ambitious effort to sequence the genes in the family's cell line, with her and her colleagues using the gene sequencing techniques they had mastered in working on the *ras* gene.

To her surprise and disappointment, Chang was notified of the grant's rejection in November. While acknowledging that the application's goal was important and its concept was interesting, the grant reviewers added, "There are a number of potential suppressor genes that might be altered. The background section does not indicate why p53 was chosen for analysis." It concluded, "The overall weakness of the proposal is that there is insufficient preliminary evidence to demonstrate that any of the approaches will definitely yield positive information."

Many scientists would have been crestfallen and moved on. But Chang, irritated by the dismissive tone of the response, took umbrage. She conferred with her lab team. Srivastava understood why the NIH reviewers thought it was a long shot, but he had an intuitive sense that they might find something interesting. "Maybe I'm naïve, but it looks very attractive to me," he told his colleagues.

Screw the NIH, the group agreed. They would pursue the project without the grant funds. Instead, Chang would have to scrounge savings from elsewhere in her lab budget and use that money to pay for this project on the side.

Spurred on by Chang—known by colleagues for always being in a hurry, racing from lab to lab—her researchers began working extra-long hours, as they had to squeeze in their search for a p53 mutation in the Southerland family genes with other projects they were obligated to work on. Like Friend's team in Boston, they found the work slow going. For months, they found nothing. Then one Friday in early August 1990, Srivastava got a call from his wife, who was taking their two young daughters to a hospital emergency room because they were experiencing bad asthma flare-ups due to allergies. Before leaving to join her, he grabbed the latest series of sequencing images he hadn't yet had a chance to look at. He'd review them at home, he decided.

Thankfully, his daughters were fine. His wife stayed with them after they were admitted to the hospital as a precaution, and he drove back to their house. While alone over the weekend, he found time to review the images he had brought home.

Srivastava couldn't believe what he was seeing. He spotted what looked like a mutation, but he wondered if it might be an error caused by the finicky sequencing equipment used at the time. Not sure of his finding, he nervously waited until Monday to show the images to Chang.

Monday rolled around, and Srivastava presented his work to Chang, saying cautiously that he might have found something interesting. Dr. Chang, who had more experience working with sequencing genes, was confident his reading was accurate. But following laboratory practices, she urged him to repeat the sequencing—not once, but several times, to make sure there wasn't anything amiss.

Chang's team was ecstatic. Their grant application had been snubbed by the NIH, but the little team that couldn't had proven it could and that their hunch about p53 had been right. "It's un-freaking-believable," declared Dr. Kathleen Pirollo, another member of the team.

It was the first week of August—amazingly, within a few days of when Malkin and Kim told Stephen Friend that they had found the p53 mutation. The one found in the family tested by Chang's lab was at codon 245, the exact spot where Friend's lab had found a mutation in samples from one of *its* five families. Just as amazing, even though the ranks of top cancer researchers were small, neither team was aware of the other's efforts or of the almost simultaneous, momentous discovery—and for good reason. Scientists typically keep their discoveries discreet until publication, to make sure the methodology and findings pass muster with peer reviewers. Even more, they want to avoid tipping their hand to rival labs—especially on a groundbreaking discovery like the p53 mutation, which would surely lead to great acclaim and fame.

22

IN MID-AUGUST, DAVID MALKIN RETURNED TO BOSTON FROM VACATION, NOW HAP-pily engaged. He and his colleagues, whose progress had slowed a bit in his absence, continued sequencing skin samples to confirm their earlier results. Then, after double- and triple-checking the results, Friend and Malkin in September spent a couple of weeks drafting a paper for publication to an academic journal, often meeting at a pizzeria in Cambridge.

Tingling with excitement over the discovery, Louise Strong—whose lab at MD Anderson in Houston had provided some family tissue samples to Friend's lab—hopped on a flight to Boston to help with the finishing touches on the academic paper, which was also reviewed by Li, Fraumeni, and others on the research team. They submitted the paper on September 24 to *Science* magazine, their top choice. First published in 1880, *Science* is the oldest and one of the most prestigious academic journals in America; it accepts for publication less than 7 percent of the articles submitted to it. The magazine is widely read not just in scientific circles, but also by journalists, who often publicize its most significant articles to a much broader readership beyond academia.

Selling *Science* on the article was a snap. Not only was Stephen Friend prominent, given his success in helping to identify the *Rb* tumor suppressor gene a few years earlier, but the coauthors on the paper included Frederick Li and Joseph Fraumeni, whose prestige had grown in recent years. Of course, the article would have to go through the usual peer review process, which often leads to some revisions; and that meant it wouldn't be published until sometime in late November. But that wasn't a concern, because there was no need to hurry—or so Friend thought.

So confident was Friend that his team was alone and had no competition that he did something he might not normally have done. He decided to discuss the breakthrough p53 finding at a public event before *Science* had set a publication date for the article. The occasion was a gathering of several hundred scientists at the annual meeting of the American Society of Human Genetics in Cincinnati in mid-October.

The invitations to make presentations were coveted, as the conference provided a platform for researchers not only to inform peers, but also to impress them with their work. At an evening session on Wednesday, October 17, 1990, Friend joined a panel on Tumor Suppressor Genes moderated by Louise Strong. He described some of the details of his lab's gene sequencing, even disclosing the location of the mutation on the p53 gene that was the culprit behind the many kinds of cancer in Li-Fraumeni syndrome families.

Not long after the Cincinnati conference, Esther Chang called William Blattner to share the good news that her team—using the tissue samples from the Southerland family that he had provided—had identified the p53 mutation causing their malignancies. He congratulated her, but what he said next took her by surprise. "Haven't you heard?" Blattner asked. "Did you know that a similar observation has been reported at a talk by Steve Friend in some meeting?"

Chang was taken aback. She had not heard, because she hadn't attended the conference. Indeed, she had already started drafting a paper she was planning to submit to *Science* magazine about *her* team's p53 discovery.

Chang delivered the news to her colleagues. They were excited—this was independent confirmation that they were right—but also chagrined;

they had thought the discovery was theirs alone. "The probability of two groups finding the same thing at the same time—although in science, it has happened, it's still rare," Srivastava confided to friends, as he and his fellow researchers became nervous that their success might not be recognized.

But Chang had a plan. She called an editor she knew at *Science* and proposed that the magazine run two articles back-to-back in the same issue—the findings of the Friend team alongside the findings of her team. In Chang's mind, simultaneous publication would only strengthen the validity of both labs' results. She even cited a precedent, in 1987, when *Science* had published her paper on radiation-resistant cells in the Southerland family along with a similar paper. Chang, who was heading off to speak at a conference in Chiba, Japan, added that her team's paper would be ready in a week for review. "Would you be willing to wait?" she asked. The editor promised to consider the idea.

Chang heaved a sigh of relief. She was optimistic that she had presented a strong case and that everything was going to work out. When Friend and his team got wind of Chang's proposal, however, they objected, viewing it as a breach of professional etiquette. Friend mistakenly suspected that Chang's lab had learned about his team's p53 discovery when word about it spread after his presentation in Cincinnati and then had raced to duplicate the results. In a frenzy, Friend and Malkin rushed to make the final revisions on their article before Chang's would be ready. To hasten their submission to the editor, Malkin hopped into his Honda and headed to the FedEx drop-off at Boston's Logan Airport. He drove directly onto the tarmac (airport security was far more lax back then) and put the article into the hands of a FedEx worker, who assured him it would be on the next plane out, to be delivered in the morning.

Meanwhile, Chang, still in Japan, was frantically trying to edit pages of the latest version of the manuscript faxed to her by her team in the United States. Then she got the bad news from the *Science* editor. The rival paper from Friend's team was almost ready, and *Science* had decided not to wait for Chang's, so the magazine wouldn't be publishing the two papers simultaneously. Scrambling, Chang cut her Japan visit short by a day, flew back to Washington, and immediately called the deputy editor at *Nature* magazine—a prestigious British journal that is a major rival of *Science*—to explain the urgency of getting her team's paper published.

The *Nature* editor told her to send the manuscript, and by working around the clock, Chang managed to polish it and submit it on November 8. The article was quickly accepted but still had to go through a final review. Now all she could do was hold her breath.

23

THE ANSWER CAME SOON. ON FRIDAY, NOVEMBER 30, 1990—JUST OVER twenty-one years after the publication of Li and Fraumeni's original, widely dismissed academic paper speculating about a genetic cause to familial cancer clusters—the medical world learned that the two pioneers had been right and that the mystery had officially been solved. The discovery of the long-elusive genetic mutation was published in *Science* magazine.

The *New York Times* recognized the noteworthy achievement by running a story at the top of its front page under a two-column headline, "Researchers Find Genetic Defect That Plays Role in Some Cancers." While only one hundred families in the world had been identified at the time as having the syndrome linked to the genetic defect, the story noted, the p53 mutation finding had the potential to advance the understanding of cancer in general. "The new work is exciting because researchers have now discovered the mutation not just in tumor cells but in every cell of the body. Carriers of the defect have what is known as a germline mutation, meaning that all cells are equally afflicted and that carriers can pass the defect along to their children," the *Times* explained, adding that Friend's team had found the defect "by studying families suffering from a rare disorder called Li-Fraumeni syndrome. . . . Over the last five years or so, scientists have been intensively studying these families for clues to the genetics of cancer." Alfred Knudson, the cancer genetics pioneer, was quoted lauding the significance of the discovery: "It's very exciting. It's the first time a gene has been identified that predisposes people to a major cancer."

The *Wall Street Journal* carried a lengthy story as well, capturing the marvel of the moment by noting that the discovery had been made "with a blend of scientific spadework and serendipity." Robert Weinberg, the prominent cancer gene researcher who had earlier helped identify the *Rb* cancer suppressor gene with Stephen Friend, told the *Journal*, "Li-Fraumeni is just the tip of a very large iceberg involving p53 and other genes like it." The story added that scientists hoped the newfound knowledge might lead to cures: "Numerous laboratories are racing to find ways to repair p53 mutations with drugs or other treatments."

The finding that p53 suppressor gene mutations were central to the syndrome explained two things that had puzzled Li and Fraumeni from the start: why the affected families suffered from so many varied cancers, and why members got cancer as early as infancy. Both, it appeared, were the logical result of having a defective cancer suppressor gene that was supposed to be—but wasn't—blocking potentially cancerous cells in myriad parts of the body.

Frederick Li's role in the breakthrough discovery came as a surprise to some members of his family. Christina Li, a younger sister of Li's who worked on Wall Street, was at her desk reading the *New York Times* when she spotted the front-page story. "Oh my God," she told colleagues, "that's my brother." She didn't know anything about Li-Fraumeni syndrome because her brother had never talked about it with her. But as she read the article, Christina thought back to a couple of decades earlier, when she had visited him in Washington, DC, and he was walking around the house grumbling that he had a theory that his colleagues didn't agree with. Now she called to congratulate him on having been right all along.

For the junior members of Friend's team, as well as the researchers from MD Anderson listed as coauthors of the *Science* article, having their names on the paper lifted them from academic obscurity. David Malkin, then thirty years old, who was the lead author, had a brief moment of celebrity in his home country. He was featured in stories in Canada's major newspapers and on the Canadian Broadcasting Corporation's popular science program *Quirks and Quarks*, and was heavily recruited by several institutions for a faculty position where he could continue researching hereditary cancers.

Similarly, Farideh Zamaniyan Bischoff (who, since arriving at MD Anderson, had married a fellow medical student and added his surname to hers) soon was offered a tenured faculty appointment at Baylor College of Medicine, a plum job, especially given that she was only twenty-seven. After David Kim returned to Stanford to finish his undergraduate degree, he began applying to medical schools—and found that admissions directors were astonished that he had participated in a huge scientific discovery before graduating from college.

Amid the accolades, Stephen Friend saluted his team with champagne at their Charlestown lab. He and Li, along with their wives, celebrated with Malkin and his fiancée over dinner at Maison Robert, one of Boston's toniest restaurants. Li, known among colleagues for his personal warmth, offered up a toast—but not to the scientific accomplishment. "You know," he said, "we're going to toast friendship, because at the end of many years from now, we won't really remember if the mutation was on codon 248 or 273, but we'll still be friends."

He also took time to make a phone call to break the news of the p53 discovery to Irma Kilius, who more than two decades earlier had helped him build a genealogy of "Family A" for its cancer history. He thanked her and said, "We have to get Darrel"—her grandson—"on the phone. I have this news to share." It took a while to track him down, because Darrel was in a laboratory toiling to finish his master's degree in materials science and engineering at Northwestern University, in Evanston, Illinois. Hearing the news, he laughed and said, "Well, I guess I'm a researcher and I'm a specimen. Now it makes sense why we've had so many of these people in our family have various types of cancers."

Louise Strong was exhilarated by the scientific achievement and proud that her team at MD Anderson had played a role. But she also found herself waking up at night thinking about the families she had treated and about the sometimes four to five generations of their members who had succumbed to cancer. She wondered how she would tell the survivors the profound—scary—reality that the mutation meant that future generations were also at grave risk. "How is it going to change their lives?" she wondered to herself and colleagues.

Nowhere in the coverage about the Harvard-led discovery was there mention of the frantic, behind-the-scenes competition of the previous few weeks with Chang's team in Bethesda. Her group's paper, though completed and submitted to *Nature* a few weeks earlier, was still undergoing review. It wasn't published until the December 27 issue, nearly a month after the *Science* paper. Outside cancer research circles, it got little notice, which was hard for Chang and her colleagues to swallow. At the end of their *Nature* article, a note was appended acknowledging the fact that they had come in second: "While this paper was being accepted for publication, similar findings in Li-Fraumeni syndrome were reported."

Bert Vogelstein, the cancer genomics pioneer who had helped identified p53 as a cancer suppressor gene, wrote an accompanying article in *Nature* lauding the findings by the two rival research teams and praising Li and Fraumeni as well: "The p53 gene has led a short experimental life, but one filled with intrigue and irony. The latest twist is reported in two papers, one in *Science* and one that appears on page 747 of this issue. . . . Two concurrent lines of investigation then brought p53 into clearer focus. . . . Enter F. Li and J. Fraumeni, who through clever medical detective work discovered a group of families devastated by cancer."

Chang second-guessed herself for not having pushed faster after Srivastava identified the p53 mutation in early August. Her team was deflated after watching all the attention garnered from the *Science* article and seeing their paper all but ignored. "If I wasn't so picky about certain things in the paper," she glumly told colleagues and friends, "then we would have been ahead."

Chang and her team also wondered whether their NIH grant application, which had been turned down in 1989, may have helped provide the kernel of the idea for Friend and his team to target p53 as a possible cause of LFS. Like all NIH grant applications, Chang's proposal was reviewed by a group of independent medical experts. One of the two dozen experts listed on the NIH letter explaining the decision to nix the grant, Chang had subsequently realized, was Stephen Friend.

Friend, who served on a number of review panels given his prominence in finding the *Rb* mutation connected to retinoblastoma, says that the impetus to switch his team's focus to the p53 gene were the articles on p53 published in 1989 by Vogelstein and others. Chang didn't bring up her suspicions to Friend at the time and or even talk to him about their rival articles.

Amid Chang's mixed emotions of excitement, disappointment, and frustration, Blattner assuaged her, congratulating her for an achievement that had contributed to a major advance in the understanding of hereditary cancers. "You were very careful about your work. Maybe it cost a week or two, but for the field and for the people whose lives are impacted, your confirmation opened the door for cancer research to see the importance of these genes," he told her.

While a mutation in the *Rb* tumor suppressor gene had been identified earlier, the p53 finding electrified the cancer research world even more. It was becoming increasingly clear that the discovery had importance far beyond these cancer-prone families. Researchers were finding that p53 mutations appeared not just in people with LFS, but the non-inherited somatic p53 mutation was found in more than half of all human cancers—bladder, cervix, colon, larynx, liver, lung, ovary, prostate, skin, stomach, thyroid, and dozens of others—contributing to, though not always the primary cause of, the malignancies.

Amid our cells' constant, everyday mutations—most of them benign—spontaneous mutations in p53 negated its power to keep cells from growing out of control and becoming cancerous. Indeed, so central was p53 to the body's defenses against malignancies that it quickly came to be known as "guardian of the genome," a phrase coined by David Lane, the co-discoverer of p53.

There were still many questions for researchers to answer: Why did some people who inherited the gene get cancer as children, while others did not until they were adults? Why did a small handful with the mutation never get cancer? What accounted for the different kinds of cancers? Perhaps most important, could the knowledge of the p53 mutations' role in hereditary cancers, combined with the increasingly sophisticated molecular biology technology, be used to target or manipulate the gene in ways to improve cancer treatment and prolong life—maybe even to defeat cancer?

For their seminal work in deepening the understanding of the role of genetics in cancer, Li and Fraumeni in 1995 together were fêted as winners of the $250,000 Charles S. Mott Prize, one of the most prestigious awards for cancer research. "The work was novel, in that it spanned a period of more than 20 years . . . laying the foundation for the development of the field of molecular and genetic epidemiology," Louise Strong said in praising their achievements. Nodding to their status as science outsiders early on, she added that Li and Fraumeni had persisted even though it was "certainly contradictory to the prevailing notion."

Without knowing it, Li and Fraumeni in 1969 had embarked on a journey that would help identify the role of one of the key genes out of the tens of thousands humans have.

24

MEMBERS OF THE EXTENDED KILIUS FAMILY HAD LONG KNOWN THAT *SOMETHING* was wrong. Now they knew *what* it was. Word filtered from Irma Kilius about the genetic mutation behind the cancers plaguing the family.

The research also explained a conundrum: why some branches of the family were cancer prone and others were not, and why some children in the same branch developed tumors and their siblings did not. The p53 defect is autosomal dominant, meaning that the mutation can be inherited if just one parent has it. But the way autosomal dominant genes work, that also means the odds are only fifty-fifty that any child will inherit a defective p53 gene from a parent with it. The fortunate children who don't inherit the defective gene can't pass it on to their own children; for the unlucky siblings, each of their children in turn has a 50 percent chance of inheriting the mutation, with a very high likelihood of developing cancer in their lifetime.

The random nature of p53 mutation inheritance had spared some while snaring others in the Kilius family. Iola Kilius Kingsley was the middle sister of Edward and Charles Kilius. Her brothers would die of cancer and both had children and grandchildren who would die of cancer. But Iola's children and grandchildren were cancer free, meaning that, unlike her brothers, she almost certainly had not inherited the p53 mutation.

This arbitrary pattern could play out even within the same nuclear family. Edward Kilius had three sons, Robert, Raymond, and Ned, but only Ned (the youngest and the father of Darrel) had cancer, dying of leukemia in 1968 after passing on the defective gene to his son.

Being cancer free for decades after birth didn't guarantee that you had not inherited the mutation. Though many Li-Fraumeni cancers occurred at early ages, some people in the studies didn't develop their first tumor until their forties or fifties. The only way for cancer-free family members to know for sure if they carried the p53 mutation—and could pass it on to any children they had—was to have a genetic test done.

But not all of them wanted to know.

First cousins Tamera (Tammy) Howard and Jennifer Godwin were especially close. They were born just eight months apart, Tammy in November 1963 and Jennifer in July 1964. Both had brothers who had died of cancer as infants—Michael Howard in 1962 and John Godwin in 1970. After Joan Kilius Howard Vance, Tammy's mom, died of breast cancer in 1969, Tammy and her other sibling, Gerald (Jerry), lived with the Godwins in La Jolla, California, for a year and a half before moving to their maternal grandmother's house in Nevada. Janette, Jennifer's mom, developed breast cancer in 1980, when she was forty-two, but survived.

Even before the discovery of the p53 genetic mutation in 1990, a doctor had advised Jennifer to consider having her breasts removed, because of the extensive history of cancer in the family, with breast cancer being among the most common in the women. "I'm an optimist. I'm not doing that," she replied. "I'm going to take my chances." Still, she and her cousins debated whether they should have children when they got older, knowing there were so many malignancies among young family members.

Both Tammy and Jennifer got married in their twenties, after first confiding their family's cancer history to their boyfriends. Despite their anxiety over passing on the mutation, each had a baby boy. Then, confronted with the unsettling news about the defective p53 gene in the family, they debated whether to get tested.

After many anguished discussions, both agreed: No. They didn't want to know.

Jennifer, who majored in psychology in college, recognized that she was in denial, but she couldn't control her feeling that not knowing was better than knowing. If she tested positive, she might worry endlessly about every niggling pain. Besides, even if you knew, how would it help? There was no way to reverse the mutation, and doctors would treat any tumors the same way they treated similar malignancies in patients without the p53 disorder. Indeed, a Dana-Farber Cancer Institute consent form that patients had to sign before enrolling in a genetics study stated, "There is no proven benefit from participating in this research. Information learned from this study may ultimately benefit your family, though that is only a possibility and cannot be assured at this time."

On top of everything, Jennifer and Tammy worried that it might be harder to get health insurance if they tested positive for the mutation. Better to be ignorant and live your life as any normal person would, they decided. "I don't want to deal with this anymore. I don't want to hear about it," Jennifer told Tammy.

This reaction was both surprising and understandable to Li, Fraumeni, and their colleagues. Dr. Judy Garber, an oncologist who had started working in the 1980s with Li at the Dana-Farber Cancer Institute, initially had expected everyone in the affected families to want to be tested as soon as possible. That way, they could find out which of their children had inherited the mutation and were at high risk and which weren't. She quickly found that a few did, but many, like Jennifer and Tammy, declined, insisting that they didn't want to know. "What do you mean you don't want to know?" Garber and her colleagues wondered. "You've been asking us for years." Some families, she learned, even dismissed the idea that the malignancies were hereditary because, over the years, they had come to firmly believe an alternate explanation.

One family was convinced that sleeping on the dirt floor in their house in Puerto Rico had exposed them to something causing their cancers, and they found the idea that it was something genetic hard to grasp.

Recognizing the trepidation of families grappling with the tragedy of multiple cancers, Li and Fraumeni began putting together a team to figure out how best to advise them. In the spring of 1991, Katherine Schneider, who had recently received a master's degree in public health, was visiting Dana-Farber when Li, whom she didn't know, approached her. "We could use a genetic counselor," he told her. "We just found a genetic mutation in p53, and we want to go back to families who have it, but we're not sure how."

The genetic counselors, oncologists, and psychologists whom Li assembled began wrestling with a slew of knotty issues over what to tell members of cancer-prone families who might have the potentially fatal p53 mutation and how to do so—considering everything from the practical (is it best to contact members individually or the extended family collectively; by telephone or by mail; and how might testing positive affect a person's ability to get health or life insurance?) to the abstract (who in a family had the right to make a decision about being tested, or being informed of test results, and what if one family member wanted to know if she had the p53 mutation but others did not?). Simply put, what was the best way to help these families without harming them?

They understood that every family was different in its ability to cope with potentially devastating genetic test results. So, after about six months of deliberation, they decided on a "three-visit" model to help assess each family. On the first visit, family members would meet with a physician, genetic counselor, and psychologist to discuss the implications of being tested. Then the family members were given a week or two to decide if they wanted to return for a second visit for a blood draw, only if they wanted to be tested. The waiting period between visits gave family members time to consider, and reconsider, their decision. "We want them to think it through, maybe talk to others. We don't want people to regret they have the information, because you can't take it back," Schneider and her colleagues agreed. On the third visit, the family member would meet with a doctor and genetic counselor to be told the results in person.

Patients often asked what could be done if they tested positive for the mutation. Other than heightening awareness about possible tumors—which most cancer-prone families already had, given their history—the information wouldn't tell doctors what to do next. Screening technology for tumors wasn't advanced at the time and, so, rarely helped with early detection, which was the best way of increasing the odds of beating cancer.

Still, Li and Fraumeni felt families should have the option of knowing. After agreeing on their testing plan, the genetics counseling team began contacting the twenty-four cancer-prone families who had been the subjects of their 1988 "Twenty-four Kindreds" paper. In the pre-internet age, this meant tracking down telephone numbers and addresses to contact all the potentially affected members of an extended family, sending out lengthy questionnaires, and then setting up initial meetings—often with many relatives in the living room of one family member's home—to discuss the implications of a genetic test.

Many families decided not to bother, seeing little benefit. In others, there were sharp disagreements. In one family with twins in their twenties, one twin insisted on getting tested, and the other adamantly refused. It was resolved when the twin who wanted to be tested promised not to divulge the results to the other twin, and their parents agreed, too.

Even as some Kilius family members had fraught discussions over whether to be tested, their deliberations at times were quickly overshadowed by the unforgiving onslaught of new cancers. Janette Kilius Godwin, Jennifer's mother, was diagnosed with ovarian cancer in 1990, having survived breast cancer a decade earlier. The latest tumor was detected early, and she again survived; despite Janette's two malignancies, however, Jennifer still declined to get tested for the p53 mutation.

Then, in the spring of 1992, another member of the extended Kilius family, Jerry Howard—Tammy's older brother, who was thirty—began getting headaches so severe that they caused nausea and vomiting. Their eldest sibling, Michael, had died of cancer as an infant in 1962, and breast cancer had killed their mother, Joan, in 1969. At first, the family thought Jerry's headaches were caused by eye strain and that he needed glasses. But when he went for an eye examination, his ophthalmologist told him, "I want you to go immediately to the hospital."

The eye doctor had spotted a swelling of the optic nerve often associated with a brain tumor, and a subsequent CT scan confirmed that Jerry had glioblastoma multiforme, a fast-growing tumor in his left frontal lobe. He underwent surgery on June 1 for "total removal of a very malignant tumor." In a sign that his long-term prognosis was bleak, the surgeons excised some frontal lobe tissue "to provide additional room for probable regrowth of the tumor."

A year later, in July 1993, Jerry's ten-year-old son, Jeremy, began suffering hallucinations. Even as Jerry was deteriorating, occasionally suffering seizures, as his tumor had returned despite treatment, he learned the terrible news that Jeremy had been diagnosed with a glioblastoma brain tumor as well. Jerry died a few months later, in November, and Jeremy just seven months after that, in June 1994, several weeks shy of his eleventh birthday.

The family was numb. Jennifer Rivas, Jerry's cousin and Jeremy's first cousin once removed, began to dread getting phone calls from her relatives, as they often meant bad news. Who would be next, the family wondered? They were terrified it would be Jaimee, Jeremy's sister and only sibling, who was eight years old at the time. Her great-grandfather had died of lung cancer at forty-eight, her grandmother of breast cancer at twenty-nine, and now both her father, at thirty-two, and her brother, at ten, of brain cancer. But her mother didn't want Jaimee tested for the p53 mutation. Why bother, she said. Knowing wouldn't matter, other than increasing anxiety.

25

MEDICAL RESEARCH OFTEN OCCURS IN OBSCURITY. THE TEDIOUS TASK OF scientists conducting experiments in labs, with no certainty of producing conclusive results, rarely generates much interest outside academic circles. But "the Race," as the search to find a mutated gene behind hereditary breast cancer came to be known, was different.

The competition began in earnest on October 17, 1990, after a late-night session of the annual gathering of the American Society of Human Genetics at the Cincinnati Convention Center. At the same conference where Stephen Friend had prematurely revealed the discovery of the p53 mutation behind Li-Fraumeni syndrome, a forty-four-year-old researcher named Mary-Claire King made an astonishing disclosure that would set off a scramble by renowned geneticists at laboratories around the world.

In the wake of the p53 mutation discovery, and of the *Rb* gene before it, scientists armed with molecular biology tools were vying to identify genetic mutations linked to a variety of cancers—skin, colon, kidney, prostate, and others. But the biggest prize of all was breast cancer, the nation's most common malignancy, afflicting more than 250,000 women a year, and among the most feared.

King had been studying breast cancer for seventeen years. She earned an undergraduate degree in mathematics at Carleton College in Minnesota in the late 1960s and then headed to Berkeley to get a graduate degree in statistics, before transferring to genetics after she wandered into a class that excited her. The campus at the time was buzzing with social activism, and King worked briefly on a project for consumer protection advocate Ralph Nader, who offered her a job in Washington, DC. But she turned it down after a friend who would become her faculty adviser, Allan Wilson, persuaded her she could have a great impact by finishing her degree. At his suggestion, King studied the genes of humans and chimpanzees for her PhD dissertation and made the surprising finding that 99 percent of their genetic makeup was shared. She was just twenty-nine when an article she coauthored with Wilson was published as a cover story in *Science*.

Not long after finishing her graduate degree, King spotted an ad for a research position working with a professor at the University of California–San Francisco medical school across the bay. He hired King and posed a conundrum for her to study: "Why are some families so severely affected with breast cancer?" With her knowledge of genetics, she surmised that some, though not all, breast cancer cases might be inherited. It was 1974, and King's supposition, as with Li and Fraumeni and their hypothesis, put her outside the mainstream; most experts said breast cancer was so prevalent that, statistically, it would be expected that an occasional family would have lots of breast cancers and that even these cases could be caused by exposure to environmental toxins.

A couple of years later, King landed a faculty job in the epidemiology department at Berkeley, where she continued pursuing her theory. Needing data to test her ideas, she persuaded the National Cancer Institute to add a few questions about family cancer history to an epidemiological study on the risk of breast, ovarian, and uterine cancer associated with oral contraceptives. Then, using the answers from some 1,500 women, she crunched numbers and spotted an intriguing statistic. In the majority of cases, the women said they didn't have any other family members with breast cancer. But about 4 percent of women answered that, yes, they had close relatives with breast cancer, and the data showed that women in these families had an 80 percent lifetime risk of getting breast cancer, versus just 8 percent for all women.

King knew it was just a predictive mathematical model—a "hypothetical" gene, she called it—but the results persuaded her that it was indeed likely that there was a breast cancer gene. "The best way to prove that it existed was to find it," she decided.

Given the limitations of molecular biology technology in the late 1970s and early 1980s, progress was slow. Adding to the difficulty, finding affected families wasn't easy, as high concentrations of breast cancer were found in relatively few families. Over time, aided by oncologists and their patients, King and her team managed to find twenty-three extended families with multiple cases of breast cancer to study. Sifting through the tissue samples of the women with breast cancer in the families was time-consuming and yielded sometimes conflicting results.

Then, in 1990, her lab had a breakthrough. A member of the team suggested arranging the families by the average age of breast cancer among the relatives. This led to focusing on a subset of families—those with many daughters, mothers, and grandmothers who developed breast cancer by the time they were forty-five. It turned out that nearly half the women in these families had early onset breast cancer, a staggering percentage, given that women rarely get breast cancer before age fifty.

It would still take months of lab work, but by targeting these families, King's team pinpointed a common defect among these women, in an area on chromosome 17, named 17q21, one of the twenty-three pairs of chromosomes humans have. While they weren't able to identify the specific gene—each chromosome can have as many as several thousand genes—narrowing the likely culprit down to a locale on a chromosome was a major breakthrough.

King was a late addition to speak at the Cincinnati conference, invited by Louise Strong, the cancer researcher at MD Anderson working with Li and Fraumeni to help identify the p53 mutation and who had helped organize the agenda. King's time slot was 10:30 p.m., and attendance was a bit sparse, both because of the late hour and because the first game of the World Series between the Cincinnati Reds and the Oakland Athletics was being played in town that evening.

King was a bit nervous, but Strong assured her the data looked persuasive. Indeed, the people who stuck around for King's presentation were riveted as she displayed slides and data showing the family trees and cancer rates and disclosed her findings about chromosome 17.

Several prominent geneticists in the audience immediately grasped the significance. Francis Collins, a renowned scientist then at the University of Michigan, who put a decal on his motorcycle whenever his lab found a new gene, approached King with the hope of collaborating with her lab. A leading French geneticist, Gilbert Lenoir, who had been looking for a breast cancer gene for several years and who had traveled to the United States for the conference, telephoned his colleagues at the International Agency for Research on Cancer, in Lyon, the next morning with the news of King's discovery; within a couple of months, his group confirmed King's findings with a different set of cancer-prone families it had been studying.

King's study was formally published in *Science* on December 25, 1990, and the *New York Times* took notice, printing a long article. Headlined "Some Genetic Pieces Are Falling into Place in Breast Cancer Puzzle," the story lauded King's work and mentioned a second paper published simultaneously in *Science* by Mark Skolnick, a geneticist at the University of Utah, suggesting that a hereditary predisposition to breast cancer may be more common than thought.

With the competition heating up to find the breast cancer gene—named *BRCA* (for BReast CAncer) by King—King agreed to team up with Collins and geneticists at several other labs to improve her chances. She and her colleagues often worked six and sometimes seven days a week, for twelve hours or more. A researcher at one of the labs collaborating with King confided, "I run marathons. I once thought I'd be an Olympic athlete. This is as intense as that."

The Race was being followed not just in the medical world, but also in the media. More than two years into the search, the *New York Times* published a profile of King and her team's effort, reporting that King believed her lab was very close to succeeding. "We're obsessed with finding the gene," she said. "I want it to happen in our lab."

"It was her reason for getting up in the morning," said Collins, who by then had become director of the National Center for Human Genome Research at the National Institutes of Health.

Confident that they were zeroing in on the genetic culprit, a graduate student in King's lab bet her brother that King's team would succeed before he finished a house his family had just started building. A year later, the family had moved into the house, but the lab was still toiling away.

Indeed, the *BRCA* gene was proving to be frustratingly elusive, even as scientists were discovering other new cancer genes—two different colon cancer genes in 1991 and 1993, a kidney cancer gene in 1993, and a skin cancer gene in early 1994. The area they were searching on chromosome 17 was large and complicated. Collins likened it to searching all of Texas to find a single house. As if that weren't hard enough, the area they were searching on chromosome 17 had what King called "messy features" that made it exceedingly hard to map. Promising genetic trails would lead nowhere. "A path that began nicely enough . . . would soon turn back on itself, yielding more a meander through a swamp than a walk from one signpost to another," as she put it. Rumors occasionally swirled about one lab or another being on the brink of a breakthrough, only to be just that, rumors.

Then, on the evening of September 13, 1994, NBC broke the news: a *BRCA* gene had been identified—not by King, the sentimental favorite, but by her rival Mark Skolnick's lab in Utah. The television network had managed to get the dramatic scoop even though the results weren't scheduled to be published until the October 7 issue of *Science*. King, though disappointed, graciously congratulated Skolnick and his colleagues, saying, "This is beautiful work. . . . These guys deserve their success."

Even so, some in the cancer research community felt Skolnick had had an unfair advantage. In 1991, he had cofounded a biotechnology company, Myriad Genetics, that tapped millions of dollars in private funding. This meant he and his team had used more advanced laboratory equipment that allowed them to sift and analyze DNA fragments faster than King's and other labs.

Still, Skolnick's victory was hardly a fluke. While not as well known at the time as King, he was a rising star in the genetics world who also had been studying families with breast cancer for more than a decade. Skolnick, then forty-four, the same age as King, had long recognized that being in Utah, home to the Church of Jesus Christ of Latter-day Saints, commonly known as Mormons, could work in his favor in hunting for genes. LDS families are typically big, often with as many as eight children, which makes for even larger extended families. They also keep extensive genealogical records, including medical records. For their breast cancer research, Skolnick and his colleagues were able to gather DNA samples from families with many cases of breast cancer. In examining the genetic makeup of the families over time, they had been able to find DNA similarities among some women with breast cancer, enabling them to accelerate their search for the *BRCA* gene by targeting a smaller segment of chromosome 17 than their rivals. Even so, Skolnick noted, "it took almost two years just to get to the right region."

The *BRCA* breast cancer gene, like p53, was a cancer suppressor gene, Skolnick and his colleagues found. When the mutated gene was inherited, the cancer-fighting power was inactivated, making carriers especially prone to tumors; as with the p53 mutation, there was a fifty-fifty chance of inheriting a defective *BRCA* gene. Moreover, they also noted that there were two, not one, distinct breast cancer genes, *BRCA1* and *BRCA2*, both of which accounted for a high percentage of early onset cancers.

Even more than the discovery of the exceedingly rare p53 mutation a few years earlier, identifying the *BRCA* genes heightened the growing awareness of hereditary cancers. Just about every major newspaper in the country reported the news, along with television and radio networks. The *BRCA* mutation, while not common, was linked to perhaps 5 percent of breast cancers. This was higher than other known cancer genes, and given the high number of breast cancer cases overall, it meant that thousands of women likely had inherited the mutation and were exposed to a greater risk and at younger ages than previously known.

But the attention also posed a difficult question for women in breast cancer families, one similar to the question facing families with Li-Fraumeni syndrome. What could you do, what *should* you do, if you had the mutation? Even cancer experts weren't sure. The last sentence of the Skolnick paper in *Science* cautioned, "Although such research represents an advance in medical and biological knowledge, it also raises numerous ethical and practical issues, both scientific and social, that must be addressed by the medical community."

The discovery of the *BRCA1* gene, for example, meant that a test soon would be available to determine if a family carried the mutation. (It was commercially feasible because the *BRCA* mutations were far more common than the minuscule number of p53 mutations in Li-Fraumeni syndrome families.) To the consternation of King and other scientists, however, Skolnick's company applied for a patent on the *BRCA* genes, and eventually was awarded one (though, years later, it would be invalidated by a U.S. Supreme Court ruling). But in the intervening years, only Myriad or its licensees could provide the screening test, which would cost several thousand dollars and, in many cases, wouldn't be covered by insurance.

Adding to King's irritation, she subsequently received a cease-and-desist letter from a Myriad attorney, insisting that she stop studying the *BRCA1* gene. This came after the University of Washington had recruited her from Berkeley, and the state's attorney general responded that she had been working on breast cancer since the mid-1970s and was conducting publicly financed research. Myriad thought better of pursuing what no doubt would have been an acrimonious, and public, legal case, and King never heard from the company again.

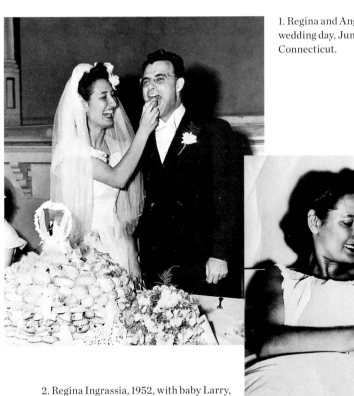

1. Regina and Angelo Ingrassia on their wedding day, June 21, 1947, Norwalk, Connecticut.

2. Regina Ingrassia, 1952, with baby Larry, the author, Laurel, Mississippi.

3. Regina Ingrassia, 1950, with baby Paul, Laurel, Mississippi.

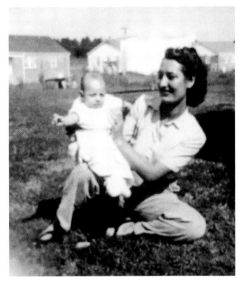

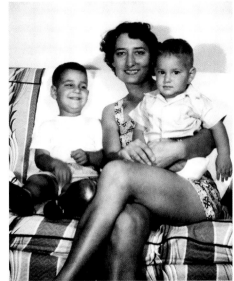

4. Regina Ingrassia, 1954, with Paul and Larry, circa 1954, Laurel, Mississippi.

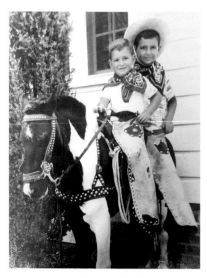

5. Larry and Paul Ingrassia, circa 1957, Laurel, Mississippi.

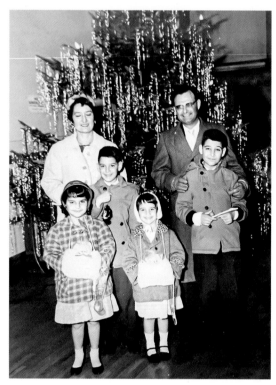

6. Regina and Angelo Ingrassia, with Gina, Larry, Angela, and Paul (children left to right), December 1960, Carol Stream, Illinois.

7. Regina Ingrassia, with Gina, Angela, and Larry (children left to right), late 1950s, Biloxi, Mississippi.

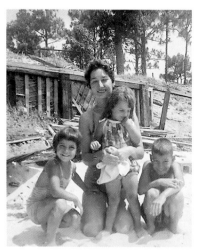

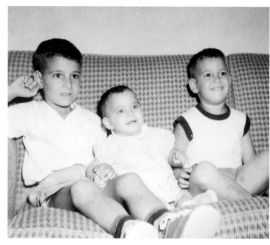

8. Paul, Gina, and Larry Ingrassia, 1955, Laurel, Mississippi.

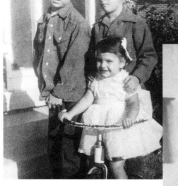

9. Paul, Gina, and Larry Ingrassia, 1956, Laurel, Mississippi.

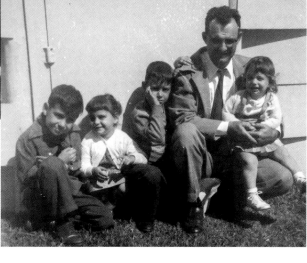

10. Angelo Ingrassia with Paul, Gina, Larry, and Angela, November 1957, Laurel , Mississippi.

11. Paul, Angela, Gina, and Larry Ingrassia, August 1960, Middletown, New York.

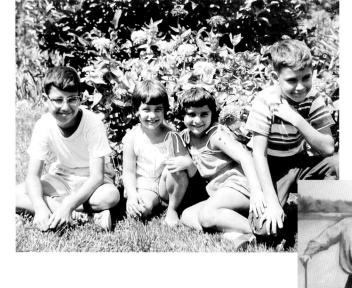

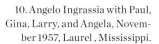

12. Larry and Paul Ingrassia, Leven Links Golf Course, Leven, Scotland, June 1998.

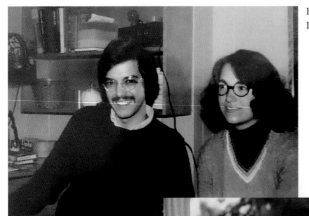

13. Larry and Angela Ingrassia, circa 1974, Champaign, Illinois.

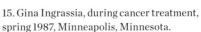

14. Angela, Angelo, and Gina Ingrassia, at Gina's wedding reception, August 9, 1980, Wheaton, Illinois.

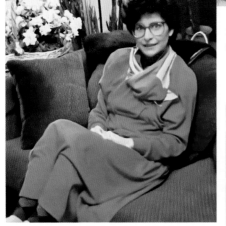

15. Gina Ingrassia, during cancer treatment, spring 1987, Minneapolis, Minnesota.

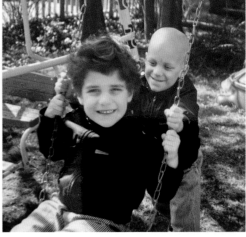

16. Twin brothers Dan and Charlie Ingrassia, 1983, Shaker Heights, Ohio.

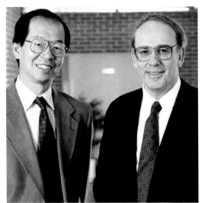

17. Frederick Pei Li and Joseph F. Fraumeni Jr., 1995, National Institutes of Health Clinical Center.

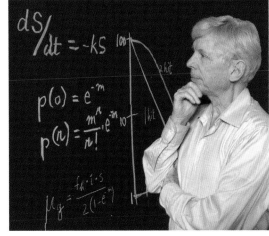

18. Alfred Knudson Jr., viewing equation on chalkboard, circa 1976 , Philadelphia, Pennsylvania.

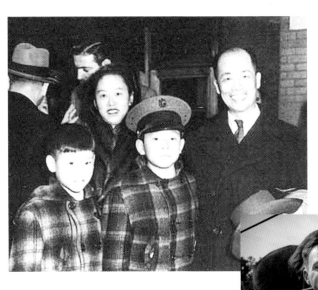

19. Frederick Pei Li, middle wearing hat, arriving in New York with his family at age seven, 1947.

20. Joshua Schiffman, 2015, Hogle Zoo, Salt Lake City, Utah.

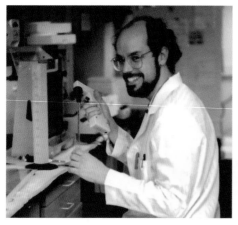

21. David Malkin, Massachusetts General Hospital lab, 1990, Boston, Massachusetts.

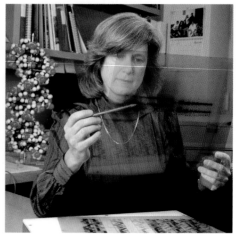

22. Mary-Claire King, 1996, Seattle, Washington.

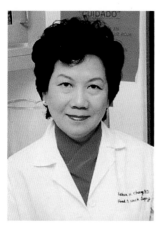

23. Esther Chang, 1994, Stanford, California.

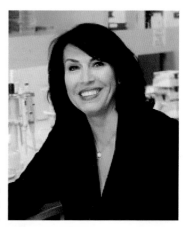

24. Farideh Zamaniyan Bischoff, 2018, San Diego, California.

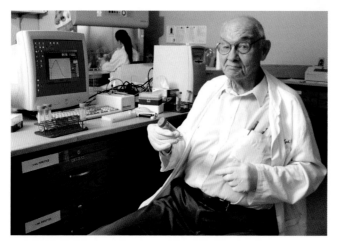

25. Henry Lynch, June 2015, Creighton University, Omaha, Nebraska.

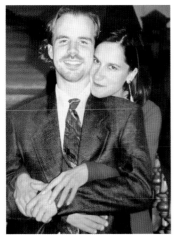

26. Darrel Kilius and Kelly Kirkpatrick, October 21, 1994, the eve of their wedding, Saratoga Springs, New York.

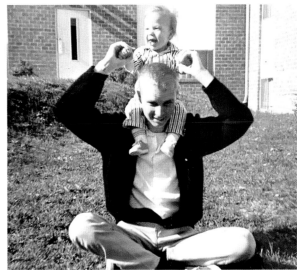

27. Ned Kilius, being treated for leukemia, with his son, Darrel, just before Darrel's first cancer diagnosis, May 1967, Baltimore, Maryland.

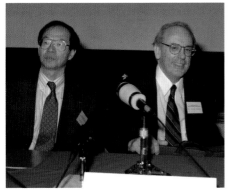

28. Frederick Pei Li and Joseph F. Fraumeni Jr., 1995, at the Charles S. Mott Prize event, awarded by the General Motors Cancer Research Foundation.

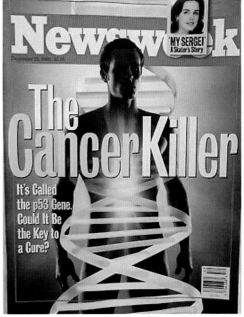

29. *Newsweek* magazine cover, December 23, 1996.

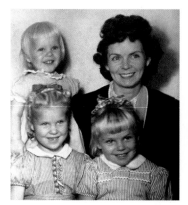

30. Jeanne Kilius, with daughters Joyce, Joan, and Janette (left to right), early 1940s, Pasadena, California.

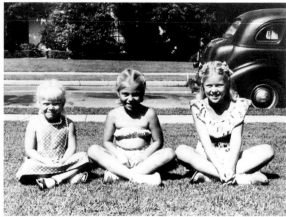

31. Joyce, Joan, and Janette Kilius (left to right), mid-1940s, Pasadena, California.

32. Jill, John, and Jennifer Godwin, circa 1968, Orange, California.

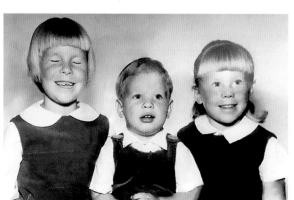

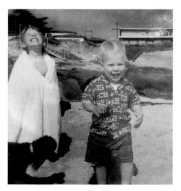

33. John Godwin, with his sister Jennifer, 1969, La Jolla, California.

F. P. LI AND J. F. FRAUMENI

Annals of Internal Medicine

- ◑ SOFT-TISSUE SARCOMA
- ◖ BREAST CANCER
- ◪ OTHER MALIGNANT NEOPLASM
- ◕ CANCER BY HISTORY (NO CONFIRMATION)

- + DECEASED
- / PROBAND
- ② 2 PERSONS

FIGURE 1. Pedigree of Family A.

34. Family tree showing cancer history of "Family A" as of 1969.

For families that were initially eager to learn what was causing cancers for generation after generation, there was a more important concern than rivalries among research labs. Would the scientific breakthroughs about inherited cancer bring breakthroughs in therapies to cure the malignancies? Without a way to fix the *BRCA* gene, or new drugs, women who tested positive for the mutation and wanted to do something basically had one option for treatment to ward off cancer: a preventative double mastectomy. *Is this the best that medicine can offer?* they wondered. Families with the inherited p53 mutation were asking the same question.

26

IN 1991, RESEARCHERS AT MD ANDERSON CANCER CENTER, LED BY LUNG SURGEON Jack Roth, began planning an experiment with cancer patients. Spurred by the knowledge that a mutated version of the p53 gene had lost its cancer-blocking powers, they wondered what would happen if they tried treating a malignancy by injecting a normal version of the p53 gene into a tumor? Would its cancer-suppressing power enable it to fight the malignancy?

By taking advantage of advances in molecular biology to modify viruses, scientists had devised a way in their laboratories to use this technique, called gene therapy. Though still in its infancy, gene therapy had already been used on patients with cystic fibrosis, which is caused by an inherited genetic mutation. Viruses are able to worm their way into cells and then instruct those cells to make more and more of the virus, which is why bad viruses can wreak havoc in otherwise healthy bodies.

But researchers had managed to insert other genes—good genes, like a normally functioning p53 gene—into a virus, taking advantage of the virus's spreading power. Their theory was that when the manipulated virus was injected into cancer cells, it could then go to work trying to fix what was going wrong.

In the wake of the news that mutations in p53 were often present in all types of tumors, the team at MD Anderson was aiming to build on a growing number of studies they and others were conducting. One experiment that got widespread attention in research circles was performed by a team at Baylor College of Medicine in Texas. The team bred genetically altered mice so that some of their offspring would be born without a p53 gene, while others in the litters would be born with the cancer suppressor gene intact. After nine months, only two of the ninety-six mice with the intact p53 gene had developed malignancies—along the lines of what the scientists had expected, as mice rarely develop cancer that young. Of the "null" baby mice, who didn't have a p53 gene but were otherwise normal, however, twenty-six of thirty-five had a malignancy by six months of age, with some developing a tumor ten weeks or sooner after birth. The researchers had anticipated a difference, but the disparity was striking—just 2 percent in the control group had developed cancer versus 74 percent of the mice without p53.

"These tumours were remarkable with respect to the variety of cell types involved, their relatively early onset and their apparent malignancy," the team reported in a paper published in the March 1992 issue of *Nature*. The cancers had appeared in various major organs—"heart, lung, spleen, liver, kidney, brain"—a result that led the researchers to conclude that "the loss of p53 function is sufficient to genetically predispose animals to spontaneous tumour development. Tumour development in these homozygous mice is reminiscent of that in Li-Fraumeni families." The findings underscored that Li-Fraumeni syndrome, though extremely rare, was starting to enter the medical establishment lexicon. Perhaps more important, the article served to confirm how central p53 often was in tumor development—not just the inherited version of the p53 mutation, but also a sporadic p53 mutation or any event that interfered with the gene's cancer-suppressing powers.

As Roth and his colleagues were seeking approval for testing p53 gene therapy on people with advanced lung cancer, they first conducted experiments on mice. They injected a common type of virus called an adenovirus, modified to deliver the p53 gene, into nude mice. The results of the mice experiments were what the researchers hoped for: the virus loaded with the working p53 gene homed to the cancer cells and "greatly inhibited" and even prevented tumor formation. If gene therapy treatment worked on malignant tumors in humans anywhere near as well as it seemed to work on mice, it could lead to the kind of dramatic breakthrough in cancer treatment that had eluded scientists for decades.

The MD Anderson researchers were far from the only ones enthused about potential p53 therapies. In 1993, *Science* magazine anointed p53 the "Molecule of the Year," noting that around one thousand academic papers about p53 would be published that year, up from just a handful a decade earlier. "These diverse avenues of research are under active investigation in many pharmaceutical companies," the magazine explained. "Indeed, the effort is worthwhile, because any therapy that restores lost p53 function would have great power to affect a diverse set of cancers." In an accompanying editorial, the magazine gushed that p53 discoveries offered the possibility of "prevention now and hope for a cure of a terrible killer in the not too distant future."

Experiments using p53 on cancer cells in test tubes and in mice are one thing; experiments with people are another. Roth and his colleagues knew that getting approval for human clinical trials wouldn't be automatic. Injecting a different modified gene into a human raised all sorts of medical questions and ethical implications that needed to be scrutinized. A cardinal rule of medicine is "first do no harm." Could a virus modified to restore p53's powers and counter cancer cells also affect a patient's other cells? If so, might that cause different, unanticipated problems? Would there be toxic side effects, as with many cancer drugs, and how bad would they be? These questions couldn't be answered easily or definitively, as that is one of the things studies are meant to determine, in addition to how well a proposed treatment works. But the aim was to make sure these issues were carefully considered and that the experiment would be conducted in a way to minimize risks. The MD Anderson scientists' proposal had to pass muster with several medical review bodies, with the highest hurdle posed by the Recombinant DNA Advisory Committee, also known as the RAC, established in the mid-1970s by the National Institutes of Health to review sensitive clinical projects. In a play on the acronym, researchers had taken to calling the committee "the Rack," after the medieval torture device, because of the painful process they often had to endure to gain its approval.

In presenting their proposal, the researchers at MD Anderson noted that patients receiving p53 gene therapy would be late-stage, terminally ill patients whose tumors couldn't be removed by surgery and had stopped responding to radiation or chemotherapy treatments. So the risk to the patients was considered low, given that they had little hope otherwise. The scientists submitted the details of their proposed study to the advisory committee in September 1992, and after many months of review it was approved by an 18–0 vote—but with stipulations and requests for additional data that took several more months to address and gather. Getting everything ready for the human trial and finding suitable patients took additional time.

The p53 gene therapy treatment finally began on February 6, 1995, on the first patient, a sixty-year-old furniture maker named Joseph Ironside from New Mexico. Ironside, who had smoked cigarettes for years and quit about a decade earlier, developed cancer in his left lung that became inoperable after the tumor obstructed an airway. Roth made multiple injections to different parts of Ironside's tumor with a retrovirus (which is similar to an adenovirus) that had been modified to carry an activated p53 gene. A week later, doctors performed a bronchoscopy to peer into the lungs and air passages. Where he had received the injections, Ironside's tumor had disappeared. To confirm what they were seeing, the researchers did multiple biopsies of lung tissue. The malignancy was indeed gone. The doctors were surprised—and encouraged.

Interestingly, while they couldn't inject the virus everywhere—the more virus injected into the body, the greater the risk of unwanted side effects—they observed that the p53 genes delivered in the virus killed cancer cells in some adjacent areas. "The magnitude of the therapeutic responses seen suggests that bystander effects may have contributed to the tumor regressions," they noted.

As in many early clinical trials testing experimental treatments, the remission was brief. The part of the tumor that had received gene therapy injections remained cancer free. But Ironside died several months later, as the malignancy grew in a part of the lung that was farther from the area targeted for treatment under the rigid guidelines of the study. Eight other late-stage lung cancer patients received similar p53 injections as part of the clinical trial, which took about a year from start to finish. Two of the patients died before they could complete the gene therapy treatment, but the tumors of two other patients disappeared or shrank, and the patients survived three to four months before dying. In several other patients, the malignancies stabilized, but didn't regress.

Still, Roth and his colleagues considered the results very heartening. Before the experiment began, Roth had said he didn't expect the treatment to reverse late-stage cancers. "We will call it a victory if we just see some shrinkage of the tumor," he noted. If the gene therapy were promising enough, Roth mused, someday it might even be used to prevent tumors by screening for early signs of cancers and delivering p53 treatment before a malignancy developed. "It would be a wonderful thing if I didn't have to treat cancer patients anymore and I could go into another field," he added. "If my services weren't needed anymore, wouldn't that be great?"

Far more research and larger clinical trials would be needed, of course, to develop new therapies that would be safe and effective for use by oncologists. But the p53 experiments by MD Anderson and other institutions seemed so tantalizing that the mainstream press soon was chronicling the gene's potential for treating cancer. In December 1996, *Newsweek* published a three-thousand-word cover story—citing the early forensic work by Li and Fraumeni—that offered new hope to cancer patients: "The Cancer Killer: It's Called the p53 Gene. Could It Be the Key to a Cure?" "This one little molecule already, with no help from doctors, stops incipient cancers millions of times every day," the article asserted. "Scientists do not have to top the elegant system that nature has engineered. They just have to harness it."

27

NANCY KILIUS GOULD HAD LITTLE INTEREST IN THE DETAILS OF THE P53 MUTATION discovery. She hardly needed an academic paper in a prestigious medical journal to tell her there was a history of cancer in her extended family. After her husband, Ned, died of leukemia in 1968 and her son, Darrel, survived his bout with cancer as a baby, she had tried to put that agonizing time behind her. She was happily married again, to a pilot for United Airlines, and had two daughters, Darrel's younger half sisters. In the back of her mind, Nancy constantly worried that Darrel's cancer might return, but more than anything, she was determined to help him live as normal a childhood as possible.

And he did. Darrel was remarkably healthy, as healthy and active as most of his friends and classmates. He carried a visible reminder of his cancer scare on his right arm, where part of his biceps had been removed. Though he always wore a long-sleeve shirt, he enjoyed baseball and swimming. He also became an accomplished pianist, composing music and winning contests. (His favorite piece to play was "Bumble Boogie," a challenging tune that requires dexterity and stamina.)

His grandmother Irma, who had helped Dr. Li build an extended Kilius family tree in the late 1960s, wanted to make sure that Darrel lived life to the fullest for however long he might have. She often took him on overseas trips, to Europe and Asia; to New York City and Washington, DC; and on an Alaskan cruise, a riverboat down the Mississippi River, and a donkey ride to the bottom of the Grand Canyon. Darrel had inherited the travel bug, which prompted him to study for a year abroad, in Chengdu, in China's Sichuan Province, while attending Pacific Lutheran University in Tacoma, Washington.

Then one day in 1989, Nancy got a phone call from Darrel, the call she had long dreaded. While studying for a master's degree at Northwestern University, Darrel, now twenty-two, had noticed a small, pencil eraser–size bump in his upper right arm, near the spot of his first tumor in 1967, but he ignored it initially. Not long afterward, he was playing a competitive game of squash and got knocked out by another player, a blow that caused a bloody nose. He went to the Northwestern University clinic, and when doctors learned about his medical history and noticed the tiny lump on his arm, they insisted he get it checked. It was a leiomyosarcoma, a rare soft-tissue cancer like the tumor that had killed his grandfather Edward. To the family's relief, surgeons were able to excise the malignancy. It didn't appear to have spread, but as a precaution, Darrel began having checkups every six months, including chest CT scans, chest X-rays, arm MRIs, and bone scans.

A top student, Darrel soon was immersed again in his studies, and he began dating a classmate, Kelly Kirkpatrick, who was pursuing a PhD. The two had started out as friends, but as time went on Kelly, despite knowing his and his family's medical history, was drawn to his energy and intellectual curiosity and how he had overcome adversity. If anyone ever wondered why she was going out with a guy who had had cancer twice by the time he was in his early twenties, Kirkpatrick would reply, "When you meet your soul mate, cancer is not going to stop you from being together."

But soon, Darrel's respite from cancer came to an end. In 1991, when he was twenty-four, a chest CT scan detected spots on his lung. It was another leiomyosarcoma. Chemo treatment put it in remission, but over the next couple of years new tumors continued popping up. Still, Darrel was determined not to let cancer rule his life. He got a job at a chemicals company in Wilmington, Delaware, and, with a colleague, applied for and was awarded a patent for a strong, composite glass fiber material used in making molded parts that was very profitable for his employer. Darrel insisted on working as much as possible during his cancer treatments, so his colleagues set up a mattress in the office to make it easy for him to rest or sleep when he got tired.

Kelly helped care for Darrel through his cancer flare-ups, and the two planned to marry, but they agreed to put off the wedding until Kelly finished her doctorate program. With Darrel ailing and Kelly having completed her studies, they set a date in October 1994, though they were worried Darrel might not be well enough for the ceremony. In the months before the wedding, lesions had been detected throughout his body (vertebrae, pelvis, femur, and shoulder), but they were zapped with neutron radiation therapy, and he managed to recover his strength.

Darrel told everyone their wedding was the best day of his life.

Not long afterward, however, more malignancies began appearing, including a lesion in his brain that was surgically removed—fortunately, without causing any brain damage. Still, one of his physicians bluntly told him, "Unless you walk out the door and get hit by a bus, this cancer is going to kill you." Darrel was devastated—and angry. "I've heard about [doctors offering] false hope. But false despair?!! Give me a break. That was the last thing I needed," he wrote about his reaction.

Darrel's tumors kept recurring. Despite the frenzy of p53 research in academic and pharmaceutical laboratories, new drugs were far from being ready. Exhausted by what he called "conventional" treatment, Darrel rejected any more chemotherapy because it made him feel miserable while offering a low chance of even slowing tumor growth. He had already become a vegetarian and now opted for alternative therapies, ranging from Chinese herbs to megavitamins to macrobiotics to acupuncture. When none of these worked, Darrel sought further treatments in Tijuana, Mexico, accompanied by his mother, on a trip paid for by his grandmother Irma. Oncologists decried the doctors peddling these alternative therapies as nothing more than quacks taking financial advantage of patients whose cancers were terminal. They reminded patients that in 1980, the actor Steve McQueen had been treated in Mexico for cancer with laetrile, an alleged alternative therapy made from apricot pits—and died soon thereafter, despite claims that he was recovering.

Darrel knew this, but he figured he had nothing to lose. So he was dejected after being turned down for treatment by one Mexican doctor. "I suspect because he is looking for patients who have a statistically higher probability of boosting his percentages" of patients who survive, he wrote. "Yet I do maintain a positive outlook and intend to keep at it and defeat this disease."

But the inherited mutation in Darrel's p53 tumor suppressor gene had dangerously reduced his cells' defenses, and the onslaught of tumors couldn't be defeated. As his condition worsened, Darrel went back to Baltimore for treatment at the University of Maryland Medical Center. On January 25, 1996, at age twenty-nine, with his wife, Kelly, and his mom, Nancy, at his side, he died in his home—a loft apartment just two miles from Johns Hopkins Hospital, where as a baby his life had once been saved.

28

EVERY CHRISTMAS EVE AFTER MY SISTERS DIED, I WOULD PULL OUT A BOX OF OLD family photos, retreat to a quiet spot in the house, and slowly sift through them. Even though it often brought a few tears, in a strange way, the ritual of reminding myself of the good times felt uplifting and life affirming. In one treasured photo, the four of us are sitting lined up in a row, oldest to youngest, Paul at eight years old, me at six, Gina at four, and Angela at two. In another, Angela, at about five, sits wearing a sleeveless striped cotton dress and smiling with missing teeth. And there is one of our mom, dressed up for an outing in earrings and with a knitted shawl, beaming while she kneels and holds up an infant Gina, standing a bit wobbly. Then, flashing forward a few decades, I would linger over a photo of Gina sitting on a swing and grinning while holding my daughter, Lisa, in 1984, when she was about the same age as Gina had been in the photo with our mom.

Holding on to the memories of the good times meant they were never really gone.

Despite these moments of contemplation over their deaths, and despite lingering concerns over Charlie's health, I didn't live in constant worry about cancer. *Nothing could be done about it,* I told myself often, *so why worry about something you can't control?* Lots of families endure all types of sadness. Ours happened to be cancer. I was a bit fatalistic and didn't seek out news about cancer or scientific advances in understanding and treating it. I don't recall my brother or me seeing the *New York Times* or *Wall Street Journal* stories about Li-Fraumeni syndrome and the p53 genetic mutation behind it, and in any case, I know we didn't discuss it. If so, I'm sure one line in the *New York Times* piece would have rung an alarm bell for us: "In these families, at least three close relatives suffer from cancer, and many more have one type of malignancy." We had four family members—Mom, Gina, Angela, and Paul's son Charlie—all with different cancers.

Maybe we didn't pay attention because Paul and I were absorbed in our careers at the *Wall Street Journal.* The paper was entering a period of heady growth, becoming the top-selling daily newspaper in the country in 1980—exceeding the *New York Times, Washington Post, Los Angeles Times,* and even tabloids like the *New York Daily News*—with circulation nearing two million and topping that a few years later.

In 1993, Paul and a colleague won a Pulitzer Prize, journalism's highest honor, for their coverage of upheavals in the auto industry, and then wrote a book about the travails of Detroit's Big Three car companies. Though some thought I must have been envious of Paul's accomplishments, I truly couldn't have been happier for my brother.

Besides, I was rising through the *WSJ*'s ranks at the same time Paul was. In the summer of 1993, I became London bureau chief, directing a staff of about a dozen reporters writing about everything from European financial markets to contentious trade battles to political news affecting economies. The following year, Paul was promoted to a senior editing job running the *WSJ*'s sister news organization, Dow Jones Newswires, and overseeing a staff of hundreds of journalists.

Paul's son Charlie was being monitored closely for a recurrence of cancer, and we knew he would need reconstructive surgery as he got older. Paul had written a moving personal story—unusual for the *Wall Street Journal*—about Charlie's first operation to reshape his face, as its growth had been stunted by the massive doses of radiation he received as a baby to save his life. It was August 1991. Charlie was just shy of his twelfth birthday and becoming more self-conscious about his appearance. "Not even his outgoing personality, athletic ability and many good friends could spare him the pain of teasing: 'Cheeky Charlie,' one boy called him," Paul wrote. Just before he was wheeled into the operating room for surgery, Charlie asked, "Mom, Dad, what happens if I don't wake up?"

The surgery took a marathon twelve and a half hours, while Paul and Sue waited anxiously at the hospital. To rebuild the cheekbone, the doctor took a piece of bone from Charlie's skull and screwed it below his left eye; then he tucked into Charlie's cheek some muscle tissue taken from underneath the left armpit; finally, he painstakingly attached tiny arteries and veins to pump blood to keep the transplanted tissue alive. When Charlie's surgery was over, Paul wrote, "His head was swollen to about twice its normal size. The stitches on his skull were thick enough for a Frankenstein mask. But he had come through in fine shape, and his recovery would be miraculously quick."

Paul and Sue balked when Charlie insisted he wanted to play on a youth football team that fall with his twin brother, Dan. They tried to talk him out of it, worried about his recently repaired face being injured. But the doctor gave Charlie the go-ahead, noting that he would be wearing a protective helmet and that "normal activities are psychologically important" for young patients. Just five weeks after the operation, Charlie was playing for the Grosse Pointe Red Barons and became his team's leading tackler.

There would be many more reconstructive surgeries to come, to balance out Charlie's face as his body grew and matured. But he was cancer free, and he did everything his brothers and friends did, often with even more exuberance.

Then, in the spring of 1997, Paul went in for a checkup for a lump in his left armpit. It had been there a while, and his doctors had told him it was nothing to worry about; it was a lipoma, a benign fatty deposit. Still, it had kept growing. Prodded by his wife, Susan, he occasionally got an X-ray to make sure it was still okay, and it had been. This time, however, something on the X-ray caught the eye of the radiologist. It wasn't the lipoma under Paul's left armpit—it was a faint spot on his opposite side, on his right lung.

A biopsy of the spot found that Paul, at forty-six, had early stage lung cancer, detected by accident. It was a different type of lung cancer, adenocarcinoma lung cancer, than our sister Gina's. The good news is that doctors thought it was operable; not having the noncancerous lipoma removed earlier had literally saved his life, as Paul wouldn't have gotten the chest X-ray done otherwise. "Detecting the tumor six months later would have been too late," his doctors told him, as the malignancy was aggressive and would have been terminal. I flew back to New York from London to be with my sister-in-law, Susan, for the surgery in May. The operation lasted about six hours, and doctors had to remove Paul's entire right lung—rather than only part of it, as they had initially hoped—because the cancer had already started invading his lymph nodes. I was standing with Susan when Paul's surgeon came out and said everything had gone well, adding, "He has a forty percent chance of survival."

My knees buckled.

The operation left a long, inflamed scar on Paul's back, where doctors had pried apart his rib cage so they could remove the cancer-ridden lung. Given the danger Paul faced if the cancer metastasized to his left lung, he soon began a grueling regimen of radiation and chemotherapy. "Paul needs to take anything they'll give him," his surgeon advised. The chemo was so nasty that Paul had to interrupt the treatment, occasionally putting off a scheduled dose for a week before resuming it. And the extra-high doses of radiation he received—to make sure any stray cancer cells didn't migrate to his left lung—so burned the lining between his pleural cavities that he had to take steroids for several years to reduce the pain and irritation.

During his recovery, Paul and I again wondered what might be causing the cancers in our family, but for whatever reason, I don't recall us pressing his oncologists for possible explanations. Even if we had, the odds are that Li-Fraumeni syndrome wouldn't have been considered; it was so rare that many oncologists treating patients hadn't heard of it. And in any case, genetic testing for the p53 and other mutations was so expensive that, for the most part, it was done only by scientists conducting research projects.

Then forty-five years old, I had never been ill enough to be hospitalized—for anything. Still, as the only one of the four siblings without cancer, I was concerned, as was my wife, Vicki. I told my doctor in London about my brother's illness and about our sisters and mom dying of cancer at early ages. *Should I get checked more often? Perhaps X-rays or other scans?* He proceeded to tell me about a colleague, a doctor who just three months after a thorough physical exam found him totally healthy was diagnosed with lung cancer and died within a year. "You can drive yourself crazy constantly undergoing tests, and something could develop right after the test," he said. "I'm not telling you not to be vigilant, but that won't necessarily help."

I wonder now: *Why didn't we push to find out more?*

Perhaps we didn't dig further because Paul—like his son Charlie—survived his lung cancer, despite the odds. Our family had now won our last two battles against cancer, after losing the first three. To give Paul something to look forward to during his often debilitating treatment, I started researching Scottish golf courses, telling him we would celebrate when he was well again by taking a trip together—our first ever by just the two of us. In June 1998, thirteen months after his surgery, he was finally feeling up to it. We began our golf tour in St. Andrews and made our way up the coast, mostly playing links courses that Paul had selected from the many I had suggested.

Even struggling at times with one lung, Paul beat me in most of the rounds we played, and on our first outing, he came within inches of making a hole in one on the ninth hole at Leven Links, a 171-yard par 3. Occasionally, he ribbed me about my failure to hit a straight drive off the tee, with my shots spraying in every direction. "You're playing military golf, Larry," he quipped. "Left, right, left, right." In the past, this surely would have irritated me, but now I just smiled. Nor did it bother me when Paul quit mid-round the only time I was winning, because walking the hilly woodlands course had left him gasping for air.

The week passed too quickly. One of my favorite memories didn't involve any of our best shots, the great meals, or the majestic scenery, but was when our baggage was going through the X-ray machine at Inverness Airport. The security guard looked at Paul, then at me, and then back at Paul and said, "You're brothers, right?"

29

JANETTE KILIUS GODWIN SURVIVED BREAST CANCER IN 1980 AND OVARIAN CANCER a decade later. Then, in 1997, she began suffering from back pains. Initially, she thought it was just aging. But when the pain didn't go away after several weeks, her daughter Jennifer Rivas urged her to get it checked. The diagnosis: pancreatic cancer, a malignancy so deadly that patients usually die within months after it is discovered.

Remarkably, treatment kept Janette, who had remarried after divorcing John Godwin and whose last name was now Laule, alive for two years. But by the fall of 1999, her chances of surviving her third cancer looked increasingly bleak. A few years earlier she had tested positive for the p53 mutation. Now sixty-one, and with her condition worsening, she forcefully renewed a request she had been making to Jennifer since then: *Please, please get a genetic test for the p53 mutation that has ravaged the family.*

It was something Jennifer had long resisted. In part, it was because cancer had been a constant and looming presence in her life since she was a young child, and she didn't want to be reminded of the family's history. And in part it was because she felt she already knew, believing that she certainly must have inherited the mutation. Her grandfather Charles Kilius; her infant brother John; her mother's two sisters, Joyce and Joan;

her cousin Jerry Howard; and his son Jeremy—all had died of cancer. And now her mom was terminally ill. Whatever was going to happen was going to happen, Jennifer believed. Getting tested wouldn't change anything. *It's in God's hands*, she often told herself.

But as her mom became more insistent, Jennifer began to reconsider. She was now thirty-five years old, and her son, Rudy, was nine. The time had come. Jennifer told her mother she would get tested. "I need to know what my chances are for living," she told herself, "for Rudy." She contacted the Dana-Farber Cancer Institute, which offered to do the test for the mutation for free—no small matter, as a genetic test cost four to five thousand dollars at the time. A nurse at her doctor's office drew a blood sample and sent it to Dr. Li's team in Boston. And then Jennifer waited nervously.

It had already been a difficult year. Months earlier, her mom had asked her to track down her older sister, Jill, who was estranged from the family. Jill had left home not long after she graduated from high school; she had begun taking drugs and drinking heavily, unable to cope with the grief over the cancers in her family that had led to the breakup of her parents' marriage in the early 1980s. Jill had mostly, and unfairly, blamed their mother, Janette, Jennifer thought.

Despite the falling-out, Janette wanted to see her daughter Jill again before she died. Jill had led an itinerant life on the beach, surfing as much as she could before leaving Southern California at some point—and she hadn't been in contact with the family for several years. Finally, Jennifer managed to locate her by contacting the Salvation Army's missing persons program, which found Jill several days later living in Sacramento, California. Jennifer was pained when she visited her sister. Now thirty-nine years old, Jill was anorexic and had developed skin cancer on her face years earlier—Jennifer suspected from a combination of possibly having inherited the p53 mutation and baking in the sun while surfing—and was scarred where part of her lip and nose had been snipped to get rid of the tumor. Despite Jennifer's pleas, Jill couldn't be persuaded to visit their mom.

In mid-December, several weeks after sending her blood sample for the genetic test, Jennifer was at work, teaching preschoolers at Tutor Time in San Diego, where she was living at the time, when the phone attached to the wall in her classroom rang. A call had come into the school switchboard for her. Her mother had been phoning often from her hospital bed, but this time it wasn't Janette on the line. It was someone from Dana-Farber in Boston. The conversation was brief: "I just want to tell you that you don't carry the genetic mutation," the voice on the other end said. "Congratulations." Jennifer was shocked. She was certain she had inherited the mutation. How could she not have? She asked the person to repeat what she had said, in case she hadn't heard right. But Jennifer was assured that, no, she did not have the p53 genetic mutation.

At the hospital that evening, Jennifer tried to tell her mom the good news, but Janette was heavily sedated for her pain and wasn't conscious long enough to understand. She would die a week later, on December 19, not knowing that her daughter Jennifer had avoided the fatal family inheritance.

Jennifer also was anxious to tell the news of her test result to her cousin Tammy Howard Delin, who had been almost like a sister since childhood. The two lived just ninety minutes from each other in Southern California and always gathered with their families for the holidays. They often headed to the beach on weekends together, and each occasionally traveled to the other's children's sports events. Tammy's son, Darren, was four years older than Jennifer's son, Rudy, and Tammy often gave Jennifer her son's hand-me-downs. Even now, they saw each other once a month and spoke on the phone frequently between visits.

But they also shared many sad memories of funerals for relatives who had died of cancer, including Tammy's brother, Jerry, and his son, Jeremy, who had died of brain cancer in the early 1990s. Though Tammy and Jennifer had decided not to get tested for the p53 mutation when they were younger, Tammy had a change of mind after Jerry and Jeremy died—and to her dismay, she learned that she had inherited it. She then developed cancer in her left breast in February 1997, when she was thirty-three, and underwent a mastectomy.

Less than a year later, in January 1998, Jennifer got a call from Tammy. "You're not going to believe this," she said, "but I got a mammogram and have cancer in the other breast." She had another mastectomy. For Tammy, it had been especially hard to tell her son, Darren, who was just ten when she had her first bout with breast cancer. "In the three preceding years, we have lost several family members to cancer. He didn't know anyone who would survive, or so he thought," Tammy wrote for a book about women with breast cancer. She tried soothing him by noting that some people do survive.

Jennifer thought Tammy would be happy to hear the news that she had tested negative for the p53 mutation. But when she called to tell her and her husband, Patrick Delin, they had a muted, awkward conversation. Tammy didn't say much. The next time Jennifer visited with her and Patrick at their house, Patrick pulled Jennifer aside and started haranguing her. "I don't see why you don't have the gene and Tammy does," he shouted. "Why does she have cancer and you don't?"

Jennifer was taken aback. Still, she understood. She had asked herself the same thing: *How come I don't have the mutation, and everybody else in my family has it?* But there was no answer.

At least Tammy had been cancer free for a while. Indeed, her doctors told her that if she survived five years, they would consider her to be in full remission. Her family nervously circled the date, and in 2002, five years after her first diagnosis, they threw a big party to celebrate. "We're clear!" they toasted.

But she wasn't, not for long. In 2003, Tammy was diagnosed with ovarian cancer. Her son, Darren, then a junior in high school, was crushed by the news that his mother was ill again. Initially, her oncologist said the tumor was small and that surgeons would be able to remove all of it. But they couldn't, and before long, the cancer had spread from Tammy's lymph nodes to her lungs, brain, and arm. For the better part of a year, she endured chemo and radiation treatment and underwent a series of surgeries, part of a desperate effort to save her.

Tammy died on October 13, 2004. She was forty years old, an age that made her the longest-lived sibling, her brothers having died at ages two and a half and thirty-two, while their mother, Joan, had died at age twenty-nine. Jill, who was Tammy's cousin and Jennifer's sister, would die of lung cancer two years later, at age forty-five. Their deaths were a stark and devastating testament to the fatal early cancers that continued to afflict Li-Fraumeni families.

In her final years, Tammy had reconnected with her father, Michael Howard, who had divorced Joan a few years after their infant son, Michael, had died. With Tammy now gone, all three of Michael's children had been killed by cancer. Years later, he made a request to his grandson Darren: "Please don't have kids, you don't understand how terrible it is to lose your whole family." Darren had pondered that very thought himself, though he wasn't yet married. But he responded by asking his grandfather, "Would you take it all back? If you wouldn't have had kids, you wouldn't, we wouldn't, be sitting here today." The question caught his grandfather off guard. "You're right," he finally responded. As sad as some of the memories were, he wouldn't have wanted to give them up.

30

"CAN THE COMMON COLD CURE CANCER?" JUST A FEW YEARS BEFORE THIS provocative headline ran over a *New York Times Magazine* story in December 1997, the question would have seemed ludicrous. But the article by one of the newspaper's top science writers chronicled the remarkable progress by a fledgling San Francisco Bay area biotechnology company, Onyx Pharmaceuticals, in creating a genetically engineered adenovirus (a version of a virus that causes the common cold) designed to attack cancer cells.

Onyx was among the most heralded of a growing number of startups to develop drugs targeting malignant tumors. Frank McCormick, its forty-seven-year-old cofounder and chief scientific officer, was a rising star in the field of molecular biology. McCormick was an adventurous risk taker, a valuable if not essential trait for an entrepreneurial scientist. He had grown up in rural England and then volunteered for the British version of the Peace Corps to teach math and science at a missionary school in Ghana in the late 1960s before attending university. While in Africa, he learned of the diseases afflicting the villagers. Back home in England, he studied biochemistry and got a PhD at Cambridge before heading to the United States, where he ended up doing postdoctoral research in molecular biology at the University of California at Berkeley.

For an innovator looking to make his mark in the early stages of the genomics revolution, McCormick had landed in the right place at the right time. The Bay Area was home to Genentech, a biotech pioneer, and to many venture capital investors looking to bankroll new ideas. In the early 1980s, to the surprise of many of his university colleagues, McCormick left academia, the safe and traditional choice for most medical researchers. The first biotech company he joined wasn't particularly successful, but venture capitalists lured him away in 1992 to help launch Onyx, figuring that his research on some important oncogenes (cancer genes that can trigger tumor growth) could help lead to the discovery of drugs to combat tumors.

Despite the demands of life at a start-up, McCormick found time to take up car racing, getting an occasional break from the intensity of lab work by climbing into a low-slung, open-cockpit formula car and careering around tracks at 140 miles an hour. "Racing is competitive and requires focus and dedication," McCormick would say, "and science does, too."

Onyx initially didn't have a specific cancer drug in mind. Rather, its goal was defined as developing "novel therapeutics including both small molecule drugs and therapeutic viruses which are based upon the genetics of human disease." Though Onyx's mission was a bit broad, the excitement about potential breakthroughs in cancer treatment attracted well-known financiers, including Kleiner Perkins of Menlo Park, California, the venture capital firm that had been among the first investors in Genentech.

In late 1992, not long after Onyx was founded, McCormick was pondering ways to battle cancer cells when a light bulb went off for him. Other start-ups, like Introgen Therapeutics in Texas, cofounded by Dr. Jack Roth of MD Anderson, were focusing on gene therapy, injecting viruses modified to contain functioning p53 genes into tumors; the idea was to kill cancer cells by replenishing patients with the p53's cancer-suppressing powers. McCormick, however, had another idea. Instead of shoring up a tumor's defenses, he would combat its *weakness*. He would also use a virus, but his approach would be different. What about injecting another kind of virus, not one containing and restoring normal p53, but an adenovirus engineered to target and attack cancer cells directly?

Typically, a specially designed virus like the one he had in mind would be thwarted after being injected, because the human body's working p53 would recognize and kill the virus before it could complete its mission of attacking the cancer cells. But McCormick's virus would take advantage of the fact that many cancerous tumors have a damaged p53, which has lost its ability to repair or destroy abnormal cells—like in cancers and viruses. That point of weakness in a tumor meant McCormick's engineered virus should survive. If the virus survived, it could rapidly replicate itself—that is, keep multiplying, which is how all viruses spread—and in the process, wipe out the cancerous cells.

It was a novel idea, dependent on intricate science, but it made sense in theory.

McCormick and his colleagues found a scientist who had developed an adenovirus that they could genetically engineer to enable it to battle only cancerous cells with mutated p53, but not healthy cells. In their initial testing of the idea, in 1995, McCormick's team injected the adenovirus into human tumor cells that had been transplanted into mice—and discovered that McCormick's hunch had been right. In the five tumors directly injected with the virus, three disappeared and two others shrank significantly. Even more, "Tumors responding completely have been followed for over 3 months without evidence of regrowth," McCormick and his colleagues reported in a paper published in *Science* magazine.

Shares of Onyx—which had made an initial public stock offering months earlier, in the spring of 1996—shot up 58 percent the day the news dropped that fall. Indeed, by then, investors had become so enamored with the prospects of biotech companies like Onyx that dozens of start-ups in the 1990s collectively received hundreds of millions of dollars to tap the expanding knowledge of genetics to develop drugs to better treat cancer and other illnesses. Teams at the National Institutes of Health, tasked with overseeing biotech medical experiments, were kept busy reviewing a steady flow of proposals for gene therapy trials.

With the financial stakes high, Onyx and other biotech companies raced to obtain patents on their lab discoveries, lest rivals try to copy, and profit from, their advances. Big pharmaceutical companies, which generally lacked the deep biotech expertise of the start-ups, took notice. Warner-Lambert in 1995 signed an agreement to invest in Onyx and collaborate in developing drugs that might come out of Onyx's labs, just one of many deals between Big Pharma firms and biotech start-ups.

After the promising results showing its adenovirus had worked on human tumors in mice, Onyx got approval from the Food and Drug Administration to begin an early stage human clinical trial in the spring of 1996. The subjects were patients with advanced neck and head cancer whose tumors had kept growing despite surgery and traditional chemotherapy or radiation treatment; head and neck tumors were considered good targets for drug trials because they could more easily be accessed for direct injections than most tumors elsewhere in the body.

Like all Phase I studies, as they are called, the goal of this experiment was to determine whether it was safe to inject the adenovirus, named ONYX-015, into humans, not to test its effectiveness, though this was measured as well. ONYX-015 had not harmed mice in the animal study, but viruses can have unpredictable and possibly dangerous effects on their hosts—in this case, people with cancer who have potentially vulnerable immune systems.

Again, the early results were encouraging. Doctors, accustomed to watching their patients steadily deteriorate, saw tumors stabilize and even shrink in many cases. "In a couple of patients we have seen some regression after a single injection. This is proof of principle that you can inject the tumor," Dr. S. Gail Eckhardt of the Cancer Therapy and Research Center in San Antonio told a reporter.

Having conceived and helped launch the clinical trials, McCormick decided to return to academia as head of the Cancer Research Institute at the University of California at San Francisco, though he remained a member of the board of directors and continued playing a key role in ONYX-015 research as a company consultant.

The Phase I study was completed in 1997. Some of the thirty-two participating patients received a single dose of the adenovirus injected into their tumors, while others were given multiple injections. None suffered major side effects, only mild flulike symptoms in some cases that quickly went away. This indicated that the adenovirus—designed to identify and target only cancerous cells, while leaving healthy cells alone—was working as planned. Though safety, not effectiveness, was the focus of this trial, researchers also found that the size of tumors was reduced by more than 50 percent in about one-third of the patients, who also experienced less pain and an improved ability to swallow.

Next came two Phase II trials, aimed at determining the best dosage for the drug. In the first of the Phase II trials, tumors in four of fourteen patients either went away or were reduced by more than 50 percent. The preliminary results of the second test, in which tumors were injected with the ONYX-015 adenovirus and patients also got traditional chemotherapy, were even better. Sixteen of twenty-six patients showed marked improvement, with the injected tumor disappearing in six patients and shrinking by more than half in another ten patients.

This "response rate" of 62 percent was nearly double the 35 percent response rate of the existing chemotherapy treatment. The cancers couldn't be said to have been cured, but the tumors either went into remission or stopped growing for relatively prolonged periods. The sixteen patients in the second Phase II trial were followed for a range of six weeks to eleven months after the trial concluded, and none of their injected tumors had started growing again. "The kind of results we are getting are as exciting as anything else in cancer therapy," McCormick said, "and we are just starting."

Some doctors with patients in the study were similarly enthused. "I have treated people for 25 years and have never seen anything quite like this before," Dr. James Arseneau, a medical oncologist in Albany, New

York, told the *New York Times*. Dr. Fadlo Khuri, an oncologist at MD Anderson Center in Houston, said, "I work in an area where you don't cure many people. You learn to relish the victories, and this one had a few more victories than usual." But he added a cautionary note that Phase III trials—randomized trials designed to compare the new, experimental therapy given to some patients with the current, standard treatment given to other patients—have larger numbers of patients and often don't deliver as good results.

Warner-Lambert doubled down on its collaboration agreement with Onyx. It bought more shares in the much smaller biotech company, increasing its ownership in Onyx to nearly 7 percent and, even more, pledged to provide forty million dollars to help pay for the last phase of clinical trials. It was a big coup for Onyx. Phase III trials are expensive because they require many more patients—Onyx was planning to enroll 300 to 360 people—and can take several years or longer to complete. The bar for delivering provable results is high because regulators scrutinize these trials in determining whether to approve a new drug or turn it down.

Even as Onyx was planning its Phase III clinical trial, however, a storm cloud began gathering over the nascent but largely unproven idea of using viruses to deliver drugs. On September 14, 1999, an eighteen-year-old patient named Jesse Gelsinger was injected with a modified adenovirus in a gene therapy clinical trial at the University of Pennsylvania. Gelsinger had been born with a rare metabolic disorder, caused by a genetic mutation, in which ammonia can build up to lethal levels in the blood. Though babies with the syndrome often suffered brain damage and died, Gelsinger had a relatively mild version and had been able to manage his condition by taking existing drugs (dozens of pills a day) and following a low-protein diet. He was otherwise healthy, and seventeen other patients were treated before him with the experimental adenovirus.

But the day after he received his injection, Gelsinger's body had an intense inflammatory reaction, and he fell into a coma. He died on September 17 after suffering kidney, liver, and lung failure. Subsequent investigations, including a congressional inquiry, found that Gelsinger had poor liver function and probably shouldn't have been enrolled in the trial; moreover, he and his family weren't informed that a couple of other patients had incurred less severe side effects, nor that two monkeys treated in earlier animal trials had died after receiving a higher dose of the adenovirus. Under the glare, the Food and Drug Administration halted all human clinical trials at the University of Pennsylvania's gene therapy institute and imposed new regulations on all gene therapy research. UPenn eventually decided to close the program, while also reaching an out-of-court settlement by making an undisclosed payment to resolve a lawsuit filed by Gelsinger's family.

Though the case didn't involve cancer or p53, and ONYX-015 was an entirely different drug, Gelsinger's death put a spotlight on the unknowns and potential risks of using viruses to deliver drugs. In the aftermath of the tragedy, Onyx expanded the list of business risks it disclosed to investors in Securities and Exchange Commission filings. "The biological characteristics of our therapeutic viruses, and their interaction with other drugs and the human immune and other defense systems are not fully understood," it noted.

Still, Onyx moved ahead and began its Phase III trial in the summer of 2000. But progress on the study was halting as the FDA began paying even closer attention to any research involving viruses to deliver drugs. One complicating factor for Onyx was producing enough of its engineered adenovirus to administer to patients in the larger clinical trial. Making prescription drugs of any type is an exacting process that involves combining chemical compounds in very precise amounts so they can achieve the desired results without any dangerous and unexpected side effects. Modifying an adenovirus for therapeutic purposes was particularly tricky, as molecules had to be attached in a specific spot on the virus so that the injection could be targeted effectively.

Making the ONYX-015 adenovirus in small batches for the limited number of patients in the Phase I and II trials was one thing; producing enough to deliver doses to more than three hundred patients in the

Phase III trial proved difficult. The contract manufacturer that Onyx had hired to produce the drug encountered recurring problems with "failed batches." At one point, Onyx had enrolled patients for trials in ten medical centers, but was able to supply the adenovirus to patients at only two centers. Adding to Onyx's challenges, oncologists at some hospitals understandably became hesitant about having patients take part in the Onyx trials after the death of Jesse Gelsinger. "Enrollment to this trial has proceeded very slowly," the company acknowledged.

The scientific obstacles of providing more than a short-term benefit to patients also proved daunting. Tumors often shrank or even disappeared when injected directly with the Onyx adenovirus, but the drug didn't work well on more distant tumors—malignancies caused by cancerous cells that had spread from the main tumor and continued to grow elsewhere in the body. Metastasis, as this is called, is what often kills cancer patients, rather than the original tumor. The hope had been that the Onyx adenovirus would replicate itself enough to also identify and attack cancer cells outside the original tumor. While it appeared to occasionally kill nearby cancer cells, McCormick and his colleagues still had not figured out a way to ensure that this would happen if the cancer had escaped to other organs.

Given the many uncertainties, Warner-Lambert withdrew from its collaboration with Onyx in September 2002. It was a devastating blow. Onyx depended on the $15 million a year it was getting from Warner-Lambert to finance the expensive clinical trials. It scrambled but failed to find a new partner, and management reluctantly decided to pull the plug on its effort to develop ONYX-015, which just a few years earlier had seemed to offer so much promise. The company laid off seventy-five employees, about three-fourths of its workforce, and refocused its efforts on developing other anti-cancer drugs—ones that didn't involve a virus. (This effort would prove very successful, as Onyx won FDA approval in 2005 for an oral chemotherapy for kidney and other cancers. With sales rising for this drug, and others in development, the company would be acquired in 2013, for $10.4 billion, by Amgen, another biotech pioneer.)

Onyx wasn't the only biotech start-up finding it hard to go from promising early stage clinical trials to a safe and effective anti-cancer drug. Texas-based Introgen Therapeutics seemed poised for success early on after creating a virus armed with a working version of the p53 suppressor gene that could be injected into a malignancy. Like Onyx, Introgen had attracted prominent pharmaceutical partners. It entered a collaboration with the European giant Aventis, which spent more than $50 million in the 1990s funding Introgen's research and then expanded the agreement by investing $14 million in the company's stock. Then, in 2005, Colgate-Palmolive also invested $20 million in Introgen, as part of an agreement to explore ways to use gene therapy technology in mouthwashes and rinses aimed at treating cancer or precancerous conditions of the oral cavity.

Despite the backing of big companies, however, Introgen faltered as it continued testing its p53 gene therapy treatment. One inherent problem, it and other biotech companies learned, is that gene therapy delivered with a virus can have limitations because of the way the human body works. Viruses, by their nature, insert themselves into cells. That's why using a modified virus in theory was a good way to deliver a gene therapy drug to attack a cancer cell. But just as the body's immune system is programmed to produce antibodies to defend against "bad" viruses that make you sick, it also produces antibodies to fight back against the "good," modified, cancer-fighting viruses meant to make you better. Indeed, the human body's antibodies get more effective over time at recognizing and fighting a specific virus.

For well-designed gene therapy viruses, this meant the first injection often would be effective at killing cancer cells. But with each subsequent injection—and multiple injections typically were needed to shrink or kill tumors—the engineered anti-cancer viruses worked less well, because a patient's antibodies started to recognize the modified virus and were produced in greater numbers to destroy it. Why not overcome the antibodies by injecting higher doses of gene therapy viruses? This was potentially dangerous, because injecting too much of a virus, even a supposedly safe one, could cause havoc in a patient's immune system, prompting it to attack healthy cells in addition to cancerous ones.

In 2008, Introgen presented the U.S. Food and Drug Administration with results of clinical trials it felt showed its p53 gene therapy drug was effective in reducing tumors and prolonging life. But the FDA declined to approve the drug, saying Introgen's application to market "was not sufficiently complete" and that there wasn't evidence that it performed better enough than existing therapies. European regulators later concluded that trials hadn't demonstrated "clinical benefit," while "several potential risks have been identified." The company filed for bankruptcy in December 2008.

The vast amounts of money spent on new cancer drugs weren't for naught. There had been many incremental advances in chemotherapy and other cancer treatments since the early 1990s that helped prolong life and slowly increased survival rates. But expectations of a breakthrough that might soon cure cancer, and maybe even fix the inherited genetic mutations in cancer-prone families like those with Li-Fraumeni syndrome, had proven overly optimistic. "The idea of gene therapy was very compelling," Frank McCormick of Onyx would say, "but no one realized how hard it would be."

31

W HAT CAN WE DO FOR THESE FAMILIES? THE QUESTION GNAWED AT DAVID
Malkin. As a young lab scientist, he had helped identify an inherited p53 mutation as the culprit behind Li-Fraumeni syndrome in 1990.
He had since returned home to Toronto, burnishing his reputation by
publishing dozens of academic papers on his continued research on p53
while also setting up practice as a pediatric oncologist.

Still, while Malkin and his colleagues were learning more about p53
every year, translating that into better treatment was proving to be vex-
ingly difficult. It pained him that many of his young patients' tumors
were discovered only when they were advanced. The patients would
undergo often excruciating treatment in a desperate effort to save their
lives—in many cases to no avail. Therapies were limited, as the much-
touted efforts to develop new p53-targeted cancer drugs had stalled.

Malkin was pondering how best to help Li-Fraumeni families when
a twenty-nine-year-old mother came to see him in 2000 at the Hospital
for Sick Children in Toronto. Luana Locke couldn't stop worrying that
her son, a healthy four-year-old, might develop cancer at any time. She
had good reason to be concerned. Toward the end of her pregnancy in
1996, Locke had been diagnosed with breast cancer, and she had a mas-

tectomy a few days after giving birth. The cancer wasn't the first in her family. Locke's sister had died in 1974 of a brain tumor when she was only nine years old; her mother died of breast cancer a few years later, when she was thirty-five; and her mother's twin sister had died of cancer, too.

Locke took tests not long after she was diagnosed with breast cancer to determine if she carried either of the two *BRCA* hereditary breast cancer genes. Both were negative, but her oncologist told her, "I am convinced there is a genetic link in your family. It's just that whatever it is has not come to light, or hasn't been discovered yet."

A few years later, while visiting her mother's relatives in Italy, Locke learned that one of her first cousins had been diagnosed with breast cancer. The family carried a cancer predisposition gene, a doctor in Milan had told them, puzzling Locke. She assumed the doctor was talking about the *BRCA* gene, which Locke knew she didn't have. "No, I've been tested, and it came back negative," she said. But the physician insisted, and when Locke returned to Toronto, she asked her oncologist if he would mind looking into what she had heard. After contacting her relatives' doctors in Italy, he found that they didn't have the *BRCA* genetic mutation, but a different mutation altogether, of the p53 cancer suppressor gene.

Like most doctors, Locke's oncologist hadn't been aware of Li-Fraumeni syndrome, perhaps understandably. Only about one hundred families at the time were known to fit the definition of classic LFS: a member with a sarcoma (a soft-tissue or bone cancer) before age forty-five who also had a parent, sibling, or child with any type of cancer before forty-five and another, second-degree relative, such as an uncle, aunt, or cousin, with cancer as well. After doing some research, Locke's doctor told her, "We actually have an expert in Toronto that deals in exactly this," and referred her to David Malkin.

After hearing Locke's family history, Malkin determined that she probably had Li-Fraumeni syndrome, and he was surprised when the first genetic test he conducted didn't find a p53 mutation. So Malkin tracked down the genetic tests for the mutation in Locke's relatives. Though most p53 mutations were concentrated in specific areas, scientists had started discovering and reporting some cases of mutations in different locations on the gene, which had prompted the Italian doctors to look outside the normal hot spots. With that information, Malkin retested Locke and, sure enough, confirmed that she had an inherited p53 mutation.

Now Locke made a plea about her son, Lucas. "I have a four-year-old, and I don't know what's going to happen to him," she told Malkin.

He could only acknowledge, "I agree with you."

Afterward, as Malkin thought about the conversation, his mind returned to an idea he had been considering for a while. If Lucas inherited the p53 mutation and had Li-Fraumeni syndrome, there was a high likelihood he would get cancer at some point. But there was no way of knowing when or where in his body, and depending on the type of cancer, there was a risk it would be caught too late to treat. Even with advances in surgery, in targeted radiation, and in chemotherapy cocktails, by the time some cancers are symptomatic they often are in late stages and can be fatal.

But what if he could do something to detect malignancies at an early, maybe even precancerous stage? Malkin asked himself. Then he wouldn't feel so helpless sitting in his office hoping for a miracle when his initial consultation came only after a child's tumor had reached an advanced stage. Like all oncologists, he knew that life expectancies increased significantly for patients whose cancers were discovered before the malignancies grew and spread.

After mulling over his idea, Malkin began sharing his plan with colleagues: we should test children in Li-Fraumeni families to see if they carry the p53 mutation—an important first step in determining which siblings were at risk, as the odds of inheriting the damaged gene are only 50 percent—and then any child who has the mutation should undergo frequent and intensive diagnostic screening to detect early stage malignancies.

To Malkin's surprise, the reaction was overwhelmingly negative. "You can't do this, David," his friends in the medical world insisted. "You can't test. You haven't proven that surveillance would help."

Malkin acknowledged that it was a radical idea. Physicians were generally discouraged at the time from even giving genetic tests to children. There was a whole host of gnarly issues. A minor couldn't give informed consent, so was it appropriate to let a parent make the decision when the child, after growing up, might prefer not knowing they carried a mutation? Would getting a positive test harm the child's ability later in life to get medical or life insurance? How would someone psychologically handle having a sword of Damocles dangling over their head every day? And how could it even help knowing that a child had inherited the p53 mutation, as there were no treatments that could do much about it?

The skeptics agreed that screening for some cancer predispositions, like for the *BRCA* genes, might make sense. But this was different. Women with the breast cancer gene could do something. Though it was a difficult decision, they could choose to have a double mastectomy before they ever developed a tumor, reducing their risk by 90 percent. But LFS patients with the p53 mutation could develop cancer in many parts of the body, so preventive surgery wasn't a viable option to ward off most future tumors.

There were other concerns. What about false positives, which were bound to crop up in frequent screenings? Tests could highlight benign as well as early stage malignant tumors. That might unnecessarily stress families and result in members undergoing invasive procedures such as biopsies that wouldn't have been done otherwise. Plus, frequent screening would be expensive, costing the Canadian national health care system thousands of dollars a year for each patient being screened.

All the concerns were legitimate, Malkin conceded, but he was undeterred. The only way to know if frequent screening would work would be to try it, he countered. And given the high risk faced by LFS patients—with 50 percent developing cancer by age forty—trying something different and unusual would be better than not trying something just because it was outside the norm. But before proceeding, Malkin called Frederick Li, who had become a mentor after they had worked together to discover the p53 mutation a decade earlier.

After Malkin explained his screening protocol, Li told him, "I know what you're going to do. You're really asking for my blessing and not my permission."

Well, yes, Malkin allowed. "I just want to make sure that I'm not totally off my rocker."

After months of consulting with other doctors and bioethicists, Malkin was ready to start his screening study with Locke's son, Lucas. But first, Lucas needed to be tested to determine if he indeed had inherited the p53 mutation from his mom. Locke and her then husband had to go through genetic counseling before Lucas could be tested, so they fully understood the implications and had a chance to back out. But Locke had already made up her mind. "I need to know," she told her husband, who was ambivalent. Ever the optimist, and knowing there was a 50 percent chance that Lucas had not inherited the mutation, she expected him to test negative. So Locke was crestfallen when he tested positive. Was there anything she could do to help protect him?

In 2000, Locke began a routine that would last for years. Every three months, she drove Lucas to SickKids Hospital for an ultrasound, blood tests, and a urinalysis aimed at screening for adrenocortical carcinoma, cancer of the adrenal glands that sit on top of the kidney; though very rare, it is one of the cancers afflicting children with LFS. He also underwent another blood test quarterly, to be screened for leukemia, and two MRI scans annually—one of the brain, to look for tumors there, and the other of the whole body, to look for bone and soft-tissue tumors.

But X-rays, or any screening involving radiation, were strictly avoided, because radiation carries a higher risk of causing mutations and thus triggering cancer in LFS patients, given that their p53 tumor suppressor gene was already damaged and thus less able to protect against malignancies. For the MRIs, the patient is slid into narrow cylinders and can't move for an hour or so while being scanned. Young patients often are sedated so they won't squiggle or become claustrophobic, though Lucas didn't need to be. For Locke, the hardest part wasn't putting Lucas through the tests or stressing about the results, as she managed to calm herself by repeating the mantra "I'm not going to worry until I know there's something to worry about." But what she never got used to was sitting in a waiting room where her son often was the only healthy child amid the many sick children and feeling guilty as she watched the other parents with anxious and anguished looks on their faces.

The first couple of years, Lucas's scans were all fine. Then, a day after one of his quarterly ultrasounds, Locke got a call. The test had spotted an anomaly in Lucas's abdomen, and doctors needed to examine him again to know what it was. That night, Locke's mind raced. She prayed that it was nothing, that it was a false positive, which Malkin had advised her was likely to pop up on occasion. But Locke couldn't help but think that identifying a tiny tumor early on would help validate the premise of the surveillance study. In a strange way, Lucas's having cancer would be bad for him but good for researchers. She knew that would give them evidence to say, *It works. We screened somebody, we caught it early, we got in there, and lo and behold, he's a survivor.*

Filled with anxiety, Locke took Lucas in for another ultrasound. This time, it was negative. He was fine, though Locke was briefly shaken.

As Lucas grew up, he began asking more questions about the frequent medical tests he was being subjected to. Locke was careful not to alarm him, so she didn't mention cancer. "We're going for a visit just to make sure that you continue to be healthy, that everything's good," she would say. "So that if there is anything wrong, then the doctor will fix it." Locke also learned to calm herself when she received the occasional calls announcing that one of Lucas's tests had highlighted something suspicious. *Here we go again,* she'd remind herself. *I'm not going to worry until I have something to worry about.* While the false positives could be unnerving, she also found them reassuring. Locke would rather deal with that than with a tumor going undetected until it was bigger.

Finding other patients to include in the study was a bit challenging for Malkin, given how rare Li-Fraumeni syndrome is. But over several years, he managed to recruit eight families; most were from Canada, but several lived in Southern California and Utah, where oncologists had learned of Malkin's study. For the study to be valid, they screened their patients using the same tests and intervals as Malkin. He was glad to include them, as the geographic diversity helped ensure that a narrowly skewed population wouldn't distort the study results. In the participating families, eighteen of the thirty-three mutation carriers opted to undergo the rigorous screening regimen.

By the end of the first stage of the study in 2010, the results were striking. Lucas Locke and his sister, Juliet, who was born in 2006 and had also inherited the p53 mutation, never developed cancer during the study period. But the frequent screening in other families in the study detected ten tumors in seven patients before any symptoms had appeared and a number of premalignant lesions that likely would have become cancerous.

In a one-year-old baby girl, an MRI brain scan detected a very early stage choroid plexus carcinoma, a type of brain malignancy that can be fatal within months, as it often isn't discovered until a later stage; and an abdominal ultrasound also discovered she had an adrenal gland tumor, on top of her kidney, when the malignancy was still small. Both were removed surgically. Without the early detection, her chances of survival would have been slim, but the little girl was still alive five years later, when the initial study concluded.

In two members of another family—a twenty-four-year-old man and his eleven-year-old sister—MRI brain scans discovered low-grade gliomas, a slow-growing brain tumor that can be terminal if it isn't caught and continues growing; both siblings underwent operations, and two years later one was disease free and the other was stable thanks to the early detection. A total-body MRI on a thirty-year-old woman found that she had fibrous histiocytoma, a soft-tissue cancer that can spread throughout the body if it isn't discovered early on, but is treatable when it is; she was still alive nine years later.

Family members who opted not to take part in the intensive screening, in contrast, fared much worse. Ten of those patients got cancer during the study, and only two had survived by the end, while all seven patients in the screening group who got cancer during the study were still alive. The findings were clear, Malkin and his colleagues helping with the study argued. In an academic article published in 2011 explaining the results, they pointedly noted that testing for the p53 mutation and intensive screening had been "discouraged for patients with Li-Fraumeni syndrome because of an absence of evidence of benefits from early detection of malignancies." Well, now there was hard data.

A few months before the paper was published, Malkin presented the preliminary findings at a conference devoted to p53 research. A rising star in the world of p53, he nonetheless was intimidated when he looked out on the audience of several hundred scientists and saw who was sitting in the front row: Arnold Levine, Sir David Lane, and Bert Vogelstein, three of the most prominent cancer researchers in the world, especially renowned for their work on the role of p53 in cancer.

At the end of his talk, Malkin watched as the crowd rose and gave him a standing ovation, for the first time in his career. Then Lane approached him and said, "This is the most impactful study we will hear in this entire meeting." Others in the audience—comprised largely of basic scientists, not clinicians who treated patients—told him they felt the research they were doing on p53 now had far more meaning. Malkin was humbled. "All of a sudden," he thought after talking with them, "they see you could actually do something for people with the mutation." Back at SickKids Hospital, he and his colleagues embarked on a second stage of the study, in the hope of proving to medical insurers that the longer-term benefits of an intensive screening regimen—now called the Toronto Protocol—were worth the high costs.

For all the accolades, Malkin understood that helping prolong the lives of Li-Fraumeni patients was just a beginning. He and others were reminded of this when he heard a talk by Oliver Wyss at a gathering of the first Li-Fraumeni Syndrome Workshop at the National Institutes of Health in November 2010. Unlike most in attendance, Wyss wasn't a prominent researcher or doctor treating cancer patients. He was among a small group of LFS family members invited to give their perspectives on living with the p53 mutation—not knowing when cancer would strike next, but knowing it almost certainly would.

Wyss started by placing a photo of his two young children, both bald from chemotherapy, on the lectern in front of him. His son, Hudson, the younger of the two, was just ten months old when he was diagnosed in 2005 with choroid plexus carcinoma, which is so rare in children that his oncologist in Los Angeles recommended a genetic test. Hudson tested positive for the p53 mutation, as did his father, though neither he nor any of his immediate relatives had cancer. This meant Oliver likely had a de novo mutation; that is, it wasn't inherited, but instead had occurred when he was conceived, which is estimated to account for 5 to 10 percent of all germline mutations.

Hudson would undergo six surgeries, fifteen different chemotherapy regimens, sixty-two radiation treatments, and multiple clinical trials, Wyss said. While their son was recovering from surgery, and was receiving chemo and radiation treatment, Oliver and his wife, Jamie, had a genetic test performed on their daughter, Abella, who was two years older than Hudson, and learned that she also had inherited the p53 mutation.

The family's oncologist, following the screening program in Malkin's study, recommended that Abella undergo a brain MRI scan, and a tiny choroid plexus carcinoma was detected in her as well. Because they had discovered it before Abella had any symptoms, the malignancy was the smallest brain tumor pediatric oncologists at Los Angeles Children's Hospital had ever seen, and it was easily removed by surgeons. Sadly, Hudson's brain tumor, which had been discovered later, kept coming back, and he underwent five more operations in an effort to beat the cancer and save his life, to no avail. He died on June 16, 2008, when he was three years old.

Abella's brain cancer never returned after her surgery. But in 2010, one of her regular ultrasound scans spotted something else—an adrenal gland cancer on her kidney. At just eight years old, Abella was battling her second cancer.

Now, after recounting his children's cancer history, Wyss politely but pointedly admonished the people in the audience, which included renowned LFS experts Joseph Fraumeni, David Malkin, and Louise Strong. It had been forty-one years since the possibility of an inherited cancer syndrome was first raised, he noted, but after years of research, the best that doctors could offer LFS families was intensive screening.

"It's not enough going on," he told them. "We cannot just be satisfied by screening. We have to find true cures to treat these genetic disorders. And again, with the highest respect to all in the medical field here, which we have the world leading experts, including the founder, we have to do more. . . . Because I'm sure, if this will be your grandchild or your child, this would not be acceptable. It is not acceptable to me. It's not acceptable to my wife. It's not acceptable to the other family members who are running out of patience. So it should not be acceptable to you."

Wyss spoke for just five and a half minutes, but years later many of the scientists remembered his speech more than any other given at the daylong gathering. They typically attended meetings where researchers presented their latest findings and congratulated themselves on all the progress they were making in understanding p53. So they were jolted when they heard that, in the eyes of afflicted families, it didn't matter much, because none of the research had stopped their loved ones from getting cancer and dying, often at early ages. As Wyss had told them, "It happens over and over and over again."

Tragically, Abella's adrenal gland tumor eventually spread, and she would die three years later, at age eleven, in December 2013. It is no consolation that she likely would have died years earlier of her first cancer if she hadn't been tested for the p53 mutation. By detecting her cancers early, the intensive screening had prolonged Abella's life, but had not saved her.

32

CHARLIE, MY BROTHER PAUL'S SON, COULDN'T GET A JOB. HE HAD JUST GRADUATED cum laude from the University of Illinois's well-regarded law school, where he had held a coveted spot as an editor on the law, technology, and policy journal. It was 2006, and the economy was booming. Charlie was invited to a lot of job interviews, but none resulted in an offer, even as some graduates with lower class rankings were being wooed by firms.

Puzzled, he sought advice from a legal recruiting firm. Not long after that, a job counselor confided to Charlie that his troubles had nothing to do with his credentials, but rather his face. Now in his mid-twenties, he had undergone multiple painful reconstructive surgeries to repair the damage done by the childhood cancer in his jaw. He looked better than ever, but the left side of his face was still a bit askew. If you knew Charlie, who had a winning personality, you paid it no mind. But law firms where he interviewed told the recruiter that they worried his appearance might hamper his ability to bring in clients.

It was unfair, though not totally surprising to Charlie, who was accustomed to drawing stares from strangers. True to his character, he refused to let the slight deter him, though he began wearing eyeglasses, which he felt would make his face look more evenly balanced.

At one point, Charlie interviewed to become a law clerk for an Illinois appellate court judge. The interviewer, Stacey Mandell, the judge's senior clerk, had been impressed by his legal writing, but she confessed that she didn't understand why he would be interested in a clerkship. "You seem supremely overqualified," she said.

Charlie replied, "I've gone out on many interviews and been close to getting jobs," he told her, "but haven't gotten offers."

He didn't elaborate, but to her, the reason was obvious: "It was discrimination based on his looks and his cancer history." She strongly recommended hiring Charlie, but the judge selected another candidate.

He ended up settling for a job that didn't excite him, working as an in-house lawyer for a benefit fund for unionized employees. But after a couple of years, he wanted something more challenging, so he was happy when Mandell contacted him and said the appellate court clerkship he had sought earlier had opened up again. This time, he got the job, quickly winning the respect of the judge and his new colleagues with his sharp wit and incisive briefs on complicated cases.

To celebrate his first year in the job, he went on vacation to Turkey in late 2009 with Susan, his mom. They had a fun time, though soon after they returned home, his stomach started bothering him. Charlie figured he had caught a bug from something he drank or ate. He wasn't concerned: in the three decades since his bout with childhood cancer, he had been the picture of health—unlike his dad, Paul, who had already had a couple of scares since his lung cancer.

In 2002, Paul had been diagnosed with "in situ" colon cancer—called stage zero because it is such an early stage carcinoma—which had been easily treated and never developed into a full-blown tumor. Then, in 2004, he developed prostate cancer. To Susan's consternation, it took his urologist twelve biopsies over a couple of months to make the diagnosis, even though Paul's prostate-specific antigen, or PSA, test, an indicator of prostate cancer, showed results that something was seriously awry. Like all of us, Susan hadn't heard of Li-Fraumeni syndrome, but she had insisted that Paul keep going back for more tests, telling him, "You have all this cancer in your family. You tell the doctor that something's going on." Fortunately, it was still early enough to treat the prostate cancer, and the malignancy, his third, was in remission.

When Charlie's discomfort persisted in the spring of 2010, he wondered if he needed to eat more fiber, had become lactose intolerant, or had developed a bad urinary tract infection. Or, perhaps, he thought, it was work-related stress; or his digestive system was simply getting thrown off by the jostling of the hour-and-a-half commuter train ride he sometimes took from his apartment in Chicago to his clerk's job in Woodstock, Illinois.

He finally decided to see a doctor, who said his abdominal pain and recurring diarrhea suggested a severe case of gastroenteritis. "We're still searching for a reason," Charlie told colleagues. His doctor put him on ciprofloxacin (better known simply as cipro), a strong antibiotic often prescribed for gastroenteritis. And for a while, that seemed to help. "This makes me wonder if I did pick up a parasite infection, which apparently causes similar symptoms to ulcerative colitis," Charlie told Mandell, now not just a work colleague but a good friend, on July 23. "I'm just glad I'm feeling better and hope it continues."

But Charlie still had bad days amid the good days, and he wondered if that meant he had a more serious underlying issue, like Crohn's disease, a chronic inflammatory bowel disease. He saw his doctor again on July 28. "He examined my abdomen and felt a lump (which he had me feel) on the lower left side. So, obviously there is an obstruction," Charlie told a colleague. The obstruction, the doctor said, perhaps was due to side effects of the cipro medication Charlie had been taking. Charlie should eat more fiber and take another round of magnesium citrate, a strong liquid laxative. If that didn't clear things up, the doctor said, then he should have a colonoscopy, a procedure typically not performed until a person reaches at least the age of forty-five. "He still wants to take it slow for some reason," Charlie emailed Mandell in exasperation.

In early August, Charlie flew to Aspen, Colorado, for a vacation with his dad and mom. When he arrived, he was feeling sick, but he attributed this to a long day of travel that began with a 5 a.m. trip to O'Hare Airport and to his body's getting acclimated to Aspen's 7,900-foot altitude. But throughout his stay, he was spending an unusual amount of time in the bathroom dealing with diarrhea, and Paul and Susan pressed him to insist on a colonoscopy when he returned home.

On August 17, 2010, more than half a year after his stomach began bothering him, Charlie got a colonoscopy and was given the devastating news that he had stage three colorectal cancer in the lower part of his colon. A CT scan confirmed the severity of the malignancy. "Not the greatest news on Charlie—he's stage 3, spread to lymph nodes. . . . I guess I thought this was really early stage," Susan wrote to us, "but Paul said the CT scan was the best the doctor said he could have hoped for after what he saw during the colonoscopy."

The obvious thoughts race through your mind: Charlie had been in pain for a while; if he didn't have such a high tolerance for pain, developed through his many surgeries over the years, would he have complained more to his doctor? If Charlie had undergone a colonoscopy months earlier, would it have caught the tumor when it was still in stage one, making it easier to treat? We knew that colonoscopies typically aren't performed on thirty-year-olds, because young people rarely develop colorectal cancer. But Charlie wasn't just any thirty-year-old. He was a cancer survivor, in a family riddled with cancer. Why hadn't that raised a red flag much earlier?

There wasn't time to ponder these questions. While the cancer was curable, Charlie was facing a potentially life-threatening tumor for the second time. His odds of recovery were at least better this time—about 60 percent of colorectal cancer patients survive at least five years—but his past history complicated matters. "As my oncologist put it (literally), the goal is to nuke the hell out of the tumor and any infected lymph nodes and then remove them," Charlie wrote to his college friends.

Underscoring his doctors' new urgency after months of misdiagnosis, on August 30, Charlie began a grueling four-week regimen of radiation and round-the-clock chemotherapy delivered through an intravenous pump, with the hope that they could shrink the tumor. If that worked, they still would need to remove part of his colon surgically.

Charlie finished his radiation and first round of chemo in mid-October, and after a brief four-week break, he started an even nastier six-month course of chemo—a cocktail of three drugs with miserable side effects. At times, he felt so cold he had to get under an electric blanket. Other times, the chemo caused bad diarrhea and extreme nausea. Paul and Susan took turns staying with Charlie at his condominium in Chicago, to help him get through the debilitating treatment.

But at least it was working. "The good news is that all the scans show that Charlie's tumor has shrunk dramatically. That is incredibly good news, actually, because it was a big and nasty tumor when they first found it in mid-August," Paul told me in late November.

Perhaps as a reminder that cancer can be beaten—and that he already had defied the odds and beaten it once—Charlie kept in his Chicago apartment a framed copy of the 1992 *Wall Street Journal* story his dad had written about his childhood tumor and subsequent surgeries. At one point, Mandell stopped by his apartment and, seeing the framed article, did a double take. She instantly remembered reading it when she was a legal secretary nearly two decades earlier, but she had never connected it to Charlie until that moment. "I've known you your entire life," she told him.

To get out the rest of the tumor, Charlie underwent surgery on January 4, 2011. The mass that doctors removed was large, though it was mostly scar tissue as a result of his radiation, along with twelve cancerous lymph nodes. "We could not have asked for a better result . . . we passed a major milestone today, and have come a long way from those very dark days of last August," Paul emailed me that night. So that Charlie could recover from the operation, doctors performed a temporary ileostomy to enable him to clear waste from his system. But temporary meant *months*, not days or weeks. As Charlie later confided in an email to friends, it meant he would have to "poop into a bag that was attached to my lower stomach for over five months. A temporary ileostomy is similar to a colostomy bag, a traditional poop bag, only it was connected to my small intestine as opposed to my colon, which made the output more liquid. The reason I had a temporary ileostomy was because we had to let my colon heal properly, particularly the internal stitches down there after part of my colon was removed and the remaining colon sewn together."

Even after the surgery, Charlie's treatment wasn't done. Next would come another four months of wrenching chemotherapy. For Charlie, as with many cancer patients after surgery, this was a tense period. Even when operations seem to go well, there is always the fear that some cancer cells have escaped and are lurking elsewhere, waiting to wreak havoc. Given the diabolical ability of cancer cells to proliferate out of control, only a few need to survive before they begin to multiply.

A few weeks after surgery, but before his chemo regimen began, Charlie had a CEA, or carcinoembryonic antigen, test, which measures substances in the blood made by cancer cells or by normal cells in response to a malignancy in the body. The test indicated that his CEA level was rising, a potentially ominous sign. "I'm nervous about the blood counts, mostly the CEA which indicates active cancer," Susan wrote in an email to my wife, Vicki. Her worry grew when Charlie's oncologist decided to put him on an especially potent—and toxic—cocktail of drugs typically prescribed for some of the worst stage four cancers. "That was a little disconcerting to hear," she added.

A few weeks later, we were all relieved to hear that the chemo seemed to be working. Charlie's CEA count was back to normal. But his recovery was far from certain. When Paul—who had been writing books since leaving the *Wall Street Journal* in late 2007 after losing out in a competition to become the top editor—was contacted in mid-February about taking a senior editor's job at Reuters news agency, he was initially reluctant. He didn't want to do anything that might keep him and Susan from spending time in Chicago helping care for Charlie.

"I've also been preoccupied with fighting another cancer crisis, not in myself but in my son Charlie," Paul told the person at Reuters who had reached out to him. Instead, he was talking about a professorship at

Northwestern University journalism school, in part because of the proximity of the campus in Evanston, Illinois, to Chicago. But a month later, Charlie's outlook had improved so much that Paul changed his mind—in part, at Charlie's behest—and started talking in earnest about the Reuters job, which he would take later that year.

But first Charlie had to clear his final hurdle—surgery to reconnect his digestive tract, so that he no longer would need the uncomfortable ileostomy bag attached to his intestines. When he finally had the operation on June 30, Charlie emailed his close friends: "I can't express how good it feels not to have that damn bag attached to me . . . having the temporary ileostomy was the total pits because it was unsightly. Although I was able to conceal it well, it required a lot of attention and was a constant reminder that I had cancer." It would still take time for his system to fully recover but, true to form, Charlie quipped that it would be relatively easy "given all the other shit, both literally and figuratively[,] I had to endure throughout the past year."

Charlie, against the odds, had beaten cancer for the second time.

33

RORY WILLIAMS SURVIVED BRAIN CANCER AS A CHILD, BUT AT SIXTEEN SHE WAS BACK in the hospital with osteosarcoma, complicated by another aggressive malignancy in her chest. Her doctors discussed how unusual it was for someone so young to already have developed three cancers.

What could be going on? they wondered. They queried her parents and learned that her mother's family had a history of different cancers—breast, lung, pancreatic, testicular, brain, and bone. "That's bad luck or something genetic," her lead surgeon told colleagues, instructing them to do some research. They came back and advised him that Rory had tested positive for a p53 mutation and had a rare genetic condition called Li-Fraumeni syndrome. "Li for what?" a second surgeon asked, and another doctor confessed, "Never even heard of it."

Rory wasn't a real person, but a character in an episode of *Grey's Anatomy*, the wildly popular hospital drama, broadcast on ABC-TV on March 6, 2014. Li-Fraumeni syndrome had gone prime time.

The writer of the episode, Tia Napolitano, was just two years old when she had a rare cancer called neuroblastoma, which develops in the nerve cells. Though she didn't have Li-Fraumeni syndrome, one thing in the episode rang especially true—a quarter century after the landmark discovery of the p53 mutation, the syndrome was still rel-atively unknown. A question about Li-Fraumeni syndrome had been added to some medical certification examinations in the early 2000s, but it was still so rare—known cases had increased, though still to only five hundred families—that even most doctors were clueless.

"The part where none of the surgeons had ever heard of Li-Fraumeni, well, that is not just possible, but probable," a woman from an LFS fam-ily wrote in a comment posted online about the *Grey's Anatomy* episode. "We have all had to explain it to doctors at some time . . . sometimes goo-gle searching it for them in the office, or bringing in papers that explain the syndrome."

The *Grey's Anatomy* episode had 8.2 million viewers. I wasn't one of them. Nor is it likely that my brother, Paul, saw the episode, as he was living in London at the time while working as managing editor of Reu-ters news agency. But later that year, in early December 2014, he received some unnerving test results regarding the prostate cancer he had devel-oped a decade earlier and that had been in remission. "Unfortunately I got bad news Friday from the doc," he wrote in an email. His PSA num-bers (a marker for prostate cancer) had tripled since August, when they should have remained stable. "More tests and bone scans to come. Bum-mer, but I will fight it . . ."

Two days later, I got a call from Paul. Perhaps triggered by the ris-ing PSA number, he told me he was taking a genetic test for a hereditary cancer syndrome at the Cancer Genetics Program at Columbia Univer-sity Medical Center in New York. He said it was called Li-Fraumeni syn-drome, after the two doctors who had discovered the condition. It was the first time I can recall hearing the name Li-Fraumeni. He explained that it was at the recommendation of his longtime oncologist there, due to his personal and family history of multiple cancers.

We spoke for only a few minutes, as he didn't know much more. But before we finished talking, I asked him for the spelling, so I could look it up. Then I jotted a brief email to myself, to make sure I had heard him correctly. My email said, in full, "Still waiting to get final results, but the doctors say they can almost guarantee that he has Li-Fraumeni syndrome, which means that a gene P-53—that usually shuts down or kills small tumors before they become big—doesn't work properly. Doesn't mean that I have it just because he has it."

A few weeks later, Paul got back the lab tests and emailed a copy to me. At the top, there was stark wording in capital letters: "RESULT POSITIVE—CLINICALLY SIGNIFICANT MUTATION IDENTIFIED." A letter from one of his doctors, a genetics expert, explaining the test results ran six pages long. But the elusive answer to the question we had been asking for decades—*why?*—was addressed in the first paragraph: "You were found to carry a mutation in the *TP53* gene that causes Li-Fraumeni Syndrome."

There it was. It wasn't a chemical our father had carried home from work on his clothes. It wasn't bad luck, or a statistical coincidence. It wasn't something that could be overcome with willpower, as our sister Gina had desperately hoped while she struggled to live. It was simply a very rare, very bad genetic mutation, hidden in our family by nature in its random complexity.

My brother was not surprised. "I actually am more relieved than upset by this, honestly," he wrote in an email. "At least we have an explanation. I wish I would have had the testing earlier, though the science was not well developed until a few years ago, and even now my primary oncologist (Dr. Stoopler) is dubious that significant benefits will come from this testing. . . . But after researching this and discussing it in detail with the genetic team at Columbia, I have concluded that any specific enhanced screening techniques and schedules that can be used on Charlie, me and others with L-F absolutely will be a significant benefit in aiding early detection, which is no small thing."

But Paul also was pained. Not by his own cancers, but the knowledge that it was something from inside him that had led to his son Charlie suffering so much.

In late 2015, I belatedly decided to get tested, too, at the behest of my children. I was sixty-three and had never developed any cancer. Still, it was possible that I had Li-Fraumeni syndrome but was among the fortunate 5 percent or so who defy the odds and don't develop malignant tumors. I needed to know because if I had the mutation, my son and daughter could have inherited it—and passed it on to their own children.

With the help of Paul's doctors, I was accepted into an academic study of how people respond psychologically to getting the results of "multiplex gene panel testing" for about two dozen different hereditary mutations, including p53. After filling out extensive forms detailing my family's cancer history, I drove to the University of Southern California Medical Center for an 8 a.m. appointment on November 16, 2015. As I was signing in at the front desk, a doctor came out to the foyer to greet me. *Isn't that nice*, I thought. I couldn't recall that happening to me before.

Then it occurred to me: I was a potentially interesting subject. How might I react if I got the bad news that I had the p53 mutation, given my family's extensive cancer history? Or, if I got good news that I didn't have the mutation, could that strain my relationship with my brother, making me regret taking the test and telling him the result?

I gave a blood sample after a genetic counselor asked if I was certain I wanted to do the test; if I tested positive for the mutation, she gently advised, it could be a traumatic, life-altering result. I nodded and shrugged. It couldn't alter all the cancers in my family. Several weeks later, at around 3 p.m. on December 8, I got a call from the genetics counselor, who said she had "very good news." The results were negative on all twenty-five genetic mutations for which I was tested, including the p53 mutation.

"You are very lucky," the doctor added, given the history of cancer in our family.

Statistically, of the four of us—Paul, me, Gina, and Angela—only two should have inherited the genetic defect. But three did, and only one didn't. I emailed my children, who expressed relief, as it meant that they and their children couldn't inherit the genetic defect. Still, as welcome as the news was for me and them, we found it hard to celebrate being spared a fate that had befallen my siblings and Charlie, my nephew and their cousin.

When I later began researching this book, and saw the family trees in the first Li-Fraumeni paper in 1969, it caught my breath. It was like looking in a mirror. Similar to us, those first four families had different cancers and multiple cancers across generations, starting at early ages, with family members dying in their twenties or thirties or forties, and sometimes much younger. And one other thing jumped out at me, as I studied the "Family A" tree: while most branches of their family had a variety of cancers over several generations, there was one branch (with squares representing males and circles representing females, all left blank) where there were no tumors for three successive generations. Surrounded by the cancers of their brothers and sisters, uncles, aunts, and cousins, this branch was cancer free.

That, I recognized, was me and my children.

It could have been easy, and understandable, after all the heartache in my brother's branch of the family, for Paul to ask why him and not me. He never once did. "Great news!!!" he responded within minutes of reading my email that I had tested negative for the p53 mutation.

Our mother and sisters almost certainly had had the mutation, though genetic testing for the abnormality hadn't been possible when they were alive. Where did it start in our family, given that neither of our mom's parents had had cancer and her sister hadn't? (All lived into their late eighties or early nineties.) Perhaps one of my mother's parents had carried the mutation, but was among the small percentage who never get cancer. More likely, it was a de novo mutation that occurred spontaneously in our mother's genes when she was conceived. We will never know for sure.

34

M Y NEPHEW CHARLIE DEVELOPED HIS FIRST CANCER WHEN HE WAS JUST TWO years old, and his second when he was thirty. His twin brother, Dan, also inherited the p53 mutation from my brother, Paul, but was spared and had no cancers by that age. My brother developed his first cancer at forty-seven. Our mom got cancer for the first time in her early-to-mid-thirties, and our two sisters, Gina and Angela, developed cancer at thirty-two and twenty-four respectively. The cancers varied not only by the age at which they developed, but also by type of cancer and where it occurred—breast, cheek, colon, abdomen, and lung. Both Paul and Gina had had lung cancer, though they were different forms of it.

One of the scariest things for families with Li-Fraumeni syndrome is that you never know when or where cancer will strike—even though the p53 mutation within a family is exactly the same in all members who inherit it. Occasionally, a Li-Fraumeni patient's second tumor will appear in a different organ a year or two later, while other patients don't develop a second malignancy for twenty years or more. Some patients have not just one or two but six or even more cancers over their lifetime—if they manage to survive their early tumors. A half dozen cancers are most common in LFS patients, but in family after family, the main pattern observed by doctors is that there is no clear pattern.

From the time Li and Fraumeni began studying the syndrome, oncologists found this baffling. Why does a mutation in the same gene, they wondered, result in so many different malignancies at random ages?

Scientists looking for answers soon began stumbling across possible clues hiding inside p53. The two teams that initially identified an inherited p53 mutation in late 1990 as the culprit behind Li-Fraumeni cancers in unrelated families had discovered abnormalities in almost the same spot on the gene. In the aftermath of the LFS inherited p53 mutation discovery, scientists working with other cancer-prone families also found mutations in similar locations.

But soon, scientists started to identify mutations outside several established "hot spots" on p53. One of the scientists who found a new variant of the mutation early on was David Malkin, the young researcher who had helped make the original p53 discovery while working in Friend's lab. In a 1992 paper in the *New England Journal of Medicine*, on a study of patients who had a second malignancy, he found that four had inherited p53 mutations—three in the same location as the 1990 families and one in an altogether different location on p53; further investigation found that the child's mother and sister had the same p53 variant.

The same issue of the *NEJM* carried an article by a separate group of scientists who had found the mutation in yet another location in a study of patients with sarcomas: of eight people found to have p53 inherited germline mutations, five were in the vicinity of the original hot spot, but three were in different locations on p53. "Diverse mutations of this gene were associated with an increased likelihood of cancer; hence, the entire gene should be considered a target for heritable mutation. It appears that the group of patients with cancer who carry germline mutations of the p53 gene is more diverse than is suggested by the clinical definition of the Li-Fraumeni syndrome. The identification of carriers could be of substantial clinical importance," according to the paper.

As more families were studied, even more variants in inherited p53 mutations emerged. In 1994, an English research team led by Jillian Birch—the first to coin the name "Li-Fraumeni syndrome," in an academic paper in the early 1980s—conducted a study of thirty-six individuals in twenty-one families with known germline p53 mutations; many were clustered near the location of the original mutation, but others had newly discovered variants. Indeed, their report noted, variants outside the initial hot spots "are likely to be underrepresented" because researchers didn't also look at other places on p53 for mutations.

Yet another paper in 1997 found even more variants, leading its author to assert, "In view of our findings that germ-line *TP53* mutations can be found throughout the entire gene . . . in Li-Fraumeni families, we consider it essential to analyze the entire gene when screening such families." That, in fact, is how doctors for Luana Locke's relatives in Italy had found their p53 mutation that her Canadian oncologists had initially failed to detect.

Tracking the many p53 mutation variants became challenging. So as their numbers grew—both inherited "germline" mutations, which people in LFS families are born with and can pass on, and spontaneous, "somatic" mutations, which occur during the normal division of human cells and can lead to cancer but that aren't inherited—scientists created and shared databases enumerating the mutations to better understand them and further research into p53. By the late 1990s, academic papers had reported dozens of different inherited p53 mutations linked to cancer. By the early 2000s, the number had multiplied to nearly 250.

The database catalogues included the type and precise location of the abnormality on p53; the diagnostic method used to identify the mutation; and detailed information on the families carrying different variants, including the total number and types of tumors, the age at diagnosis (and at death, if a patient had died), and the generation of the family members who developed cancer. The hope was that as scientists accumulated more and more data on variants, the growing volume of information might help unravel the mystery of why patients with inherited p53 mutations got different cancers at different ages.

In many cases, only a handful of patients or families carried a specific mutation variant. This was hardly surprising. Given the often deadly nature of inherited p53 mutations, and the fact that many patients developed cancers between infancy and their twenties, some families didn't produce enough children to pass the mutation on for multiple generations; that's why the Kilius family was unusual and why only about five hundred Li-Fraumeni families had been identified a decade after the mutation was discovered.

But there was a particularly notable exception. In the late 1990s and early 2000s, researchers in Brazil began taking notice of patients with p53 mutations. One of the researchers was a medical student named Maria Isabel Achatz, who initially came across an unusual case while in her fifth year in Santo André, a municipality about twenty miles southeast of São Paulo. After she treated a woman who had developed five tumors over the years, Achatz visited the library and found articles describing patients just like hers with something called Li-Fraumeni syndrome. But when she relayed her suspicion to faculty advisers, they expressed skepticism. Knowing the rarity of LFS families worldwide, they responded, "You think you found one here?" Still, the case left such a lasting impression on Achatz that she decided to focus her studies and research efforts on oncogenetics.

Then a group of Brazilian researchers led by an oncologist published a paper in 2001 documenting an unusually high number of childhood cases in southern Brazil of adrenal cortical carcinoma, in the adrenal glands on top of the kidneys—one of the signature pediatric cancers in Li-Fraumeni families. Almost all the patients had the same p53 mutation variant, located outside the previously identified hot spots that accounted for the preponderance of known p53 mutations. Still, the Brazilians were cautious about identifying the cases as Li-Fraumeni syndrome, noting that "there was no history of increased cancer incidence among family members." They also suggested the mutations they found might have been caused by environmental carcinogens, as extensive use of pesticides for farming in the region "may be implicated in the origin of this abnormality."

By the time these cases were reported, Achatz had finished medical school and was a doctor trainee at A.C. Camargo Cancer Center in

São Paulo. In her first year or so, she came across more cases like the cancer-ridden woman she had seen as a medical student. The number of families Achatz saw that displayed all the characteristics of Li-Fraumeni syndrome—thirty—was staggering. Granted, the cancer center drew patients from all over a heavily populated country, but it was odd, given the low number of LFS families worldwide. *Either I'm overdiagnosing those families or we have a special situation in Brazil*, she thought to herself.

Recognizing the potential significance of Achatz's observations, her boss suggested that she present a summary of her findings to a cancer conference in Paris in late 2002. While there, she met a Belgian researcher, Pierre Hainaut, who had helped launch a database of p53 mutations years earlier. Hainaut proposed to Achatz that they collaborate in researching her Brazilian families, using gene sequencing techniques to map any p53 mutations in relatives who had cancer.

Back in São Paulo, Achatz collected fresh blood samples and returned to Hainaut's lab in Lyon, France, to study them. To her surprise, however, in the DNA from the blood samples she had collected, only three of the forty-five patients tested positive for mutations in the regions on p53 where researchers most often looked for abnormalities. Achatz was embarrassed and wondered if she might have misdiagnosed the patients; perhaps many of them didn't have LFS, despite their extensive family cancer histories.

But Hainaut proposed sequencing the DNA from the samples again to look at other spots on p53. This time, most of the patients tested positive—but at codon 337, the location where the other Brazilian doctors had identified mutation a few years earlier among children with adrenal cortical tumors, rather than the area around codon 248, where the initial mutation linked to LFS had been identified a decade earlier. The variant in almost all the Brazilian families was the same, and subsequent research would determine that it was almost exclusive to southeastern Brazil, concentrated in a relatively narrow geographic band that stretches 1,500 miles. Many of the families with the mutation traced their lineage to early Portuguese settlers to the region. Achatz and other

Brazilian researchers theorized that they had inherited what is known as a founder mutation, which likely originated with a *tropeiro*, a merchant who traveled along a trade route in the seventeenth and eighteenth centuries and may have slept with a number of women along the way, passing onto offspring this particular p53 mutation that he carried, perhaps as a de novo mutation.

As Achatz and her colleagues expanded their research over the years into the families that carried this p53 variant, they determined that it was far more common than the p53 mutations linked to Li-Fraumeni syndrome elsewhere. As many as 1 in every 375 people in southern and southeastern Brazil carry the mutation, compared with an estimated 1 in 7,000 in the United States.

How could this be, given the lethality of LFS? To understand, they compiled extensive records and analyzed medical histories of the family members who had inherited the Brazilian mutation. What the researchers found was surprising: this particular p53 variant had what scientists call a lower penetrance, or percentage of people who develop cancer. While Brazilian family members with the mutation get malignancies far more often than the overall population, in general, they have a significantly lower lifetime risk than people with most other p53 mutation variants—60 percent get cancer versus 90 to 95 percent of people with other p53 variants.

Moreover, they found, people with the Brazilian variant often develop cancer at a later age. "Only 15%–20% of the p.R337H [the Brazilian variant, named after the fragment of p53 where it is located] carriers develop cancer by 30 years of age, compared with 50% in carriers of classic mutations," Achatz and her colleagues determined. While breast cancer is the most common malignancy among women with virtually all p53 mutations, for example, women with the Brazilian variant typically develop it around age forty, compared with age thirty-two for women with the classic variants. Together, this means that people carrying the Brazilian mutation live longer, so they have more time to reproduce and pass the mutation on to the next generation . . . and on and on—which explains the higher rate of LFS in Brazil's southern region.

While differences in the cancer histories of patients with the Brazil-ian and classic p53 mutation were particularly stark, they reflected what other researchers were finding in other variants they identified—which by 2016 had reached 360. Researchers started thinking in terms of a Li-Fraumeni *spectrum* rather than a single Li-Fraumeni syndrome.

Underscoring the complexities, the traditional definition of what constitutes Li-Fraumeni syndrome has evolved. In most cases, people with LFS have a p53 mutation. But in some instances, they are diagnosed either with LFS or with the related Li-Fraumeni-like syndrome (LFL), based on their having a similar personal and family cancer history even though they may have tested negative for the p53 mutation.

Depending on the p53 variant, some LFS patients seemed prone to develop more varieties of tumors; or to get their first cancer at earlier ages; or to experience shorter or longer periods between their first and second malignancy; or to be especially susceptible to a certain type of cancer, such as brain, breast, or colorectal tumors. Even minor differ-ences in the same p53 variant could result in major differences in cancer histories, as illustrated by researchers who found that patients carrying one version of the Brazilian mutation got their first malignancy, remark-ably, an average of seventeen years later than patients with a similar ver-sion of the same mutation.

While researchers could discern trends, however, the data also showed that in family after family, members with the exact same mutation type developed different cancers at different ages. What would explain that?

One obvious possibility: each family member, even when living in the same household, is exposed to different environmental factors that can set cancer in motion. One child might attend school near a chemi-cal factory, while an older sibling might go to a different school across town. Or one might play soccer on a field near a river that carries runoff from farms, while another might play basketball indoors. Their differ-ent experiences throughout their childhood and teenage years could be almost limitless.

Hoping to shed light on the interplay of external and genetic factors, a group of researchers, including p53 pioneer Arnold Levine, conducted a study designed to exclude the possibility of different environmental exposures. They couldn't run a controlled experiment like this with people, of course, so they did it with mice. Male mice with the same p53 mutation—thus predisposing them to cancer—were crossed with seven different strains of females that had functioning p53 genes. The mice were kept in the same laboratory environment, free of contaminants. By the end of the experiment, the majority of the mice had developed tumors—but of varying types and at different ages on average. The rate of cancer incidence ranged from about 30 percent in one strain of mice to just over 70 percent in another strain. Some strains developed virtually all their cancers within thirteen months, while others got tumors more slowly, with a majority of their malignancies appearing between thirteen and twenty months. Some had higher rates of bone cancer, while others had more lymph system tumors or skin tumors.

The conclusion: "The genetic background of mice carrying *Tp53* mutations"—that is, each strain's different genetic makeup other than p53—"has a strong influence upon the tissue type of the tumor produced and the number of tumors formed in a single mouse." Even while scientists observed broad patterns, the variety of tumors within the mice strains indicated that other, unknown genetic factors likely play a role in the types of frequencies of malignancies, which is why it is hard to predict cancer occurrence.

Similarly, all members of human families, while sharing many genes, have slightly different genetic backgrounds. Some siblings have blond hair and blue eyes, while others have brown hair and eyes. One brother can grow to be six feet tall, while another brother can grow to six feet, five inches, and yet another can top out at five feet, ten inches. One sister can be left-handed while all her siblings are right-handed. The possibilities are endless, and the genetic differences cumulatively can interact in ways that are beyond the understanding of scientists—and might explain why family members with the same p53 mutation can have very different cancer histories.

Even as they accumulated knowledge about p53 variants and Li-Fraumeni families—by 2015, scientists had found a thousand different mutation variants—researchers still couldn't predict with much certainty who would develop what kinds of cancers and at what ages. "It has been almost 25 years since the discovery of *TP53* as the defective gene in LFS," David Malkin, who had taken the mantle from Li and Fraumeni to become one of the preeminent authorities on p53 mutations, wrote in a paper he coauthored in 2015. "Nonetheless, the answers to these questions have been slow to emerge."

35

LATE ONE AFTERNOON IN THE SPRING OF 2014, JAIMEE HOWARD FINNELL'S FOUR-year-old daughter, Taylin, told her she was seeing a purple dot in front of her eyes, though she knew it wasn't really there. The remark sent Finnell into a panic, her mind flashing back two decades earlier to her own childhood.

Finnell had never forgotten that her older brother, Jeremy, began hallucinating when he was ten years old. She had accompanied him with their mom to the hospital, where he underwent a scan and was diagnosed with brain cancer. Finnell, just eight years old at the time, was especially frightened because their dad, Jerry Howard, was himself already being treated for brain cancer that had been discovered a year earlier. Finnell could still vividly recall once being home alone with her dad and calling 911 when he suffered a grand mal seizure while sitting in a recliner. His body jerked violently, and he lost consciousness, scaring her so much that she hid in the kitchen until the ambulance arrived, so she wouldn't have to watch him.

Both Finnell's dad and Jeremy, her only sibling, would suffer agonizing declines before dying, her dad at age thirty-two in 1994 and her brother the next year, just a month before his eleventh birthday. So it was hardly surprising that Finnell freaked out when Taylin mentioned seeing a purple dot.

Was that the first symptom of a brain tumor, like her brother's hallucination? Was Taylin going to be the latest member of Finnell's family to be stricken with and succumb to cancer, following not just her father and brother, but also other members of the extended Kilius clan from which she came—her dad's sister, Tammy, and their baby brother, Michael; her grandmother Joan Kilius Howard; her great-grandfather Charles Kilius; her great-great-grandmother Cora Stansberry Kilius; and various great-aunts and cousins at ages ranging from two to forty-eight.

Finnell had tried to put the family's tragedies in the past. At some point—she didn't remember exactly, perhaps when she was twelve or thirteen—her aunt Tammy had told her about a cancer-causing gene in the family. While the Kilius family had been central to the research by Li and Fraumeni that led to the discovery of the p53 mutation, over the years most members had fallen out of touch with the National Cancer Institute as so many in the earlier generations died off.

Now twenty-nine years old, Finnell assumed she would get cancer someday. But she hadn't so far, and as she grew up, she hadn't been interested in learning more about Li-Fraumeni syndrome. Perhaps it was because her mother discouraged her from getting tested for the p53 mutation, telling Finnell that even if they found out she had inherited the mutation from her dad, there was nothing doctors could do.

Though Finnell didn't know much about the hereditary mutation, she did know there was some risk of passing on the genetic disorder. For many young couples, the big questions are when to have children and how many. For couples in families with an inherited cancer syndrome, the biggest question often is whether to have them. The decision is deeply personal of course, and fraught. There is a 50 percent chance that a child will inherit a p53 mutation if one parent has the abnormality—which means that there is also a 50 percent chance they won't inherit the damaged gene.

For some people who know they have the mutation, the 50 percent risk is too high. Especially for those who suffered from their own child-hood cancers or watched as young siblings or cousins underwent treat-ment, the fear that cancer could strike their own children anywhere and anytime is unbearable. My nephew Charlie, who knew all too well the travails of childhood cancer, confided to family and friends that he didn't plan on having children because he wouldn't want them to go through what he went through. Researchers have found that people with Li-Fraumeni syndrome worry not only about passing on the mutation, and their children suffering from cancer, but also about getting cancer them-selves and dying and leaving their children without a mom or dad.

To avoid passing on the mutation, some parents choose in vitro fer-tilization, or IVF. With IVF, the fertilized embryos can be tested for the p53 mutation before implantation in the mother's womb, and any embryo carrying a genetic abnormality can be rejected. But IVF is expensive, as much as $20,000 to $30,000, a cost that some insurers don't cover—and even then it typically has a success rate of only 20 to 25 percent. For many couples wanting to start a family, that means it isn't a realis-tic choice. And for many of them, the desire to have children outweighs the 50 percent risk that their babies will inherit the p53 mutation. While new treatments for cancer are developing slowly, a breakthrough, these couples reason, could come at some point. If that happened after they had decided not to have children, they feel they would regret the deci-sion—so they go ahead.

Despite the risks, Jaimee Finnell and her husband, Sean Finnell, couldn't contemplate the idea of not having kids. Jaimee had always wanted to be a mom, and that outweighed the fear of passing on a genetic mutation. "I'm not going to let anything stop me or change my mind," she would confide to friends who knew her family's cancer history. In 2007, a year after they married, they had their first daughter, Gracee; in 2009, they had Taylin, their second baby girl. After starting their family, they bought a house in Rancho Cucamonga, an exurb east of Los Angeles in the foothills of the San Gabriel Mountains.

Then Taylin saw the purple dot.

Though it was late afternoon when Taylin told her mom about the dot, Finnell immediately called the family physician in a panic. She took Taylin in the next morning, and after Finnell explained her family's cancer history, the doctor scheduled an MRI brain scan. To Finnell's relief, it was negative. (It turned out that Taylin needed eyeglasses, which may have been the reason for the purple dot.) Still, Finnell was unnerved by the episode. For her own peace of mind, she told doctors she wanted both her daughters to take genetic tests to determine if they had inherited the p53 mutation that causes Li-Fraumeni syndrome.

There was a hitch, however. Finnell herself had never been tested, and her girls could have inherited the mutation only if she had it. Given the then-high cost of genetic testing—typically, several thousand dollars or more—doctors advised that health insurance wouldn't cover the expense of tests for her daughters unless she first tested positive. So, after two decades of telling herself there was no point in getting tested, Finnell now had a compelling reason. For moral support, her cousin Darren Delin—her aunt Tammy's only child and Jaimee's closest relative—agreed to get tested at the same time, as he had never had it done, either.

On May 5, a week or two after sending in their blood and skin samples, they both got the results. Finnell had inherited the p53 mutation; Delin had not. She was happy for her cousin, but she couldn't help wondering, *Why do I have to have it? It doesn't feel fair.* While Finnell had told friends for years she was sure she had the mutation, actually testing positive for it alarmed her. What might it mean for her daughters?

"LFS has taken out everyone on my dad's side of the family. I have one cousin left and myself . . . that's it," she wrote the next day in a post on a Li-Fraumeni syndrome support group on Facebook. "I have two daughters, ages 4 and 6. They will be getting tested soon as well. It scares me to death to think about my girls losing their mother or me having to lose one of them. Trying to stay positive but looking at my family tree doesn't make that very easy to do."

A month later, Finnell and her husband got more bad news: Gracee and Taylin both tested positive for the p53 mutation. Jaimee posted, "My

4 and 6 year old are also mutants. Even though I pretty much 'knew' this would be the case, it still shook me to the core."

Even as she worried about what the future held for her young daughters, Finnell turned her attention to doing whatever she needed to do to stay healthy as long as possible while they grew up. Knowing that many of her female relatives had died of cancer between twenty and forty-five, she decided, after consulting with her doctors, to undergo a prophylactic double mastectomy and hysterectomy as a precaution against future cancers. "I don't want to take any chances," she told her husband and her doctors. "Boom. Just take it all out. I don't want anything risky in my body." Women with Li-Fraumeni syndrome have an 80 to 90 percent chance of developing breast cancer in their lifetime, and often at an early age, between twenty and forty—like my mother, Regina Ingrassia, and many of the Kilius family women. The risk for LFS patients, in fact, is even higher than for women who inherit the *BRCA* gene, who have a 50 to 60 percent of getting breast cancer and who typically get their first tumor at an older age, between forty-five and fifty-five. Having a hysterectomy was a logical choice for Finnell, too. She wasn't planning on having more children, and ovarian cancer is also one of the fairly common malignancies for women with Li-Fraumeni syndrome.

On June 23, just six weeks after learning she had the p53 mutation, Finnell underwent surgery. A week later, she was shocked to learn the results of the pathology report: tissues showed she had a tumor in one of her breasts that hadn't been detected in any of her presurgical tests. Though small, it was a very aggressive type of cancer, one that often can be fatal. "I feel like this is a shit storm that is never ending," Finnell wrote on Facebook. But at least the tumor had been caught at an early stage. As a precaution, Finnell underwent chemotherapy treatment to zap any stray cancer cells that might have spread from the breast tumor.

Li-Fraumeni syndrome had exacted a cruel toll on at least six generations of the extended Kilius family. Now one member with the p53 mutation, Jaimee Howard Finnell, had caught a break. Call it luck or fate or divine intervention—if she had decided not to have children, if her daughter Taylin hadn't seen the purple dot, if Finnell hadn't belatedly gotten herself tested for the p53 mutation so she could get her daughters tested, her breast cancer would not have been caught until a later stage. By then, malignant cells could have metastasized from her breast, and Finnell might have died within a year or two.

Instead, after twenty-six rounds of chemotherapy over thirteen months, Finnell's doctors declared her cancer free in August 2015.

36

ON OCTOBER 8, 2015, THE *JOURNAL OF THE AMERICAN MEDICAL ASSOCIATION* RAN A long article on what seemed like an odd topic for a top academic publication, an article that other journals in fact had turned down: "Potential Mechanisms for Cancer Resistance in Elephants and Comparative Cellular Response to DNA Damage in Humans." Or, translated into plain English, why do elephants rarely get cancer, and what might that mean for people who get cancer? The answer would lead researchers to an unlikely place in their long and largely futile search for drugs to treat genetic mutations that might help Li-Fraumeni families: elephants' p53 genes.

The study was the brainchild of a pediatric oncologist at the University of Utah, Joshua Schiffman, himself a cancer survivor. At fifteen, he had developed Hodgkin lymphoma, a type of blood cancer that initially had been diagnosed by his father, who was himself an oncologist. (Schiffman refers to his treatment as his summer of R and R, "rest and radiation.") The experience motivated Schiffman to become a doctor, though his initial plan was to practice medicine rather than to conduct research.

Then, on call one weekend in 2004, at the start of his career and doing a fellowship at a Stanford University oncology lab, he saw a four-year-old girl named Danielle with leukemia. He learned it wasn't her first cancer. Danielle had survived a brain tumor when she was two, and both her father and her father's brother had died of brain cancer. "This is very strange," Schiffman told a colleague, who responded, "It sounds like Li-Fraumeni syndrome." It was the first time Schiffman had heard of the condition, so he investigated further. He learned about LFS, probed Danielle's family history, and tested for the p53 mutation—and sure enough, Danielle and her family had it.

Danielle's case prompted Schiffman to shift his career path. Over time, he focused his work on Li-Fraumeni families, and in 2008 he took a job at the Huntsman Cancer Institute at the University of Utah in Salt Lake City, with the agreement that he both conduct research and treat LFS patients; he was inspired in part by David Malkin in Toronto, whom he had met and with whom he would eventually collaborate by including many Utah families under his care in Malkin's Toronto Protocol studies, which determined that intensive screening to spot early cancers could prolong the lives of patients with inherited p53 mutations.

Schiffman became intrigued by elephants in August 2012, while attending a conference on evolutionary medicine at the Mount Desert Island Biological Laboratory in Maine. He had wandered into a lecture where the speaker, Carlo Maley, a biologist specializing in cancer and evolution, remarked that elephants almost never develop cancer. Elephants, Maley noted, are seventy to one hundred times bigger than humans, which means they have far more cells constantly dividing and mutating than people do. Because mutations can trigger malignancies in all mammals, logic has it that elephants should be riddled with cancer. Why aren't they? Maley said it was unclear, but he added that elephants have forty copies of the p53 cancer suppressor gene, while humans have just two.

After Maley's presentation, Schiffman approached him. "What if we could take blood from an elephant and compare it to the blood from my Li-Fraumeni patients and truly understand if this extra p53 is what's protecting elephants from cancer?" he asked. Maley replied that it might be a great subject for a scientific paper, assuming Schiffman could figure out how to get fresh elephant blood that wasn't contaminated.

A few weeks later, Schiffman took his three young children on a Sunday outing to Utah's Hogle Zoo, not far from their house in Salt Lake City. They arrived shortly before the start of one of the twice-daily elephant shows. As Schiffman sat with his enthralled children listening to the zookeeper talk about how he trained elephants, he kept thinking about how much elephant blood was right in front of him.

Then the keeper said, "African elephants have big veins in the back of the ears to fan the blood and keep them cool. And did you know, kids, once a week we draw blood from our elephants from those veins in the back of their ears to make sure they're healthy." Schiffman could hardly contain himself. At the end of the show, with his children in tow, he raced to speak with the keeper. "I'm a cancer doctor, and I have a question for you," Schiffman blurted out. "How do I get some elephant blood?"

It took him months of work to design a study, get approval, and find funding. But soon, his colleagues would trek once a week about a mile from their lab at the cancer center to the zoo to draw fresh blood with sterile needles from its African elephants and rush it back to the lab. To broaden the study, Schiffman worked with Ringling Bros. and Barnum and Bailey Circus to provide blood from its Asian elephants. The research team conducted lab tests by subjecting elephant skin and blood cells to radiation and chemicals known to cause DNA damage that could lead to malignancies—and they found something surprising. Elephants not only have more p53, but their p53 causes apoptosis (that is, it destroys mutated cells that could become cancerous) at a significantly higher rate than human p53 does.

Rather than first trying to repair mutated cells, which human p53 does, elephant p53 instead moves more quickly to simply kill them. "It's as if the elephants said, 'It's so important that we don't get cancer, why even try to stop the cell and repair it, when we can just kill it and start over again.' That seems to be the safest way to make sure that mutations that can cause cancer won't be passed on," Schiffman concluded. (Another research group working independently subsequently found that elephants have another safeguard against cancer: compared with p53 in other close mammal relatives, elephant p53 can induce cells to die when there isn't as much damage to DNA in them, thus thwarting potentially cancerous cells at an earlier stage, before they can proliferate and spread.)

Excited about their findings, Schiffman began pitching a paper to top academic journals, including *Science* and *Nature*, only for editors to reject it or even decline to read it. Finally, he made a personal appeal in a telephone call to an editor at the *Journal of the American Medical Association*, which also had initially declined the paper.

"I know this study sounds crazy, but we think it's relevant for people who get cancer and it would be amazing for your readers," Schiffman said.

"Okay," the editor replied, "we'll take a risk."

Not only would the article become one of the journal's most popular articles of 2015, but Schiffman had a moment of celebrity beyond the cancer research world. *Newsweek* ran a cover story devoted largely to his team's study, with a photo of him standing by an elephant at Hogle Zoo, and *PBS NewsHour* ran a long segment a few months later.

Many cancer scientists found the paper interesting, albeit quirky, but they weren't sure of its practical application. A few months before the elephant study was published, Schiffman gave a presentation about it at a pediatric oncology conference in Israel. He concluded by lamenting, "It's too bad there's no way to take the p53 from an elephant and deliver it to a person, because then maybe we could treat or even one day prevent cancer."

Afterward, Avi Schroeder, an Israeli scientist in the audience, reached out to him. Schroeder worked in the new field of developing microscopic nanoparticles—specifically, lipid nanoparticles designed to encase and carry drug molecules into cancer cells. Nanoparticles were just beginning to emerge as a promising vehicle for delivering therapeutics while limiting toxicity. They are much smaller than the adenoviruses and retroviruses that were used, largely unsuccessfully, to inject gene therapy drugs into tumors in the 1990s. Another advantage: nanoparticles have what is called low "immunogenicity." This means they are less likely to cause an immune response that produces antibodies to kill the nanoparticle—and, along with it, the drug it is delivering.

Schiffman and Schroeder quickly teamed up to cofound and raise money for a biotech company named Peel Therapeutics. (*Peel* is Hebrew for "elephant.") Peel hopes to design nanoparticles that can safely deliver EP53 (elephant p53) into human tumors and work the way it does in elephants. There are plenty of skeptics in the cancer research world who say the idea of putting an elephant gene into a human body, with all the uncertainties involved, is a bit far-fetched. Even Schiffman concedes he isn't sure if it will succeed: "I don't promise my patients it will happen, because I don't want to have them disappointed. But if I didn't believe this would work, I wouldn't be trying it."

If Peel's efforts fail, it would hardly be surprising, given that 90 percent of all new drug trials don't succeed—including numerous efforts to create a major new p53-related drug, despite the initial enthusiasm. As scientists have studied p53, they have learned that its complexities make it difficult to target with chemical compounds that would bind to it in the right way and in the right place to have the desired effect on tumors. Also, the ideal p53 drug would "reactivate" the cancer-suppressing powers that a mutation had switched off, but that is harder to accomplish than devising a compound to turn it off (much like it is harder to revive a wilted, dying plant than it is to stunt a plant's growth by killing it with a herbicide).

Finally, almost all new drug compounds have potentially negative side effects, which is why early stage drug trials are designed to first determine a drug's safety. Only then do scientists conduct next-stage trials to determine how well the drug works. The higher the dosage—which often is needed to fight aggressive cancer cells—the higher the risk of side effects. In 1999, researchers at pharmaceutical giant Pfizer identified a synthetic compound that seemed to have the ability to turn back on the cancer-suppressing powers of some p53 mutations, slowing the growth of tumors in mice. Their work suggested that "this class of compounds may be developed into anticancer drugs of broad utility." But researchers subsequently determined the compound had an unwanted toxic effect on cells in lab tests, so Pfizer didn't pursue efforts to develop a drug.

A team of scientists at Karolinska Institutet, a Swedish medical university, has been more persistent. In 2002, they reported promising test tube results with a molecule, known as PRIMA-1, or APR-246, that, like the Pfizer compound, is aimed at restoring the cancer-suppressing functions of mutant p53 genes in a tumor and that triggered cell death in mice and in human cancer cells in the lab. "The identification of a small molecule able to restore biochemical and biological function to mutant p53, resulting in significant tumor suppression in vivo, opens exciting prospects for future cancer therapy," they asserted. Confident about the prospects, some of the scientists helped found a biotech company, Aprea Therapeutics, to develop a drug. Nearly two decades later, they haven't succeeded—but they haven't given up, either.

After getting promising results in Phase I and II trials, Aprea received regulatory approval for the final hurdle, Phase III trials, but the results were discouraging. Of 154 patients with a rare type of blood cancer, myelodysplastic syndromes, Aprea found that 33 percent of the patients' cancers went into remission when treated in combination with a chemotherapy drug; but that was not considered significantly better than the 22 percent remission rate for patients receiving only the chemo drug. Disappointed but undeterred, the company is testing its molecule in combination with other chemotherapy drugs on other malignancies, including leukemia and solid tumors such as lung cancer.

After decades of frustration over trying to develop drugs that target the gene, researchers are far from losing interest in p53—in fact, they are keener than ever to understand its intricacies, and they are steadily making progress. Each year, multiple conferences devoted to p53 research draw hundreds of scientists from academia and companies trying to develop drugs. A group dedicated to p53 research in 1983 began holding an International p53 Workshop, and their eighteenth gathering, in 2022 in Israel, drew hundreds of attendees to listen to more than fifty presentations on a dizzying array of esoteric topics—such as "Structural Studies on Reactivation of Tumor-related p53 Mutants by a Small Molecule"; "Unexpected Roles for p53, MDM2 and MDMX in Cell Survival and Cell Death"; and "p53 in Control of Endogenous Retrobiome and Inflammation."

The research has led to a better understanding of the intricate structure of p53, which in turn has given scientists new ideas for chemical compounds to use—along with new delivery methods like nanoparticles—to create drugs aimed at countering the mutated form of p53 found in so many different cancers. As a result, the number of clinical trials involving p53-related drugs has risen steadily over time, from fewer than ten from 2000 to 2005 to thirty in a similar period over six years through 2022.

Arnold Levine, who helped identify p53 in 1979, is one of the scientists pursuing new p53-related drugs. He predicts that someone will be successful in the 2020s. A company he cofounded in 2013, PMV Pharma, has some promising experimental drugs that have shown success in shrinking or killing a variety of cancers—including ovarian, prostate, lung, and breast. But there's a catch, Levine hastens to add. The compound works on a particular p53 mutation variant. Given that there now are upward of one thousand different known p53 mutations, developing a one-p53-drug-fits-all therapy is unlikely, as any drug created might be able to treat only tumors associated with a relative handful of variants, or perhaps even just one. And this is true of most p53-targeted drugs. "That's a depressing thing if you think about it, because there isn't one drug that's going to work in every case, right. And so, it's the reason why it's been so hard," he says. "It's a thousandfold complicated matter."

37

I N JANUARY 2017, I WROTE AN EMAIL TO MY BROTHER, PAUL, WHO HAD RETIRED ABOUT six months earlier—as I was soon planning to do myself, not long after I turned sixty-five that summer. "Just occurred to me that this is the 20th anniversary year of your [lung] cancer surgery, right? We should plan a celebratory golf trip somewhere—maybe Scotland, or maybe the Pacific Northwest—in the fall, after I am retired. You think?"

It took him all of twenty minutes to reply: "Yes!! Scotland perfect. And for your 65th!" We vowed to soon start planning an itinerary to play some of the seaside links courses we hadn't had time for on our earlier trip, maybe Royal Dornoch, north of Inverness, or Royal Troon, south of Glasgow on Scotland's west coast.

Though Paul still was concerned about his prostate cancer coming back, he otherwise was feeling fine. At times, he had taken drugs to block male hormones (which has been shown to prolong the lives of men with prostate cancer) and had also become a vegan (as studies have found that plant-based diets might protect men from prostate cancer). He exercised regularly and, after learning he had Li-Fraumeni syndrome, began traveling to MD Anderson in Houston for an annual full-body MRI. It had been more than a decade since his last cancer.

Then, in March 2017, while we were still plotting our golf holiday, Paul sent me an ominous email following his latest trip to Houston: "The full-body MRI I had at MD Anderson in Houston spotted something suspicious on my pancreas. . . . Probably nothing, but best to check." The next week, his doctor in Florida, where he was now living, performed a biopsy, and Paul got on a plane to see his oncologist in New York to plan treatment. While still on the flight, he got an email from his wife, Susan: "It's not cancer! It's chronic pancreatitis. They took several slides of the biopsy—all came back negative." Though a dangerous condition that can cause diabetes, pancreatitis is not terminal. Paul responded with an ecstatic email: "GREAT NEWS!!! . . . Chronic pancreatitis never looked so good . . . !"

Alas, we had celebrated too soon. The results were wrong—a false negative—because the biopsy material had come from a part of the pancreas that didn't register cancer cells. A follow-up scan and a second biopsy confirmed that Paul had yet another new and different cancer, an adenocarcinoma, which typically forms in glandular tissues in internal organs like the pancreas.

It felt especially unfair, as Paul had so recently retired and had more time to indulge his hobbies. He played golf every chance he had and sent me emails recounting his rounds (whenever he played well, anyway). He was an avid fly fisherman, hand-tying his own flies and fishing with throwback bamboo rods from L.L.Bean; he loved to go casting on trout streams in Montana and in the Everglades. And he had continued his love affair with the auto industry, working part-time as a writer and consultant for the Revs Institute, an automotive history center near his home in Naples that has a fabulous classic car museum, and appearing frequently on CNBC to weigh in on the car world. As if that weren't enough, he was thinking of writing his fourth book (perhaps about self-driving cars, or the Ford family history).

Paul's prognosis was scary, but he also was a bit lucky. Pancreatic cancer often is fatal within a short period of time, with patients rarely living more than six months, as there are no symptoms until it is too late to treat. But thanks to Paul's adherence to the regular Toronto Protocol screenings, his malignancy was caught early. The tumor was small and confined to the tail of his pancreas, making it operable. He seemed to have beaten the odds again.

The surgery on March 20 went well, albeit with complications, as the surgeon nicked a blood vessel, which resulted in significant internal bleeding and a second surgery two days later. Most important, there were no signs of cancer cells in my brother's lymph nodes, reducing the fear that the malignancy might spread. To be safe, Paul's oncologist prescribed a five-month course of chemotherapy treatment beginning in May. It wouldn't be fun, but he had been through the drill before.

But Paul's relief over his successful surgery and promising prognosis quickly disappeared. In early April, while out running, his son, Charlie, felt an ache in his right hip. Also a serious cyclist who was very fit, Charlie shrugged it off as a strained muscle, along with "being on the wrong side of 35," as he put it in an email to friends. But the nagging injury persisted. A month later, while he was walking home from the subway after a late night at his law firm, the pain became so excruciating that it took him half an hour to cover just three blocks.

Hoping not to worry his parents—with Paul still recovering from his surgery, and his mom, Susan, having undergone double knee replacement surgery in March—Charlie decided to get it checked before saying anything to them. What his doctors found was unnerving: a bone tumor in his hip socket that measured fourteen centimeters, about five and a half inches, meaning it was too large for surgery. Instead, his doctors would first have to try to shrink the malignancy with chemotherapy and radiation.

Charlie was at his law office when he got the news. Thanks to his experience working for an appellate court judge, he had landed a job in 2015 at a well-regarded downtown Chicago firm where he focused on defending clients in complicated aviation liability cases. Charlie asked Austin Bartlett, a senior colleague who had become a mentor, to come to his office. Visibly upset, Charlie was crying. He explained the diagnosis to Bartlett, and then said, "Austin, how am I going to tell my parents?"

Paul and Susan were devastated, but like Charlie, they were hopeful. And why not? He had already beaten cancer twice, so why not a third time? Ever the optimist, Charlie told friends, "The good news is that it's a primary tumor and not related to or metastasis of what I had in 2010. And it's localized and early stage. . . . The bottom line is that this appears to be very treatable in the long run, but we're not sure of the specific course of action. In the end, this will be just another bump in the road." Paul, though worried, wrote, "This at first read does not seem as bad as the rectal cancer diagnosis he got in 2010."

Paul and Charlie were now both battling potentially life-threatening cancers and undergoing chemotherapy treatment. Paul's treatment was postsurgical, meant to kill any stray cancer cells that might have escaped from his pancreas. Charlie's was presurgical, making it especially critical that it was effective at shrinking the tumor before surgeons could go in to cut out most or all of it.

While Paul's chemo was doing its job, Charlie's wasn't working as well as hoped, despite a couple of nauseating months. The tumor in his hip had stopped growing, but it hadn't shrunk much, so Charlie's doctors considered a different chemotherapy cocktail. Radiation that could have killed the cancerous cells was, unfortunately, not a good option. Oncologists have long known that radiation can trigger cellular mutations that, in turn, can lead to cancer; that's why patients wear lead vests while getting X-rays, and why technicians leave the room for a protected area. But the risk of radiation was much higher for someone like Charlie, with Li-Fraumeni syndrome. Because of the mutation he had inherited in his p53 cancer suppressor gene, his body had less natural ability to protect against radiation causing cells to begin growing out of control and becoming malignant.

This was the ultimate tragedy of Charlie's colorectal cancer not being diagnosed in early 2010, when he first saw a doctor about his bowel irritation, and of our not learning about Li-Fraumeni syndrome until 2015.

Given our family's cancer history, he should have undergone a colonoscopy when his bowel problems didn't quickly go away. That would have detected his colorectal cancer at a much earlier stage and almost certainly meant he would have needed far less radiation to treat that tumor.

While there was no knowing for certain, Charlie's doctors suspected that the heavy doses of radiation he had received back then, in the vicinity of where he now had developed bone cancer, may well have caused his latest malignancy. "All part of Li-Fraumeni. . . . I am worried sick. Can't stand it," my brother emailed me.

With the tumor in his hip stubbornly resisting chemo, Charlie was in so much pain that he needed crutches to walk; he missed the wedding of our daughter, Lisa, outside Seattle in late July, because traveling such a long distance would have caused him agony. In early August, Charlie began another course of chemotherapy with the hope that it would shrink the tumor, while his dad was also getting a weekly chemo infusion at the same hospital, Northwestern Memorial, in downtown Chicago.

The next month was impossibly difficult for Charlie and the rest of the family. As debilitating as chemo is physically, waiting to find out if it is working can be even harder psychologically.

Charlie's new chemo didn't work. Surgeons scheduled an operation for October 31, advising Charlie that there was a chance they would be able to remove the tumor—but most likely, they would have to amputate his leg and his hip. Not getting out all the cancer would be a short-term death sentence. After all the suffering Charlie had gone through, from his childhood cancer to his many reconstructive surgeries to colorectal cancer to his hip cancer, this was almost too much even to contemplate.

As the day of the surgery approached, Paul wrote, "This is the Big Show. There is no getting around it, so we might as well get on with it." When I talked to my brother on the telephone the day before Charlie's surgery, he sobbed several times.

The surgery began at 8 a.m. and didn't end until an exhausting nine hours later, at nearly 5 p.m. The tumor was so large that the surgeons, as they had forewarned, had no choice but to take Charlie's leg and hip.

I cried when my brother called with the news. More than the rest of us, Charlie had braced himself for the worst, and he took in the news stoically when he woke up from the anesthesia ninety minutes after the operation. Then, no doubt wanting a small bit of normalcy, Charlie, a devoted Chicago Cubs fan, insisted on watching the sixth game of the World Series between the Los Angeles Dodgers and the Houston Astros. The next morning, he emailed friends. "Losing the leg is tough, but I view it as a new beginning rather than a loss of a limb. As I told my parents, I will adapt and all will be good." Even with powerful drugs, he would be in lots of pain, and for a long time. Still, Charlie now had a chance.

But first would come intensive rehab. Just getting in and out of bed or standing on his remaining leg was an exhausting feat initially. In a sign of Charlie's determination, he told Paul he wanted to buy special gear so he could resume cycling and golfing. His twin, Dan, also a lawyer, relocated from Florida and moved in with his brother to help during the lengthy recovery.

Then, while Charlie was doing rehab and continuing to undergo chemotherapy, a scan in February detected a tiny spot on his lung, and a biopsy confirmed that it was malignant, most likely an offshoot of the bone tumor. It seemed a minor setback, as the tumor began shrinking after doctors prescribed an oral, take-at-home drug. But Paul took the news hard. "As if the leg amputation was not enough, plenty enough, the spread of cancer to his lung is really tough. But I beat lung cancer 21 years ago," he told a friend.

Despite everything, Charlie's hard work began to pay off. For weeks after the surgery, he could stand for only a brief period, but he slowly began building his strength and walking on crutches, initially around his condo and then for short distances outside. In early May, he walked around the block on his crutches. For most of us, that is an everyday event we don't even think about; for Charlie, it was a monumental achievement, something he hadn't managed to do since October, before his surgery. He started working a few days a week from home, writing briefs on legal cases, and by May, he was fit enough to go into the office for a few hours on occasion. He seemed to be making a remarkable recovery. And why not? Hadn't he always?

But there were still troubling signs, as well. Charlie increased his dosage of painkillers, even though he had a high tolerance for pain and didn't like taking them. He was on so many medications that his mom, Susan, created a spreadsheet to keep track of them all. He developed a urinary tract infection that required hospitalization. Then his kidney was swelling, perhaps a side effect of the stent that was delivering his chemotherapy. He needed blood transfusions because his blood count at times was falling too low for him to keep receiving the chemotherapy drugs. Worst of all, by midsummer he had another small bone tumor, in what remained of his hip area, and neither it nor the lung tumor, while stabilized, were shrinking any longer. Though the battle was exhausting him, his oncologists were reluctant to change his chemo regimen. "There aren't many options left—so he needs to stay on this combination as long as he can tolerate it and it's working," his mom, Susan, confided to us.

By fall, the tumors were growing again. The chemo that had seemed to work for a while no longer was, so his doctors switched to another therapy. His weight had fallen to 116 pounds, down about one-third. He began taking time-release morphine to ease the unrelenting pain. "We need a miracle," Paul wrote me.

Instead, the excruciating news kept coming. The malignant mass in Charlie's lung was starting to clog up one of his bronchial tubes, which carry oxygen from the windpipe to the lung. The tumor was potentially life-threatening, so even though surgery would provide only a temporary reprieve, Charlie underwent an operation to clear the tube

But nothing seemed to keep the tumors from spreading for long. By early 2019, Charlie was in a fight for survival, and Paul and Susan were desperate to try anything and everything. They had heard of a relatively new and very expensive immunotherapy drug, called Keytruda, which works by helping a patient's immune system recognize and fight cancer cells. The drug wasn't a cure for cancer, but clinical trials found that it modestly improved survival rates. When Charlie's insurance company balked at covering the cost, he filed an appeal. But feeling they couldn't wait for an answer, Paul and Susan paid out of pocket—$17,500 for the initial dose, though his next two doses were provided free on a compassionate basis—in a desperate effort to save their son.

Even as his condition deteriorated, Charlie remained characteristically optimistic. In early February, he told a cousin visiting him, "I just know I will hear the words, 'Your cancer is cured.'" He renewed his Chicago Cubs tickets package that he shared with friends.

A week later, early on the morning of February 17, 2019, I was awakened by a call from my brother. Choked up, Paul could barely get out the words.

"He's gone."

38

C "AN'T STOP CRYING . . ."

That was the subject of an email my brother, Paul, sent me on February 26, 2019, barely a week after Charlie had died. The email otherwise had no words, just a photo of the urn containing his son's ashes: "Charlie Ingrassia. September 18, 1979–February 17, 2019." He had lived thirty-nine years and five months. For a long time after Charlie died, Paul broke into tears every time we talked. He felt especially close to Charlie, as they both had been through so many cancers. They both had experienced the anxiety of waiting to hear test results. The daunting recovery that came after major surgery. The violent reaction to chemotherapy, the nasty side effects of radiation. The relief and joy of being proclaimed cancer free, and the shattering moment when they were diagnosed with another cancer and braced themselves because they knew what they were in for. "It will take me a very long time to come to grips with this," Paul told friends.

In mid-April, while still grieving, Paul did something unexpected, something I didn't think much of at the time. He revisited our early childhood, taking a trip by himself to Laurel, Mississippi, where our parents had moved a year or so after getting married in 1947 and where all four children had been born and lived until we moved to the Chicago suburbs in 1960. "I call it my Rip van Winkle trip," he quipped in an email.

He reveled in the visit, snapping photos of the hospital where we were born, the small white house at 763 North Park Street where we grew up before moving north, the Catholic church and school we attended, and two of the city's recent mayors, whom he bumped into in the town center. "Just down the street from the Confederate Monument in Laurel, a black man and a white woman saw me taking pictures and waved me over to introduce themselves. The man is the current mayor, Johnny Magee, and the woman is one of his predecessors, Susan Boone Vincent." Much of what Paul saw was familiar, but the fact that this city in the Deep South had a black mayor (and a woman mayor before him) was a testament to how much things in Laurel had changed—when we lived there in the 1950s, it would have been inconceivable for either of them to be elected mayor.

I never asked Paul why he had made the trip. But maybe, in the wake of Charlie's death, he had sensed even more that life was fleeting and that he shouldn't put off things he wanted to do. When he visited me and Vicki on a business trip to Los Angeles in early May, he spoke nervously about his fears that his prostate cancer might recur. He was adhering more strictly than ever to his vegan diet, hoping that would help. So, despite all the fabulous restaurants in Los Angeles to choose from, we went for dinner to a new vegan pizzeria nearby, with nondairy toppings like macadamia ricotta and cashew mozzarella rather than real cheese, along with what Paul joked was his favorite cocktail, a "vegan martini."

Then, in mid-June, Paul saw his oncologist in New York and called to tell me that a scan had detected something suspicious in his lung. It might be something, it might be nothing; he was going back in a few days for tests to learn more. Not waiting, he did some quick internet research and sent me a note with a link to an academic article about pancreatic cancer reappearing in the lungs. The top of the article had a sobering line, noting that "the 5-year survival rate remains poor even in patients with early stage disease who are surgical candidates." That would be like Paul, whose pancreatic cancer was discovered early and removed in

March 2017. Looking for something positive, Paul focused on a section lower in the article, which described five patient cases. "All five patients developed lung metastases at approximately two years after the initial first treatment approach and they are still alive (29, 35, 39, 39 and 48 months respectively from initial diagnosis). At the time of this report, all patients still appear to have stable disease." Paul's initial diagnosis had been twenty-seven months earlier.

"Definitely encouraging," I emailed him after reading the article, trying to be optimistic.

"Yep!" his reply came back.

But a couple of days later, on June 18, an unsettling email from Paul popped into my in-box. "My PET scan at Columbia yesterday found that there are some small spots on the lung 'lighting up,' which generally means some sort of cancer. There also is a larger spot in the lymph nodes where the two bronchial tubes split off. Also lighting up was my thyroid," he wrote. He added, "There are lots of treatment options in all of this, so let's see how it unfolds."

The following week, he had a bronchoscopy that confirmed a tumor in the lymph node next to his windpipe. "It's unclear just what the origin and nature of this cancer is. More specifically, is it a new lymphoma? Or a metastatic pancreatic cancer? Or something else? The docs need/want to know more before beginning treatment. . . . The oncologist said there is 'some urgency' to dealing with the lymph-node mass lest it grow big enough to obstruct my windpipe," he explained.

We were all alarmed, but Paul assured a friend in an email, "I will be ok. My mind is at peace . . . and I have lots of fight left in me."

In early July, shortly before doctors planned to perform another biopsy to determine what type of cancer he had, Paul and Susan took a trip to Montana to stay with friends at their ranch. For Paul, it was a respite where he could enjoy fly-fishing for trout for a few days. He sent friends a photo of himself wearing waders and standing on the bank of a stream, showing off a fifteen-inch rainbow trout he had caught, "before all the fun begins next week."

In the photo, Paul, who had always beaten cancer, looked great, like he was on just another of his many fishing jaunts. For all his smiles, however, this time felt different. He seemed weary. Maybe it was because Charlie had died four months earlier. Maybe it was because he felt his luck—if you can call having several cancers and surviving them luck—at some point would run out. Maybe it was the fact that the initial indications, while tentative, seemed troubling. To help Paul brace for the ordeal ahead, our cousin Anne Ingrassia Federwisch sent family members T-shirts with "FIGHT LIKE CHARLIE!" emblazoned across the front, borrowing a phrase Paul often used as a tribute to Charlie's never-give-up attitude.

The biopsy on July 12 confirmed a malignancy in Paul's lung, but there would be still more waiting for a pathology report on the tissue. Paul and Susan came to stay with us at our weekend house in Westhampton, New York, and then he and I headed back into Manhattan on July 18 to meet with his oncologist. Paul was still worn down from his hospital stay and biopsy of a week earlier. His doctor's message was sobering. The tumor in Paul's lung had metastasized from his pancreatic cancer. It was not curable, he said, though it appeared to be treatable. But the doctor's body language wasn't good; he paused frequently while trying to answer Paul's questions, and he seemed to be grasping for what the best treatment might be.

Twenty years earlier, after the discovery of the genetic mutation behind Li-Fraumeni syndrome, there had been predictions of p53 gene therapies that would greatly improve treatment and prolong the life of cancer patients. Yet we were still waiting. Instead, Paul's oncologist said the standard source of treatment for his tumor was a very harsh cocktail of chemotherapy drugs that make most patients violently ill. When Paul asked the doctor if he should go through with it, given how hard it would be, the doctor said absolutely. There was no guarantee it would work, his oncologist added, but Paul had virtually no chance otherwise.

The next morning, Paul had coffee with his close friends at Reuters—Stephen Adler, Alix Freedman, Michael Williams, Amy Stevens, and Gina Chua, all former colleagues at the *Wall Street Journal* who, like him, had joined Reuters and helped turn around the moribund newsroom, winning a growing number of journalism prizes, including Pulitzers. As they reminisced about the good times, Paul got teary-eyed. He thanked everyone for being good colleagues and friends and told them he was determined to beat cancer again. But as he hugged everybody on his way out, they sensed it might be the last time they saw him.

Paul confided to me that this cancer might do him in. He figured he had at least six to nine months, and if the treatment worked, perhaps as long as two to three years. He was eager to begin treatment as soon as possible, but his chemotherapy was delayed as laboratory technicians studied his tumor to determine if it would respond to a targeted immunotherapy drug. If so, it would be a less harsh and potentially more effective treatment.

But not all malignancies can be targeted with immunotherapy. A week's delay became two, then three. Upset with the delay, Paul wrote me, "I really do want to start with chemo tomorrow. . . . I have had enough waiting."

On the morning his treatment finally began, on August 7, Paul sent us all a "chemo selfie": him trying to smile while hooked up to an IV delivering the drugs. But the chemo was every bit as debilitating as advertised. After two rounds over the first few weeks, Paul was constantly sick—so sick that the doctor suggested eliminating the most toxic chemo.

At the end of August, I traveled to Naples, Florida—racing to catch an earlier flight that would land before Hurricane Dorian shut down airports—to help Paul through the third round. A couple of hours after I arrived, we drove to a local TV studio so Paul could do a live satellite interview with CNBC-TV about the auto industry. It was vintage Paul: though exhausted by the treatment, he didn't want to miss an opportunity to critique the industry he had followed for much of his career.

He had a break of a few days before the next round of chemo would begin, so we headed out to the golf course—he was so drained physically that we played only a few holes—and then did some fly-casting on a pond near his condo. As we enjoyed our time hanging out together, Paul said again, matter-of-factly and without tears, that he planned to keep fighting, but that he was ready to go if it was his time.

Sadly, it was. The night before his next chemo round was to begin, I had to rush him to a hospital emergency room, as he was having a hard time breathing. He was released the next day and came home. But at around five o'clock the following morning, he was again gasping, even more than the night before. This time, Susan called an ambulance. It seemed to take forever to arrive, though it was only about five minutes. The medics raced Paul to the nearest hospital, where he was put on a ventilator and heavily sedated.

Paul had always been an optimist, a survivor. He frequently said he would always "Fight like Charlie!" But in the brief periods when he was alert while in intensive care, he began calling a few friends without telling us. "I want you to know that I love you and appreciate our friendship, because I don't know how much longer I'll be in this world," he told Pat Massenberg, one of his closest colleagues at Dow Jones Newswires for more than decade. Pat got off the phone crying and said to her husband, "Paul just said goodbye to me." But Paul made one final call to her a few days later. "Susie and Larry just left the hospital," he told Massenberg, "but there's one person still here. It's Charlie. He's sitting in the chair and he keeps getting closer and closer to me."

Paul, my brother, my best friend, my last sibling, died a few days later, on September 16. Until nearly the end, I had not imagined this could happen—not so quickly, anyway. We had hoped for a year or two, but got only a few months. His body was riddled with cancer, as the chemotherapy had failed to contain the malignancies in his lung, trachea, and thyroid. He was sixty-nine, far too young but still much older than his son, our mom, and our sisters. I sent an email to his legions of friends: "We will miss you, Paul. May all the drives you hit be straight and all your putts fall. May all the fish you hook be big. May all the cars you drive be fast."

39

THE STORY OF LI-FRAUMENI SYNDROME AND, MORE BROADLY, OF CANCER research isn't one story, but two. It is both a heartbreaking story of family loss and an inspiring story of scientific achievement.

Thanks to the pioneering work beginning in the 1960s by Joseph Fraumeni Jr., Frederick Li, and a remarkable cohort of others, the world knows vastly more about hereditary cancers—indeed, cancers of all types—than ever before. These intrepid researchers journeyed into the scientific unknown and returned with a deeper knowledge of what causes cancer, how to detect it, and how to treat it. The journey has been long and meandering, as scientific journeys frequently are, especially journeys undertaken to gain knowledge about what goes on and can go wrong inside our very selves. And of course it still isn't over. The human body, this physical thing we inhabit, which we might think we know well, has mind-boggling complexity made even more complicated by the many external things it interacts with day by day, month by month, year by year.

It should be of little wonder, then, that from decade to decade, the focus on, and the occasionally fierce debate over, the causes of cancer has shifted. For a long time, it was viruses. Then it was the environment. Then heredity. And myriad other things, including diet. The proponents of different theories were all right, it turns out. "One of the major advances we've had as a result of cancer research is deep recognition of the complexity of cancer. It's not one disease, it's lots of different diseases. Every single cancer is different when you look at it on a genetic level," Harold Varmus, cowinner of a Nobel Prize in 1989 for his cancer research, noted when he stepped down as director of the National Cancer Institute in 2015.

Viruses aren't the primary cause of cancer, as long thought, but they do trigger 10 to 15 percent of malignancies. A wide variety of environmental factors—everything from smoking to radiation to exposure to the sun's rays to dozens of chemical carcinogens—account for perhaps 65 to 70 percent of cancers. What might broadly be called poor health factors, such as body fatness, physical inactivity, and alcohol consumption, cause another 15 percent, give or take. Hereditary syndromes—of which more than fifty have been discovered by researchers in the past few decades—account for 5 to 10 percent of cancers. And sometimes cancer is caused not by one thing but by an interacting combination of factors, in ways still not fully understood, that result in normal cell division and mutation spiraling out of control, causing cells to become malignant.

Li-Fraumeni syndrome accounts for a tiny proportion of hereditary cancers, with *BRCA* and Lynch syndrome far more common. Despite the rarity of LFS, its role in helping to illuminate the central role of p53—in preventing cancer in its natural state and accelerating it when mutated—has given the syndrome an outsize importance in furthering the understanding of malignancies and the search for ways to combat them. The guardian of the genome, p53 has become the most studied gene in the human body. Before 1990, when Stephen Friend's and Esther Chang's laboratories independently identified p53 mutations as the culprit behind Li-Fraumeni syndrome, fewer than 100 papers were published annually on the gene, a number that quickly rocketed above 2,000 annually by the mid-1990s. Since 2011, at least 5,000 new articles have been published every year on p53, with a cumulative total of more than 115,000. The growing knowledge of the intricacies of cancer, together with continuing advances in molecular biology, has slowly, but steadily, improved both the early detection and treatment of malignancies.

This has given researchers a much more robust tool kit to design drugs that attack cancer cells, resulting in a variety of new targeted therapies that are more effective at hunting down and thwarting malignancies, sometimes in combination with existing chemotherapy drugs. These new treatments include a variety of immunotherapy drugs, such as growth signal inhibitors that can restrict cancer cell division by fortifying the body's own immune system to fight malignancies; and anti-angiogenesis drugs that can diminish the creation of new blood vessels needed by invasive, voracious tumors to grow faster. Though these are significant leaps forward, they aren't miracle drugs. My nephew Charlie was treated with Keytruda, a growth cell inhibitor, in the last month of his life, to no avail. Moreover, these new therapies are hugely expensive, costing tens or even hundreds of thousands of dollars, which is the main reason that spending on cancer drugs in the United States soared 60 percent, to $61 billion, in 2017 compared to five years earlier.

The result has been a revolution in cancer treatment. Cancer is still a dread and deadly disease, but the five-year survival rate after diagnosis has risen to 67 percent from 50 percent in 1977 and just 35 percent in 1946. For some types of cancer, the five-year survival rate is much higher, as with prostate cancer, which has increased to 98 percent from 68 percent in 1977; breast cancer at 90 percent, versus 75 percent; and leukemia, up to 60 percent from 34 percent. But it lags in others, with the five-year survival rate for brain cancer still just 30 percent, up from 22 percent; for lung cancer, at 18 percent versus 12 percent. Pancreatic cancer—which killed my brother, Paul, and remains one of the deadliest cancers because there rarely are symptoms until it is in its late stage—even now has a five-year survival rate of only 8 percent, up from 2.5 percent.

Families with inherited cancer predispositions have benefited from these advances in cancer treatments. And they also have benefited from vastly improved and cheaper genetic screening. In 2016, when I took a test to see if I carried the p53 mutation and a couple of dozen others that cause cancer, it would have cost several thousand dollars if I hadn't been accepted into a study that researchers were conducting, which meant there was no cost to me. Less than a decade later, the cost of the same multi-gene panel test had fallen to about $250.

But if we are—finally, haltingly—winning the war on cancer launched in 1971 by Richard Nixon, it may end up being a hundred years' war. The admonition by Oliver Wyss, whose two young children died of cancer, to leading researchers at the National Cancer Institute in 2010 was still true more than a decade later: the progress still isn't enough for Li-Fraumeni families fearing constantly that their children might develop cancer almost anywhere and at any time. Better five-year survival rates mean a lot less if you get cancer when you are under forty—as many LFS patients do—than if you have already lived a long life, into your sixties or seventies, when the odds of getting cancer in the general population increase. Even some leading scientists understand the frustration. "Since 1970, there's maybe 50 percent improvement in cancer survivors. Given all the effort, it's not great," Nobel Prize–winning biologist Leland Hartwell has acknowledged.

When I began researching this book, I joined several Facebook groups for LFS families. For many of them, social media offers a community of like-afflicted families, a community that can serve as both a vital support group and a source of information—and one they almost certainly can't find in the place they live, because the syndrome is so rare that there are so few families like them. Even now, many of their doctors have limited experience with Li-Fraumeni syndrome.

To scroll through their posts is to visit an alternative universe, where the carefree, everyday world has been left behind and where fear constantly hovers. Newcomers to this exclusive club—a club no one wishes to belong to—often express anguish and confusion. They occasionally refer to themselves as *mutants*, a word that might sound like a pejorative if used by others, but is an eye-winking, inside joke when used by members of the club. Many seek practical medical and personal advice. How to tell children that they have tested positive for the p53 mutation? What's the best way to monitor for breast cancer recurrence after a mastectomy? Who offers good health insurance for people with conditions like LFS?

> One young man wonders: "Any singles here who have dealt with when to tell someone about your cancer/LFS when you start dating them? First date? After a few? When there's talk about a committed relationship?"

> A woman newly diagnosed with LFS asks: "Does anyone understand the genetic reports? I got my report today which said I am 'heterozygous for a likely pathogenic TP53 c.743G>A p.(Arg248Gln) variant. In addition, next generation sequence analysis shows no evidence of an exon deletion or duplication in this gene.' Does anyone know what this means?"

To many, it is a relief to be able to connect with others who have already gone through what they are starting to go through, explaining that they still find doctors who blurt out "Lee Frow what?" when they first see a patient with the p53 mutation.

But most often the people who belong to the Facebook groups share their heartbreak, and seek solace in their shared grief, with husbands and wives telling of losing their spouses and children—sometimes within months—and parents looking for guidance on how to cope with the pain of a fourth or fifth cancer diagnosis for a teenage child.

> A mother writes: "LFS is robbing me of my family. And no one understands what LFS is and can't comprehend what you're saying. . . . I'm dying on the inside."

> Another woman writes: "I just received confirmation yesterday that I have the mutation. . . . My father died of brain cancer at age 40 (I was 10), his mother died of breast cancer at 39, his sister died of some form of abdominal cancer. Then at age 35 my brother was diagnosed with lung cancer (never smoked) and died a year later leaving behind young kids.

I made it past 40 and thought, 'Whew, I made it.' However 2 years ago at age 45 I was diagnosed with breast cancer. I am the first to survive cancer in our family."

"Does anyone else have a hard time following the [screening] protocols due to anxiety. . . . I have my oncology appointment in 5 hours and haven't slept a wink. I was supposed to get a prophylactic mastectomy last winter and chickened out at the last minute. I just feel like nobody in my life understands what I am going through since getting this [LFS] diagnosis."

"We were told today my daughter's cancer (3rd battle) is not curable this time. It has spread to her lungs and lymph nodes. . . . They gave us a timeline of 6–12 months total. . . . My husband wants to run to all corners of the world looking for something more! I feel like we would be chasing something that doesn't exist. . . . [At] what point do you transition to quality of life? And what does that look like?"

Sometimes there are pleas of desperation, like parents who heard about patients successfully treating tumors with an animal deworming medicine, and asking whether it might halt their child's cancer, only to be gently advised by others in the group that it wouldn't.

Occasionally, I refrain from looking at posts for a while. I understand it is therapeutic for these families to know they aren't alone in the suffering, that there are other families just like theirs. But at times I find it too painful. In the stories about their moms and dads, their siblings and their children, I see my mom and sisters and brother and nephew.

Then I go back and am touched by the heartfelt messages of encouragement and support for one another. "Does anyone have positive LFS stories?" one woman asked. Dozens of people quickly posted uplifting responses—of going long periods between cancers; of detecting tumors early, when they were treatable; of children who tested negative for the p53 mutation.

"When I was 28, I had an astrocytoma (brain tumor). The maximum positive outlook for my particular tumor was 8 years survival. 7 years later, I had a recurrence. Now, over 13 years later I am still here!"

"I'm 51, I have had 2 cancers (breast and then lung) both in my 40s when I found out I was LFS. Only needed surgery, no chemo for both. Cancer free now for 3 years. Screening has saved my life."

"My mother LFS, 70 years old, 5 different cancers, still alive!!! My aunt 77 years old, LFS, 1 cancer, still alive as well."

"Despite my circumstances, I choose to carry on. My mother died of breast cancer at age 30. I was 10. I've had breast cancer twice. The first time I was barely 30 with a 3 year old and a 6 month old. The second time it was metastatic, I was 40. I'll be in treatment for the rest of my life. I'm 42. I lost my sister to breast cancer, she was 38. She had melanoma at age 23 and had a 3 year old die of neuroblastoma. We still live, we still enjoy life. No matter what that life looks like, or how long it is."

40

SOMEDAY, HUMANITY MAY RECALL A PRIMITIVE TIME WHEN DOCTORS COULDN'T treat people born with debilitating or life-threatening genetic disorders simply by injecting them with a drug to fix the mutation, just as we now look back to periods in history when surgeons operated on patients without anesthesia to ease the pain and without antiseptics to prevent deadly infections. We may consider it astonishing, and tragic, that there was a time when medical science was so limited that people who seemed otherwise healthy, but who had inherited a mutation predisposing them to serious illness, couldn't be helped until symptoms signaled something had already started going awry.

That day may come—in a few years, if we are lucky. Though more likely, it will take a decade or two or perhaps even longer, if we aren't. If that day does come, as many genetic researchers predict it assuredly will, it will arrive in large part because of a groundbreaking discovery in 2012 by two women scientists. Jennifer Doudna, an American, and Emmanuelle Charpentier, who is French, led collaborating research teams that developed a blueprint for correcting genetic mutations that cause not just cancer conditions like Li-Fraumeni syndrome but a variety of inherited diseases.

Doudna and Charpentier identified a way to use something called CRISPR—an acronym for "clustered regularly interspaced short palindromic repeats," which are DNA sequences encoded in our genes—to "edit" genes, including genetic mutations. CRISPR technology enables scientists to create molecules that enter a cell; target and snip out a specific segment of a gene's DNA, such as a mutation known to cause an illness; and replace it with a strand that corrects the mutation. It is akin to a word processing program on a personal computer that can find and edit typos or inaccurate lines in text.

When Doudna and Charpentier published an article describing their findings in *Science* on June 28, 2012, it got surprisingly little notice outside academic circles at first. Perhaps it was the dense title: "A Programmable Dual RNA-Guided DNA Endonuclease in Adaptive Bacterial Immunity." Perhaps it was that the paper, while noting the discovery "could offer considerable potential for gene-targeting and genome-editing applications," didn't allude to practical medical uses, not once mentioning "disease," "illness," or "mutation," much less "treatment" or "drug" or "therapy." Or perhaps it was that the far-reaching promise of what they were describing seemed more like science fiction than science. The *New York Times*, which typically jumps quickly on major medical news, failed to take note until nearly two years later, on March 3, 2014, when it belatedly published a story not on its front page but in its Science section, headlined, "A Powerful New Way to Edit DNA."

By then, investors had begun to grasp the potentially momentous nature of the discovery and were pouring hundreds of millions of dollars into biotechnology start-ups, including companies founded by Doudna and Charpentier, with the goal of using CRISPR to develop new therapies to treat inherited ailments, including cancer.

In 2020, in recognition of CRISPR's importance, the two women were co-awarded the Nobel Prize in Chemistry—a mere eight years after their discovery, an astonishingly short time to win the prestigious honor. "Emmanuelle Charpentier and Jennifer Doudna developed a chemical tool that has taken life sciences into a new epoch," the Royal Swedish

Academy of Sciences declared. "They have made us gaze out onto a vast horizon of unimagined potential and, along the way—as we explore this new land—we are guaranteed to make new and unexpected discoveries."

Doudna herself has spoken expansively about the potential of CRISPR to fix a vast host of ills: "It's kind of a profound thing because if you really think about it, it really means altering human evolution on some level." In time, she has said, CRISPR could "eliminate sickle cell anemia, or eliminate cystic fibrosis, or have someone not have to suffer from Huntington's disease anymore or worry about getting it when they get older."

If the history of medical science tells anything, however, it is that progress can be achingly slow. So it has been with CRISPR. Taking what works correctly some of the time in a laboratory and making it work all the time, and safely, in a human body is proving challenging. In some early experiments, researchers found that CRISPR changed a segment in a gene that it wasn't meant to change. Using the word processor analogy, a new word or line that was meant to replace an existing word or line in a paragraph actually and wrongly changed similar wording in a different paragraph. When that happens in a written document, an incorrect insertion can result in an unfortunate and perhaps embarrassing alteration in the meaning. But in a living being, if a gene is wrongly changed, or a wrong gene is changed, the consequences can be potentially dire.

Science doesn't stand still, of course. As more researchers have worked to advance the discovery by Doudna and Charpentier, they have found ways to improve the precision of CRISPR editing, reducing the chances of a mistake. But even when nothing goes awry, achieving the hoped-for result can be elusive. The efficiency of early CRISPR therapies tested on human embryos—that is, the chances of a successful repairing of a targeted mutation—can be low, sometimes under 10 percent. This has frustrated researchers, because it means higher doses have to be injected for a CRISPR therapy to work, and higher doses of almost any drug increase the risk of the body's having a toxic reaction.

Still, scientists have made enough progress in fine-tuning CRISPR technology to win the approval of regulators for a number of clinical tri-als using experimental CRISPR therapies to see how well they work for genetic conditions such as sickle cell anemia; for an inherited blood dis-order known as beta thalassemia; for a life-threatening condition known as hereditary angioedema, which causes severe swelling of various parts of the body; and for transthyretin-mediated amyloidosis cardiomyopa-thy, an inherited disorder that can cause heart failure.

In 2019, one of the earliest CRISPR biotech start-ups, Editas Medicine—whose founders include Doudna—collaborated with phar-maceutical giant Allergan to begin the first clinical trial on humans in the United States using CRISPR gene editing. Its experimental medi-cine was designed to treat a rare inherited mutation that occurs in just one out of thirty thousand newborn babies. The condition, which causes degeneration of the retina and results in blindness or severe impairment of vision, is called Leber congenital amaurosis type 10 (LCA10). In the study, doctors injected directly into cells in patients' eyes a CRISPR mol-ecule designed by Editas to snip out the mutated, defective strand of the gene and replace it with a segment that restored the normal function of the eyes' photoreceptor cells, so the retina could sense light.

Early results were promising. For the first time, some patients who volunteered to take part could make out the shapes of people nearby, recognize and maneuver around obstacles, and see colors. Though they didn't regain full vision, the procedure was nonetheless life-changing for them. But a year later, as the CRISPR therapy was tried on more patients, there was sobering news. Of fourteen patients undergoing treatment, only three had "clinically meaningful" improvements in their sight. The therapy had improved the sight of patients with a particularly rare type of the mutation causing the condition, but it didn't work well on other variations of the LCA10 mutation. Editas put a positive spin on the results, saying the clinical trial demonstrated "proof of concept." But the company, though not giving up, put the study on hold while considering its options.

Scientists also are beginning to experiment with CRISPR to correct mutations linked to cancer, including defects in p53. In one laboratory experiment using the latest gene-editing technology, the p53 mutation in a type of breast cancer cells was snipped and replaced with a segment that restored the gene's cancer-suppressing powers. The desired correction was achieved, albeit in just 7.6 percent of the treated cells. While encouraging, "a major caveat is that, to have clinical benefit, successful conversion must be achieved in the vast majority of cancer cells. Time will tell whether this is feasible in humans," concluded two scientists who reviewed this and other efforts to use CRISPR on p53.

Another study of tissues with p53 mutations from a Li-Fraumeni syndrome patient found that defects could be repaired with CRISPR gene editing. But a second study on LFS mice with bone cancer found that CRISPR didn't restore p53's cancer-suppressing abilities even though it repaired the mutated segment of the gene. "Overall, these results highlight the feasibility of precision gene editing in mutant p53 systems and shed light on the complexities of germline p53 mutant signaling in both normal and cancer cells," concluded the author of the study, a PhD student under David Malkin.

Given the many challenges, no one can predict how long it will take to sufficiently improve CRISPR editing of p53 and other cancer gene mutations to make effective clinical solutions. Even if the scientific hurdles are cleared, there are other complicating issues. The price of CRISPR-engineered drugs could be staggering. In the best-case scenario, proving that a new CRISPR therapy is both safe and works will likely take years of clinical trials on large numbers of patients, at a cost of hundreds of millions of dollars. Many of the mutations that CRISPR drugs will target could be rare, meaning a therapy might potentially help a limited number of patients. So to recoup the cost of developing a drug, pharma companies will likely charge hundreds of thousands of dollars for each patient using the drug—a price that insurance companies are likely to balk at paying.

Possibly even more daunting are the ethical questions gene editing raises. Early CRISPR drug experiments have been limited to fixing somatic mutations—that is, mutations in an individual patient's genes, rather than a germline mutation in an embryo before a child is even born with the defective gene. In theory, editing out a germline mutation, such as the inherited p53 mutation variants linked to Li-Fraumeni syndrome, might be preferable. Not only would that protect newborns from the higher lifetime risk of cancer that comes with an inherited p53 mutation, but editing the mutation out of their genetic makeup would mean they wouldn't have the mutation to pass on to their children. And the cycle of devastating cancers in generation after generation in Li-Fraumeni families would end.

The idea of editing germline cells, however, has sparked a fierce debate. Given the complexities of human genetics, and the many unknowns, how can scientists be sure that changing one gene won't affect another gene at some point, perhaps many years later? Moreover, editing the genes in an embryo has also raised the specter of CRISPR designer babies. If doctors start to edit germline genes in embryos to eliminate mutations that cause debilitating or potentially fatal medical disorders, what is to prevent the temptation to edit genes in embryos so that a child will be smarter, taller, more athletic . . . or blond? Once perfected, how could CRISPR technology be restricted so it would be used only to make people better, rather than to make better people?

How and when these questions will be answered is far from clear. But the fact that we are asking them underscores how much our knowledge and understanding of cancer genetics have advanced in the half century since two young epidemiologists at the National Cancer Institute became curious about seemingly unrelated malignancies in cancer-prone families. And while these are difficult questions, just asking them gives a glimmer of hope that someday, perhaps not for this generation but for the next, science will find a way to free families from the pain of Li-Fraumeni syndrome and other inherited disorders.

41

MY EYES WELLED UP THE INSTANT I SAW THE SUBJECT LINE ON THE EMAIL THAT HAD just appeared in my in-box: "I have never forgotten your sister."

Only a few hours earlier, I had sent a LinkedIn message to a retired doctor, wondering if by chance he happened to have treated my sister Angela forty years earlier. Susan, my sister-in-law, had remembered that the last name of Angela's physician was Locker, but nothing more. I searched online and found an oncologist in his seventies, Gershon Locker, who had spent his career in the Chicago area. Was he Angela's doctor? And even if he was, what were the chances he might recall one patient he treated many years earlier out of the thousands he had cared for?

"I realize you may not remember my sister Angela's case, as this was decades ago," I wrote. "But if you do, I'm hoping to speak with you."

I wasn't sure if I would hear back. So his quick response floored me: "The day after your sister died, I received a beautiful flowering plant (at home). . . . Not only do I remember her, so does my wife. I was in tears then and I am now," he responded.

I sat silently for a few minutes to gather myself. Then I sent Locker a note, and we set a time to chat on the phone a couple of days later.

"I was a basket case when I got that flower," he told me. "That's not something you ever forget." How Angela had gotten his home address he didn't know. Locker was just thirty-three years old at the time, but even after all the years, he said, "I can almost see her. I remember her room on the ninth floor. She never complained, ever."

When we are gone, we live on in memories. Those memories can remain surprisingly vivid for a long time through the people whose lives we have touched, however briefly. I was moved that Locker still treasured memories of Angela. But I know memories invariably can fade and even be lost, when the people whose lives we touched are themselves gone. So, while this is a book about scientific discovery begun by two tireless doctors, it is even more a love letter to my family, written to preserve memories for my children, and their children, and the children after them. Because I will be gone someday as well, and I don't want these memories to be gone with me.

Many of my family memories came flooding back to me on July 10, 2021, a day I had marked on my calendar long before it arrived. It wasn't my birthday, or wedding anniversary, or any other special event. It was the date that I would become, at sixty-nine years and thirty days, the longest-living member of my family—one day older than my brother when he died and decades older than my mother and two sisters (and ten years older than my dad, who died of a heart condition). In the United States, life expectancy is nearly eighty years. In my family, not including me, the average life span was forty-five. But somehow, I had lived seven decades without once being seriously ill or being hospitalized, not for a single night.

I'm occasionally asked if I feel survivor's guilt. Maybe it is strange, but I don't. After all, it's genetics. With a fifty-fifty chance of inheriting the mutation, the odds were that two of us would not. Though three of us had, and one hadn't, that was out of my control. Like me, Paul and Susan's oldest son, Adam, was fortunate and didn't inherit the p53 mutation, either. Charlie's identical twin, Daniel, did inherit the mutation, but—in a reminder of the starkly different experiences even of siblings who inherit the same p53 mutation—he never developed cancer before dying of unrelated causes at age forty in the summer of 2020.

If I do feel guilty, it's for not probing more about what was going on. As a journalist, that's what I have always done—and what I didn't do in perhaps the most important circumstance of my life, one involving my family. While my family members were getting cancer after cancer, I was working at the *Wall Street Journal* and the *New York Times*, which extensively covered the genetics revolution and the growing evidence of hereditary cancer syndromes. And yet I never paid attention. Why not? I rationalize it by saying that we had an explanation for our family cancers, that we were certain they had something to do with our dad having worked with chemicals that may have been carcinogenic. But maybe that was just an excuse not to dig further.

Occasionally, a wave of melancholy envelops me, and I feel an emptiness inside. I miss that my wife, Vicki, and my children never knew my mom. I miss not knowing what it is like to grow into old age with my brother and sisters and to share memories that only siblings know about. I miss laughing at inside family jokes and gathering at holidays or going on vacations together. Once, on the anniversary of my sister Gina's death, I wrote to her husband, Michael Nystuen, just to let him know how much I missed her. His poignant reply captured my feelings: "I ponder the life not lived, both hers and mine. The adventures we had, and those adventures we had planned but never realized."

Every now and then, I come across people who haven't spoken with their siblings in years, much less seen them. They explain that there was a falling-out over something or other—a perceived slighting of a spouse, a disagreement over how to handle their parents' estate, or maybe an argument over politics that ended in a shouting match. I listen quietly and nod, all the while thinking to myself that I find it incomprehensible: *Why can't they find a way to reconcile? Don't they know how lucky they are that their siblings are alive?*

So on the date I had circled on my calendar, July 10, 2021, to commemorate my parents and siblings, I was determined to do something that would make me feel viscerally alive, to experience the wonder of the world. I considered hiking in the stark beauty of Joshua Tree National Park, sea kayaking in the Pacific Ocean, soaring high in a hot-air balloon, or hiking in a forest of giant sequoias, which can live for three thousand years. In the end, I decided to take a flight in a tiny two-seat gyrocopter— think of a flying contraption not much bigger than a large motorcycle— over the Southern California coastline. Or, as my wife, Vicki, put it, "So you're going to celebrate becoming the longest-living member of your family by putting your life at risk?" Admittedly, a good line, but I was undeterred.

At eight in the morning that day, I got into my car in Venice, California, and began driving to a small airport in Chino, an hour inland, where my gyrocopter flight would take off. It was a blistering hot day, with the temperature heading toward a high of 99 degrees. I thought back to my last visit with my brother in Florida, in September 2019, just before he was scheduled to start the third round of particularly nasty chemotherapy for the pancreatic cancer that had metastasized to his lungs. One afternoon, when we walked out of his condominium, the humidity and heat were oppressive.

Paul turned to me and said, "Don't you just love it!"

"No, it's awful," I replied.

We didn't know at the time that he would die just a couple of weeks later. Only later would I come to realize that maybe Paul wasn't commenting on the weather that morning. He was really saying, "Isn't it great to be alive?"

Paul had lived much longer than he expected when his first cancer was discovered in 1997. "I often think my biggest lifetime achievement is simply having a lifetime," he once had deadpanned in a speech accepting the prestigious Gerald Loeb Lifetime Achievement Award for business and financial journalists in 2016. He and I often talked about the many ways we were blessed. As grandchildren of poor immigrants from southern Italy, we had done things we never dreamed of doing and had gone places we had never dreamed of going while we were growing up.

As I continued my drive to Chino, I recalled many happy quotidian memories. Our eighteen-hour family road trips from Chicago to New York every summer to visit family. Puzzling over the deep-dish Sicilian pizza with anchovies our grandmother Ingrassia cooked for us when we were little. Begging her to make us her "cake of bianca," for *biancomangiare*, an Italian dessert of milk thickened into a gelatin and interspersed with layers of thinly sliced cake and chocolate flakes. Curiously peeking behind her house into the defunct-but-still-standing outhouse my dad's family used for years before they had indoor plumbing. Eating steamed clams with my sister Gina at our grandmother Iacono's and scurrying up and down the steep rock cliff behind the house. Attending Christmas midnight Mass with the family in Chicago's bitter cold. Going pheasant hunting with our dad. Mowing lawns for neighbors with my brother (for the princely sum of twenty-five cents in the early 1960s) and delivering newspapers house-to-house in the snow. Taking Angela, while she was sick, on an outing to the Minnesota Zoo. Driving up the coast of Maine with Paul and his family and lunching at lobster shacks along the way. Fly-fishing with Paul and our teenage sons on the Au Sable River in northern Michigan, and rushing through the water to rescue our boys when the currents flooded their hip-high waders and started carrying them downstream. Golfing with Paul in Scotland . . . and England, New Jersey, North Carolina, and Long Island.

WHEN I ARRIVE AT DUSTY CHINO AIRPORT AT AROUND 9 A.M., THE PILOT OF THE two-seat gyrocopter hands me a "release of liability and waiver of rights" form that I must sign before we take off: "I acknowledge that Aviating is an action sport and recreational activity involving travel in three dimensions and such activity is subject to mishap and even injury to participants. I understand I may suffer a broken limb, paralysis, or fatal injury while participating in the activity of Aviating." Hmmm. I guess Vicki's quip wasn't that far off target.

Soon we are in the air, speeding at a couple of thousand feet in the sky over the empty, parched brown Santa Ana Mountains and past densely packed tracts of housing on our way to the Pacific. By the time we reach the coast, the morning haze has lifted and the brilliant sun sparkles on the white-capped waves, the color of the water alternately emerald green or dark blue depending on the depth. Steep cliffs plunging into the sea interrupt broad, sandy beaches. Dozens of surfers dot the water, their pastel surfboards looking like confetti floating gently on the waves from my perch high above the ocean. I feel an exhilarating rush of adrenaline and, yes, one or two stomach-churning ones, too, as the gyrocopter dips and spins.

I contemplate what my mom and dad, and my brother and sisters, would have made of my jaunt. I'm pretty sure they would have rolled their eyes and then smiled, happy that I was doing something just a little bit wacky on this day.

For them, and for me. For us. Because they couldn't.

Notes

CHAPTER 1

1   **According to family lore**: Unpublished memoir by Anthony Ingrassia, an uncle of the author's.

2   **Starting as sharecroppers**: Email to the author from Anthony Ingrassia, November 12, 2016.

2   **As one of my dad's cousins**: "A Supreme Life," eulogy for Angelo John Ingrassia by John Ingrassia, a son, March 2013.

2   **The two married within**: Author interviews with Dorothy Coppola, an aunt of the author's mother, October 31 and November 14, 2020, and family records.

3   **At work, Dad made a name for himself**: United States Patent and Trademark Office, patent numbers US2666037A, US2744047A, and US3135625A.

3   **Once, after she had undergone**: Email from Marion Smith, the author's aunt, January 1, 2020.

4   **"I felt real sad"**: Letter from Elizabeth Iacono, the author's grandmother, to his mother and father, September 30, 1962.

5   **In another letter, written by my mom**: Letter from the author's mother, Regina Ingrassia, to her parents, dated October 30, but without a year; judging from the family activities mentioned, the author calculates that it was 1966 or 1967.

5   **During one of the periods**: Both letters in this paragraph were written by the author's mother to his grandmother.

6   **The malignancy, I later learned**: Regina Ingrassia death certificate, March 31, 1968, in the author's possession.

7   **She was one of 318,500 Americans**: C. Percy, L. Garfinkel, and D. E. Krueger, "Apparent Changes in Cancer Mortality, 1968," Public Health Reports, Centers for Disease Control and Prevention, September–October 1974, stacks.cdc.gov/view /cdc/65021.

CHAPTER 2

8   **Christmas 1966 was a happy time**: Information in chapter 2 about Ned and Nancy Kilius, and on the cancer diagnoses and treatment of Ned and their son, Darrel, is based on author interviews with Nancy Kilius Gould on December 2, 2021, and February 20, 2022.

9   **Ned's prognosis**: Estimate based on "Five-Year Survival Rates by Year of Diagnosis," chart for the period 1960–63, Leukemia and Lymphoma Society, https://llsorg .prod.acquia-sites.com/facts-and-statistics/facts-and-statistics-overview/facts -and-statistics.

10   **The surgeon did a biopsy**: "Key Statistics for Rhabdomyosarcoma," American Cancer Society, https://www.cancer.org/cancer/rhabdomyosarcoma/about/key-statistics .html.

CHAPTER 3

13   **"I would be interested in cases"**: Letter from Dr. Frederick Li to Dr. Avrum Bluming, July 14, 1967, in "Li-Fraumeni Syndrome Family" case files at the Dana-Farber Cancer Institute, Boston, Massachusetts. Unless otherwise stated, letters and medical records regarding the extended Kilius family are from files at Dana-Farber; members of the family approved granting the author access to these files.

14   **Li was a bit of a whiz kid**: Information in chapter 3 about the Li family history and Dr. Frederick Li's early years come from the author's interviews with family members, including Dr. Elaine Shiang, Dr. Li's widow, on April 15, 2020, March 19, 2021, and November 19, 2021; and his sisters Virginia Li, on March 26, 2021; Angela Li-Scholz, on April 19, 2021; and Christina Li, April 11, 2021; and from Virginia Li, *From One Root Many Flowers* (New York: Prometheus Books, 2003).

14   **"Tongues wagged about the fact"**: Li, *From One Root Many Flowers*, 220.

14   **He was known at the University of Rochester Medical School**: Frederick Pei Li obituary, Legacy.com, published in the *Boston Globe*, June 13, 2015, https://www .legacy.com/us/obituaries/bostonglobe/name/frederick-li-obituary?id=9172210.

15   **He selected all the dishes**: Author interview with Dr. Avrum Bluming, a fellow Bellevue Hospital intern and friend of Dr. Li's who attended the dinner, on November 12, 2021.

15   **Less than two months after joining the NCI**: "Dr. Robert Miller Oral History 1995," interview with the head of the Clinical Epidemiology Branch of the National Cancer Institute, April 19, 1995, https://history.nih.gov/display/history /Miller%2C+Robert+1995.

15   **But, recognizing that the odds**: Author interview with Dr. Avrum Bluming, friend and colleague of Dr. Li's.

16   **Fraumeni's father belonged to a riding group**: "Paul Revere Rides Again in Boston," *Life* magazine, May 5, 1941; and author interview with Dr. Joseph Fraumeni Jr., on March 25, 2021.

16   **Congenial and soft-spoken**: Author interviews with Dr. Shelia Hoar Zahm, a former colleague of Dr. Fraumeni's at the National Cancer Institute, on April 22, 2021; and with Arthur Fraumeni, brother of Dr. Fraumeni, on April 10, 2021.

16   **He graduated near the top of his class**: Unless otherwise stated, the account of Dr. Fraumeni's high school and college years and his medical training in chapter 3 come from the author's interviews with Dr. Fraumeni.

17   **A pediatrician by training, Miller had worked**: Jeremy Pearce, "Robert W. Miller, 84, Who Studied A-Bomb Effect, Dies," *New York Times*, March 29, 2006, 20.

17   **"There are no Nobel Prizes for epidemiology"**: "Genetics of Human Cancer: An Epidemiologist's View," presentation by Robert W. Miller, at the Genetics of Human Cancer conference in Orlando, Florida, in December 1975, the proceedings of which were published in J. J. Mulvihill, R. W. Miller, and J. F. Fraumeni Jr., eds., *Genetics of Human Cancer* (New York: Raven Press, 1977).

17   **Upon arriving at the NCI in 1961**: Author interview with Dr. John Mulvihill, former chief of clinical genetics for the National Cancer Institute, April 15, 2021.

17   **His philosophy was that**: *New Yorker* magazine cover, September 11, 1971.

18   **In addition, after Fraumeni joined**: Author interview with Dr. Fraumeni; and "Dr. Robert Miller Oral History 1995."

18   **Why the two were related was unclear**: Robert W. Miller, Joseph F. Fraumeni Jr., and Miriam D. Manning, "Association of Wilms's Tumor with Aniridia, Hemihypertrophy and Other Congenital Malformations," *New England Journal of Medicine* 270 (April 1964).

CHAPTER 4

19   **Rous had all but stumbled into studying cancer**: Peyton Rous Biographical, https://www.nobelprize.org/prizes/medicine/1966/rous/biographical/.

20   **One day, a farmer brought to Rous's laboratory**: "Discovering the First Cancer-Causing Virus," Rockefeller University, 1910–2010 Hospital Centennial, https://centennial.rucares.org/index.php?page=cancer.

20   **He solidified his renown as a distinguished scientist**: "Discovering the First Cancer-Causing Virus"; and Jane E. Brody, "Peyton Rous, Nobel Laureate, Dies," *New York Times*, February 17, 1970, 43.

21   **"Numerous facts, when taken together"**: Nobel lecture by Peyton Rous, "The Challenge to Man of the Neoplastic Cell," December 13, 1966, https://www.nobelprize.org/prizes/medicine/1966/rous/lecture/.

21   **Rous's confidence in what was known**: Clarke Brian Blackadar, "Historical Review of the Causes of Cancer," *World Journal of Clinical Oncology* 7, no. 1 (February 2016).

21   **What is believed to be the first historical mention**: "Understanding What Cancer Is: Ancient Times to Present," American Cancer Society, https://www.cancer.org /cancer/cancer-basics/history-of-cancer/what-is-cancer.html#.

21   **Several hundred years later, a Roman physician**: Guy B. Faguet, "A Brief History of Cancer: Age-Old Milestones Underlying Our Current Knowledge Database," *International Journal of Cancer*, 136, no. 9 (August 2014): 2024.

21   **Hoping to improve understanding of the dread disease**: Faguet, "A Brief History of Cancer," 2027.

22   **It was the first time a possible environmental carcinogen**: "An Act for the Better Regulation of Chimney Sweepers and Their Apprentices 1788," chap. 48 of Chimney Sweepers Act 1788, Education in England, http://www.educationengland.org .uk/documents/acts/1788-chimney-sweepers-act.html.

22   **Nearly a century later, in 1866, a French surgeon**: Anne J. Krush, "Contributions of Pierre Paul Broca to Cancer Genetics," *Transactions of the Nebraska Academy of Sciences* 7 (1979): 125–29.

22   **with U.S. cancer deaths rising**: Siddhartha Mukherjee, *The Emperor of All Maladies* (New York: Scribner's, 2011), 25.

23   **NCI pamphlets published in the late 1930s and 1940s**: David Cantor, "The Frustrations of Families: Henry Lynch, Heredity, and Cancer Control, 1962–1975," *Medical History* 50, no. 3 (July 2006): 279–302.

23   **An American Cancer Society video**: *The Traitor Within*, produced for the American Cancer Society by John Sutherland Productions, 1946, https://www.bcdb.com /cartoon-video/148194-Traitor-Within.

23   **Potential environmental carcinogens**: Ernst L. Wynder and Evarts A. Graham, "Tobacco Smoking as a Possible Etiologic Factor in Bronchogenic Carcinoma," *Journal of the American Medical Association* 143, no. 4 (May 1950): 329–36; and Richard Doll and A. Bradford Hill, "Smoking and Carcinoma of the Lung; Preliminary Report," *British Medical Journal*, 2, no. 4682 (September 1950): 739–48.

23   **Funding for the program accounted for more than 10 percent**: Mukherjee, *The Emperor of All Maladies*, 175.

23   **"Family studies revealed occasional instances"**: Alfred G. Knudson Jr., *Genetics and Disease* (New York: McGraw-Hill Book Company, 1965), 241.

CHAPTER 5

24   **All told how forensic investigations**: Berton Roueché, *Eleven Blue Men and Other Narratives of Medical Detection* (New York: Little, Brown, 1953).

25   **Fraumeni, with Robert Miller, had come across**: "Clinical Patterns of Familial Cancer," presentation by Dr. Fraumeni at the Genetics of Human Cancer conference in Orlando, Florida, December 1975; and American Association of Cancer Research Oral History Project interview of Joseph Fraumeni by Jeffrey Womack, May 3, 2019 (hereafter cited as "Fraumeni interviewed by Womack").

26   **A graduate of UCLA with a business degree**: Irma Kilius Swan obituary, *Ventura County Star*, April 3, 2008.

26   **Though Ned's and Darrel's doctors at times felt**: Author interview with Nancy Kilius Gould, daughter-in-law of Irma Kilius Swan.

26   **The very evening that she returned**: Letter from Irma Kilius to Li dated September 21, 1967.

27   **When doctors diagnosed Michael**: Michael C. Howard medical records, St. Bernardine's Hospital, San Bernardino, California, 1962.

27   **There are only five cases**: "Investigative Approach to Familial Cancer: Clinical Studies," presentation by Dr. Li at the Genetics of Human Cancer conference in Orlando, Florida, December 1975.

27   **Before age ten, only 0.17 percent**: Mary C. White et al., "Age and Cancer Risk," *American Journal of Preventive Medicine* 46, no. 3 (March 2014): 58.

CHAPTER 6

29   **The letters typically began**: Letters written by Dr. Li to various hospitals and state public health departments.

30   **Li contacted hospitals in Reno, Nevada, and Cleveland**: Joyce Kilius Ciafardone correspondence and medical records, Cleveland Clinic Foundation and St. Mary's Hospital, Reno, Nevada.

30   **"I realize that it is somewhat unpleasant"**: Letter from Dr. Li to Irma Kilius, November 2, 1967.

30   **"We realize [Ned's] condition is terminal"**: Letter from Irma Kilius to Dr. Li, November 7, 1967.

30   **"Our records only go back 25 years"**: Response from Bethesda Hospital, Cincinnati, Ohio, to letter dated May 27, 1968, from Dr. Li requesting medical records for extended Kilius family members from the 1940s.

31   **When Li contacted the firm**: "Investigative Approach to Familial Cancer."

31   **While Li and Fraumeni couldn't locate**: Letter from Irma Kilius to Dr. Li, September 11, 1968, and death certificates and other records listing dates of death.

31   **By November 1967, Li was able to advise**: Letter from Dr. Li to Dr. Robert Wainer, U.S. Public Health Service Hospital, Baltimore, Maryland, November 2, 1967.

31   **As Li wrote to one family member**: Letter from Dr. Li to Larry Kent, son of Walter Kilius, November 28, 1967.

31   **The only son of Walter Kilius**: Letter from Larry Kent, son of Walter Kilius, to Dr. Li, December 11, 1967.

32   **He wrote to Joyce's mother, Jeanne**: Letter from Dr. Li to Jeanne Kilius Durand, February 12, 1968.

32   **In part, Li and Fraumeni felt it would be helpful**: Author interview with Dr. Fraumeni.

33 **Nancy Kilius, numb and distraught**: Author interview with Nancy Kilius Gould.

33 **"Patient has a miserable family history"**: Medical history workup for Joan Kilius Vance, St. Mary's Hospital, Reno, Nevada, September 2, 1968.

33 **"Last night was the first time"**: Letter from Irma Kilius to Dr. Li, September 12, 1968.

33 **Joan underwent a radical mastectomy**: Joan Kilius Vance medical records, St. Mary's Hospital, Reno, Nevada, 1968.

34 **In a letter to Irma Kilius, Li explained**: Letter from Dr. Li to Edward and Irma Kilius, January 10, 1969.

34 **On several occasions, Li asked family members**: Letter from Dr. Li to Jeanne Kilius Durand, mother of Joan Kilius, June 12, 1969; and author interview with Dr. Fraumeni.

34 **In mid-1969, about thirty members**: The account of researchers taking blood and skin samples from extended Kilius family members came from interviews on November 18, 2020, and September 19, 2021, with Jennifer Rivas, a daughter of John Godwin and Janette Kilius Godwin, who was at the gathering and provided samples to NCI researchers.

35 **"I can recall my father-in-law telling us"**: Letter from Irma Kilius to Dr. Li, November 7, 1967.

35 **Li and Fraumeni began sifting through the records**: Frederick Li, "Cancer Families: Human Models of Susceptibility to Neoplasia—The Richard and Hinda Rosenthal Foundation Award Lecture," presented May 25, 1988, at the 79th annual meeting of the American Association for Cancer Research, New Orleans, Louisiana, and published in *Cancer Research* 48, no. 19 (October 1988): 5381–86.

37 **Indeed, some of the family members**: Author interview with Jennifer Rivas, daughter of John Godwin and Janette Kilius Godwin.

37 **When it was published**: Frederick Li and Joseph Fraumeni Jr., "Soft-Tissue Sarcomas, Breast Cancer and Other Neoplasms: A Familial Syndrome?," *Annals of Internal Medicine* 71 (October 1969): 747–52.

37 **Fraumeni and Li had sweated and argued**: Author interview with Dr. Fraumeni.

37 **"I never paid much attention to epidemiology"**: Speech by Dr. Louise Strong, MD Anderson Cancer Center, at the National Cancer Institute symposium on "Li-Fraumeni Syndrome: Discovery and Future Challenges," May 2014, https://www.youtube.com/watch?v=xHVZBFkzcVA&list=PLYKy4VbxNln6fm6yecgv5ujOSbjDTvtF4; and author interview with Dr. Strong, October 22, 2020.

38 **"Why are you studying genetics?"**: Author interview with Dr. Fraumeni.

38 **In November 1969, John Godwin**: Letter to Dr. Li from Dr. J. M. Quick, Santa Ana, California, November 17, 1969.

38 **Initially, John's physicians had told his mother**: The account of John Godwin's illness is based on the author's interview with Jennifer Godwin Rivas, his sister,

and his medical records from St. Joseph Hospital and Children's Hospital of Orange County, Orange, California.

38   **For more than a year, they insisted:** Author interview with Jennifer Godwin Rivas, sister of John Godwin, September 19, 2021.

CHAPTER 7

39   **The article listed more than a dozen cases:** Henry T. Lynch, Anne Krush, and Rose Faithe, "Medical Genetics in Nebraska," *Nebraska Medical Journal* 49 (August 1964): 406–11.

40   **Two years later, in 1944:** Gina Kolata, "Dr. Henry Lynch, 91, Dies; Found Hereditary Link in Cancer," *New York Times*, June 13, 2019, A23.

40   **A towering figure at six feet, five inches tall:** Author interview with Dr. Patrick Lynch, son of Dr. Henry Lynch, June 25, 2021; and Cantor, "The Frustrations of Families," 279–302.

40   **After Lynch started teaching:** Author interview with Dr. Patrick Lynch.

41   **With the help of Anne Krush:** Henry T. Lynch, Thomas Smyrk, and Jane F. Lynch, "Molecular Genetics and Clinical-Pathology Features of Hereditary Nonpolyposis Colorectal Carcinoma (Lynch Syndrome)," *Oncology* 55, no. 2 (March–April 1998): 103–8.

41   **She knew of another family:** Cantor, "The Frustrations of Families," 279–302.

41   **Warthin was one of the first to speculate:** Dr. C. Richard Boland and Dr. Henry T. Lynch, "The History of Lynch Syndrome," *Familial Cancer* 12, no. 2 (April 2, 2013): 145–57.

42   **Despite noting this uncertainty:** Dr. Henry Lynch et al., "Hereditary Factors in Cancer: Study of Two Large Midwestern Kindreds," *Archives of Internal Medicine* 117, no. 2 (February 1966): 206–12.

42   **Though his article had been peer reviewed:** Cantor, "The Frustrations of Families," 279–302.

42   **Lynch quickly agreed and began taking:** Dr. C. Richard Boland interview with author, July 8, 2021; and Lynch, Smyrk, and Lynch, "Molecular Genetics and Clinical-Pathology Features of Hereditary Nonpolyposis Colorectal Carcinoma (Lynch Syndrome)."

42   **Among the few others to show serious interest:** Author telephone interview with Dr. C. Richard Boland, July 8, 2021; and C. Richard Boland, *Cancer Family: The Search for the Cause of Hereditary Colorectal Cancer* (Bloomington, IN: Author-House, 2015), location 1520 on ebook on Kindle app.

43   **"Gee, you know I've got a family":** Author interview with Dr. Patrick Lynch.

44   **Then Lynch, along with:** Author interviews with Dr. Patrick Lynch and Dr. Thomas Smyrk, former colleague of Dr. Lynch at the Creighton University School of Medicine, July 7, 2021.

44 **Given that many of the family members**: Lynch, Smyrk and Lynch, "Molecular Genetics and Clinical-Pathology Features of Hereditary Nonpolyposis Colorectal Carcinoma (Lynch Syndrome)."

44 **Frustrated, but accustomed to rejection**: "Damon Runyon Alumnus Henry T. Lynch, MD, Father of Cancer Genetics, Dies at 91," Damon Runyon Cancer Research Foundation, June 10, 2019, https://www.damonrunyon.org.

CHAPTER 8

45 **At its peak, the Ann Landers advice column**: Margalit Fox, "Ann Landers, Advice Giver to the Millions, Is Dead at 83," *New York Times*, June 23, 2002, 1.

45 **Instead, she urged readers**: "About Ann Landers," Creators Syndicate, https://www.creators.com/author/ann-landers; and Fox, "Ann Landers, Advice Giver To the Millions, Is Dead at 83."

45 **Lederer didn't mention**: "Catalyst for the National Cancer Act: Mary Lasker," Lasker Foundation, https://laskerfoundation.org/catalyst-for-the-national-cancer-act-mary-lasker/.

46 **Like Lasker, Farber had a keen sense**: "Who Was Jimmy?" The Jimmy Fund, https://www.jimmyfund.org/about-us/about-the-jimmy-fund/einar-gustafson-jimmy-was-inspiration-for-the-jimmy-fund/; and Douglas Martin, "Einar Gustafson, 65, 'Jimmy' of Child Cancer Fund, Dies," *New York Times*, January 4, 2001, C17.

46 **So, on December 9, 1969**: "Catalyst for the National Cancer Act: Mary Lasker."

46 **"Cancer is a disease which can be conquered"**: "Report of the National Panel of Consultants on the Conquest of Cancer," November 27, 1970, https://cancerhistoryproject.com/primary-source/report-of-the-national-panel-of-consultants-on-the-conquest-of-cancer/.

47 **U.S. senator from New York Jacob Javits**: Richard Rettig, *Cancer Crusade: The Story of the National Cancer Act of 1971* (Princeton, NJ: Princeton University Press, 1977); and Harold M. Schmeck Jr., "Senate Approves a Special Agency to Combat Cancer," *New York Times*, July 8, 1971, 1.

47 **Rejecting the moonshot analogy**: Quoted in Norman C. Sharpless, "Working Together to End Cancer as We Know It: 50 Years of the National Cancer Act," lecture by National Cancer Institute director, Yale Cancer Center, November 2, 2021, https://cancerhistoryproject.com/article/norman-e-sharpless-calabresi-lecture-nov-2-2021/Lasker Foundation.

48 **By the time of Rauscher's appointment**: Mukherjee, *The Emperor of All Maladies*, 355.

48 **Under his guidance, a pie chart**: Author interview with Dr. John Mulvihill.

48 **True to Miller's contrarian nature**: Author interview with Dr. John Mulvihill.

CHAPTER 9

49   **Even as genetics continued to get short shrift**: Alfred G. Knudson Jr., "Mutation and Cancer: Statistical Study of Retinoblastoma," *Proceedings of the National Academy of Sciences* 68, no. 4 (April 1971): 820–23.

49   **Knudson had attended college**: Alfred G. Knudson Jr., "A Personal Sixty-Year Tour of Genetics and Medicine," *Annual Review of Genomics and Human Genetics* 6 (March 2005): 1–14.

50   **"How can these little kids"**: Interview with Dr. Knudson by Richard Klausner, for the 1998 Lasker-DeBakey Clinical Medical Research Award, Lasker Foundation, http://www.laskerfoundation.org/awards/show/tumor-suppressor-genes-as-a -cause-of-cancer/#alfred-g-knudsonjr. (hereafter cited as "Knudson interview by Klausner").

50   **In keeping with the prevailing wisdom**: Knudson interview by Klausner; and Dr. Alfred G. Knudson Jr. interview, MD Anderson Oral History Interview Collections, March 5, 2013, https://openworks.mdanderson.org/mchv_interviewsessions/54/ (hereafter cited as "Knudson Oral History Interview").

50   **"A hereditary tumor that could be found"**: Dr. Alfred Knudson Jr., "Reflections on a Life," Kyoto Prize Lecture, November 11, 2004, https://www.kyotoprize.org/wp -content/uploads/2019/07/2004_B.pdf.

51   **Knudson asked himself**: Knudson interview by Klausner.

51   **For clues, Knudson determined that he needed**: Ezzie Hutchinson, "Dr. Alfred Knudson and His Two-Hit Hypothesis," interview, *The Lancet Oncology* 2, no. 10 (October 2001): 642–45.

52   **This gave him forty-eight cases of children**: Knudson, "Mutation and Cancer."

53   **Like many breakthroughs, it was greeted**: "Knudson's 'Two-Hit' Theory of Cancer Causation," Fox Chase Cancer Center, https://www.foxchase.org/about -us/history/discoveries-fox-chase-research/knudsons-two-hit-theory-cancer -causation.

53   **Genetics might still be outside the mainstream**: Author interview with Dr. Fraumeni.

CHAPTER 10

54   **At family gatherings of the extended Kilius clan**: Author interview with Jennifer Rivas, member of extended Kilius family.

54   **Edward's doctor removed five malignancies**: Letters exchanged by Dr. Li and Dr. Robert T. Carson Jr., Oxnard, California, December 30, 1969, and February 2, 1970.

54   **After examining him, doctors initially diagnosed**: Edward W. Kilius medical records, St. John's Hospital, Oxnard, California, October 5, 1971.

54   **Irma Kilius, who continued to send updates**: Letter from Irma Kilius to Dr. Li, September 19, 1971.

55 **"The patient has a very, very strong familial history"**: Dr. John R. Hartman, Edward W. Kilius case history, October 21, 1971.

55 **"We have been told by doctors"**: Letter from Irma Kilius to Dr. Li, September 19, 1971.

55 **Irma's fears for her husband**: Edward W. Kilius medical records, Pleasant Valley Hospital, Camarillo, California, August 4 and 11, 1975.

55 **"He suffered just two days"**: Letter from Irma Kilius to Dr. Li, August 23, 1976.

56 **In late 1969, a younger cousin**: James W. Daugherty medical records, Christ Hospital, Cincinnati, Ohio, December 30, 1969.

56 **His father, Henry**: Henry Daugherty death certificate, March 5, 1941, Ohio Division of Vital Statistics.

56 **Henry's only sibling**: Berneda Ernst medical records, Miami Valley Hospital, Dayton, Ohio, various dates, and death certificate, May 13, 1958, Ohio Division of Vital Statistics; and Phyllis Ernst Prine medical records, Miami Valley Hospital, Dayton, Ohio, various dates, and death certificate, August 16, 1964, Ohio Division of Vital Statistics.

56 **Then, in February 1973**: James Daugherty medical records, Christ Hospital, Cincinnati, Ohio, April 27 and June 27, 1973.

56 **Less than two years later, James's only child**: Author interviews with George Robert Armour, husband of Debra Daugherty Armour, January 25, 2023, and February 15, 2023; Debra Daugherty Armour medical report, Christ Hospital, Cincinnati, Ohio, July 8, 1975; and letter from Irma Kilius to Dr. Li, August 23, 1976.

57 **"You may be interested to know"**: Letter from Dr. Li to Dr. Cornelia Dettmer, Christ Hospital, Cincinnati, Ohio, October 14, 1975.

57 **His father, also named John**: Author interview with Jennifer Rivas, a daughter of John Godwin and Janette Kilius Godwin.

58 **She insisted they drink**: Author interview with Jennifer Rivas, a daughter of John Godwin and Janette Kilius Godwin.

CHAPTER 11

59 **There was Ernst Wynder**: List of Participants, Joseph F. Fraumeni Jr., ed., *Persons at High Risk of Cancer: An Approach to Cancer Etiology and Control* (New York: Academic Press, 1975), ix–xii, based on proceedings of a conference in Key Biscayne, Florida, December 10–12, 1974.

59 **Over two and a half days**: Temperature during the conference from WeatherUnderground.com, https://www.wunderground.com/history/daily/us/fl/miami/KMIA/date/1974-12-11.

60 **"The question is no longer"**: All quotations in chapter 11 from attendees at the conference in Key Biscayne are from Fraumeni, *Persons at High Risk of Cancer*.

61 **Disney World had opened four years earlier**: Author interview with Dr. John Mulvihill, former chief of clinical genetics for the National Cancer Institute, who helped organize the conference.

61   **But no one minded, because a who's who**: List of "Contributors," in Mulvihill, Miller, and Fraumeni Jr., *Genetics of Human Cancer*, xv–xviii.

61   **As word about the conference spread**: Author interview with Dr. John Mulvi-hill.

62   **As the conference unfolded, some researchers**: All quotations in chapter 11 from attendees at the conference in Orlando, Florida, come from transcripts of presentations and discussions in Mulvihill, Miller, and Fraumeni Jr., *Genetics of Human Cancer*.

63   **On January 1, 1974, she had begun studying**: Mary-Claire King interview with the Breast Cancer Research Foundation, July 7, 2014, https://www.bcrf.org/qa-dr -mary-claire-king/.

64   **He conceded that this wasn't the same**: Dr. Fraumeni presentation on "Clinical Patterns of Familial Cancer," in Mulvihill, Miller, and Fraumeni Jr., *"Genetics of Human Cancer*; and Fraumeni interviewed by Womack.

64   **Six years later—just in time for the opening**: Frederick P. Li and Joseph F. Frau-meni Jr., "Familial Breast Cancer, Soft-Tissue Sarcomas, and Other Neoplasms," *Annals of Internal Medicine* 83, no. 6 (December 1975), 833–34.

CHAPTER 12

66   **In the early 1970s, Fraumeni was helping**: Author interview with Dr. Fraumeni.

67   **The man responded, "Absolutely not"**: Author interview with Dr. Fraumeni.

68   **It asked about everything**: Mulvihill, Miller, and Fraumeni Jr., *Genetics of Human Cancer*, 489–93.

68   **Fraumeni had become especially well versed**: Fraumeni interviewed by Wom-ack; and Anna M. Lee and Joseph F. Fraumeni Jr., "Arsenic and Respiratory Cancer in Man: An Occupational Study," *Journal of the National Cancer Institute* 42, no. 6 (June 1969): 1045–52.

68   **Then, in the 1970s, Fraumeni**: Robert Hoover et al., "Cancer by County: A New Resource for Etiologic Clues," *Science*, September 19, 1975; Robert Hoover and Joseph F. Fraumeni Jr., "Cancer Mortality in U.S. Counties with Chemi-cal Industries," *Environmental Research* 9, no. 2 (April 1975): 196–207; and Deborah M. Winn et al., "Snuff Dipping and Oral Cancer Among Women in the Southern United States," *New England Journal of Medicine* 304 (March 26, 1981): 745–49.

68   **"We've got a family"**: The description in chapter 12 of efforts to find cancer-prone families to include in research being done by Dr. Li and Dr. Fraumeni came from the author's April 15, 2021, and April 26, 2021, interviews with Dr. Margaret Tucker, who, as a medical student, worked for Dr. Li and who later led the National Cancer Institute's research program on familial cancers.

69   **Tucker couldn't place his face**: Author interview with Dr. Margaret Tucker.

CHAPTER 13

72   **But when it was still there**: Angela Ingrassia's initial diagnosis and interaction with her doctor come from the author's May 7, 2021, interview with Anita Borsdorf Messerschmidt, a close friend of Angela's.

74   **Angela was single and just starting**: The description of Angela Ingrassia's college years is based on the author's interviews with her University of Illinois classmates Susan Bonner, on August 11, 2021; Mary Schuch, on September 20, 2021; and Nancy Adams, on September 27, 2021; and on Angela's correspondence with Schuch in the summers of 1978 and 1979.

75   **"My goal is to enable you"**: Author interview with Dr. Gershon Locker, Angela's oncologist, June 30, 2022.

75   **"Why didn't Angela go to the doctor"**: Author interview with Anita Borsdorf Messerschmidt.

76   **"She looks like a little old man"**: Author interview with Mary Schuch.

77   **Angela had never had a serious boyfriend**: Author interview with Anita Borsdorf Messerschmidt.

78   **As the holidays approached, Angela jotted**: Angela Ingrassia handwritten note to herself, December 20, 1980.

CHAPTER 14

79   **So when they noticed on Thanksgiving**: Unless otherwise noted, the description in chapter 14 of Charlie Ingrassia's diagnosis and treatment comes from the author's interview with Susan Ingrassia, Charlie's mom and the author's sister-in-law, January 25, 2021; an email from Susan on July 23, 2021; and other conversations while the author was researching this book.

81   **The goal, as Paul put it**: Paul Ingrassia, "Weeks After Dr. Jackson's Surgery, Patient Is Back on the Football Field," *Wall Street Journal*, November 13, 1992, A11.

CHAPTER 15

83   **Again, they found a stunning increase**: Frederick P. Li and Joseph F. Fraumeni Jr., "Prospective Study of a Cancer Family Syndrome," *Journal of the American Medical Association* 247, no. 19 (May 1982): 2692–94 .

84   **Debra Daugherty Armour, from the Ohio branch**: Author interview with George Robert Armour, husband of Debra Daugherty Armour; and Debra Daugherty Armour autopsy report, dated April 16, 1981.

84   **Another young cousin from the Daugherty branch**: Thomas Prine death certificate, State of New Mexico, June 23, 1973.

84   **"For a while I thought the bad news"**: Letter from Irma Kilius Swan to Dr. Li, April 11, 1980.

84   **Janette's husband, John, had become angrier**: Author interview with Jennifer Rivas, a daughter of John Godwin and Janette Kilius Godwin.

85   **Lab tests of the skin tissues**: Li, "Cancer Families," 5382 and 5384.

86   **"Cancer surveillance should begin in childhood"**: Li and Fraumeni Jr., "Prospective Study of a Cancer Family Syndrome."

86   **That same year, English cancer researchers**: A. D. J. Pearson et al., "Two Families with the Li-Fraumeni Cancer Family Syndrome," *Journal of Medical Genetics* 19 (March 1982): 362–65.

CHAPTER 16

88   **Bishop went to Gettysburg College with the plan**: "J. Michael Bishop Biographical," https://www.nobelprize.org/prizes/medicine/1989/bishop/biographical/; and J. Michael Bishop, *How to Win a Nobel Prize: An Unexpected Life in Science* (Cambridge, MA: Harvard University Press, 2004), 41.

88   **But as an undergraduate, he switched**: Bishop, *How to Win a Nobel Prize*, 57.

89   **After being rejected twice**: "Harold Varmus," Biographical Overview, The Harold Varmus Papers, National Library of Medicine, https://profiles.nlm.nih.gov/spotlight/mv/feature/biographical-overview; and Bishop, *How to Win a Nobel Prize*, 57.

89   **Bishop agreed, later recounting**: Gina Kolata, "2 Doctors Share Nobel Prize for Work with Cancer Genes," *New York Times*, October 10, 1989, C3.

89   **The study Bishop and Varmus published in 1976**: D. Stehelin et al., "DNA Related to the Transforming Gene(s) of Avian Sarcoma Viruses Is Present in Normal Avian DNA," *Nature* 260 (March 1976): 170–73.

90   **One of the studies**: D. I. Linzer and A. J. Levine, "Characterization of a 54K Dalton Cellular SV40 Tumor Antigen Present in SV40-Transformed Cells and Unaffected Embryonal Carcinoma Cells," *Cell* 17, no. 1 (May 1979): 43–52; and D. P. Lane and L. V. Crawford, "T Antigen Is Bound to a Host Protein in SV-40 Transformed Cell," *Nature* 278 (March 1979): 261–63.

90   **"The role of this protein"**: Lawrence K. Altman, "Scientist Wins Prize for Work on Cancer Gene," *New York Times*, March 15, 2001, B6.

92   **This knowledge added support**: Jerry E. Bishop and Michael Waldholz, *Genome: The Story of the Most Astonishing Scientific Adventure of Our Time—The Attempt to Map All the Genes in the Human Body* (New York: Simon and Schuster, 1990), location 2680–2701, Kindle ebook app.

92   **The effort to identify it began in 1985**: Interview with Robert Weinberg for the Cold Spring Harbor Oral History Collection, June 3, 2016, http://library.cshl.edu/oralhistory/interview/scientific-experience/scientific-research/retinoblastoma-gene/ (hereafter cited as "Robert Weinberg Oral History").

92   **Friend had majored in philosophy**: George Anders, "Disrupter—Stephen Friend," *Fast Company*, October 31, 2001.

93   **"I know I gave this to my son"**: Author interview with Dr. Stephen H. Friend, June 27, 2021.

93   **The method was at the time rudimentary**: Richard F. Seldon, "Analysis of DNA Sequences by Blotting and Hybridization," *Current Protocols* 104 (1987): 1269–80.

94   **"That's all very good"**: Interview with Robert Weinberg for the Cold Spring Harbor Oral History Collection.

94   **Building on existing research**: Robert Weinberg Oral History; and Thaddeus P. Dryja et al., "Molecular Detection of Deletions Involving Band q14 of Chromosome 13 in Retinoblastomas," *Proceedings of the National Academy of Sciences* 83, no. 19 (October 1986): 7391–94.

95   **In the October 16, 1986, issue of *Nature***: Stephen H. Friend et al., "A Human DNA Segment with Properties of the Gene That Predisposes to Retinoblastoma and Osteosarcoma," *Nature* 323, no. 6089 (October 1986): 643–46; and Harold M. Schmeck Jr., "Scientists Find Gene That Blocks the Growth of a Form of Cancer," *New York Times*, October 16, 1986, 1.

95   **Sure enough, in 1987, a team of researchers**: W. F. Bodmer et al., "Localization of the Gene for Familial Adenomatous Polyposis on Chromosome 5," *Nature* 328, no. 6131 (August 1987): 614–16; and Harold Schmeck, "Cancer of Colon Is Believed Linked to Defect in Gene," *New York Times*, August 13, 1987, 1.

95   **Even up to that point**: Author interview with Dr. Thomas Smyrk, former colleague of Dr. Lynch at the Creighton University School of Medicine, July 7, 2021.

96   **"Why have we pursued studies"**: Frederick P. Li, "Keynote Lecture: The Familial Syndrome of Sarcomas and Other Neoplasms," Princess Takamatsu Cancer Research Fund Symposium, Tokyo, Japan, 1987, https://europepmc.org/article/med/3333495.

96   **Li and Fraumeni's original premise was strengthened**: Frederick P. Li et al., "A Cancer Family Syndrome in Twenty-Four Kindreds," *Cancer Research* 48, no. 18 (September 1988): 5358–62.

96   **"We have conducted laboratory studies"**: Li, "Keynote Lecture: The Familial Syndrome of Sarcomas and Other Neoplasms."

CHAPTER 17

97   **The two had met in the late 1970s**: Unless otherwise noted, details in chapter 17 on the personal life and cancer diagnosis and treatment of Gina Ingrassia, the author's sister, come from interviews on February 11 and 12, 2022, and February 17, 2023, with her husband, Michael Nystuen.

100   **Their friend Leslie**: Author interview with Dr. Leslie Baken and Mike Schock, close friends of Gina Ingrassia's, February 11, 2022.

101   **"I'm searching for the whys"**: This quotation and others from Gina Ingrassia in chapter 17 come from entries in a diary she kept in 1987 that was provided to the author by her husband, Michael Nystuen.

101   **So her friends Mike and Leslie**: Author interview with Dr. Leslie Baken and Mike Schock.

104 **Now anyone who hadn't seen her**: Author interview with Julie Nelson, a friend of Gina Ingrassia's, February 13, 2022.

105 **"Family history is remarkable"**: Autopsy report for Gina Ingrassia, Abbott-Northwestern Hospital, Minneapolis, Minnesota, July 23, 1987.

105 **In the 1970s and '80s**: Blackadar, "Historical Review of the Causes of Cancer"; and "Chemicals, Cancer and You," Agency for Toxic Substances and Disease Registry, U.S. Department of Health and Human Services, https://www.atsdr.cdc.gov/emes /public/docs/Chemicals,%20Cancer,%20and%20You%20FS.pdf.

105 **The response he received began**: Letter to Michael Nystuen from Richard Jagels, associate professor, College of Forest Resources, University of Maine, February 19, 1988.

CHAPTER 18

108 **In early 1989, he visited Dr. Li**: Author interview with Dr. Stephen H. Friend.

108 **The son of two physicians**: Unless otherwise noted, the account in chapter 18 of Dr. David Malkin's career and his work with Dr. Stephen Friend in identifying the genetic mutation that causes Li-Fraumeni syndrome is based on the author's interviews with Dr. Malkin, May 4, 2021, and Dr. Friend, June 27, 2021.

109 **In March 1989, after learning**: Letter from Dr. Li to Dr. James Fox, Winnetka, Illinois, who was treating Darrel Kilius for a cancer recurrence, March 6, 1989.

110 **So he started taking classes**: Author interview with Margaret G. Dreyfus, a research colleague of Dr. Li's at Dana-Farber Cancer Institute, December 13, 2021.

CHAPTER 19

111 **In the summer of 1986**: Unless otherwise noted, the account of Dr. Farideh Zamaniyan Bischoff's research at MD Anderson Cancer Center is based on the author's interviews with her on April 22, 2021, and with Dr. Michael Tainsky, Dr. Zamaniyan's faculty adviser, May 4, 2021.

111 **Shortly after Zamaniyan arrived**: Dr. Louise Strong et al., "The Li-Fraumeni Syndrome: From Clinical Epidemiology to Molecular Genetics," *American Journal of Epidemiology* 135 (January 1992): 190–99.

113 **But Louise Strong had a long relationship**: Author interview with Dr. Fraumeni.

CHAPTER 20

115 **A team of researchers in Toronto**: Alain Lavigueur et al., "High Incidence of Lung, Bone, and Lymphoid Tumors in Transgenic Mice Overexpressing Mutant Alleles of the p53 Oncogene," *Molecular and Cellular Biology* 9, no. 9 (September 1989): 3982–91.

116 **David Malkin learned about the article**: Unless otherwise noted, the account in chapter 20 of the research to identify the genetic mutation that causes Li-Fraumeni syndrome is based on the author's interviews with Dr. Malkin.

116 **A few months later, *Nature* published**: Janice M. Nigro and Bert Vogelstein, "Mutations in the p53 Gene Occur in Diverse Human Tumour Types," *Nature* 342 (December 1989): 705–8.

116 **This built on another article**: Suzanne J. Baker et al. and Bert Vogelstein, "Chromosome 17 Deletions and p53 Gene Mutations in Colorectal Carcinomas," *Science* 244, no. 4901 (April 1989): 217–21.

117 **Explaining the project to Kim**: Author interview with Dr. David Kim, July 6, 2021.

118 ***Don't screw up***: Author interview with Dr. David Kim.

118 **All told, they examined tissues**: David Malkin et al., "Germ Line p53 Mutations in a Familial Syndrome of Breast Cancer, Sarcomas and Other Neoplasms," *Science* 250, no. 4985 (November 1990): 1233–38; and Dr. Sharon Savage, "Inheritable Cancer," presentation, Demystifying Medicine Lecture Series, National Cancer Institute, Tuesday, March 19, 2019, https://videocast.nih.gov/summary.asp?Live =30280&bhcp=1.

CHAPTER 21

120 **Dr. Esther Hwei-ping Chang, a diminutive**: Unless otherwise noted, the account of Dr. Esther Hwei-ping Chang's personal history, early career, and research work is based on the author's interviews with Dr. Chang, June 9, 2021; September 16, 2021; January 26, 2022; and August 10, 2022.

121 **While pondering where to focus**: William A. Blattner et al., "Genealogy of Cancer in a Family," *Journal of the American Medical Association* 241, no. 3 (January 1979): 259–61.

121 **"Whatever this defect is"**: Author interview with Dr. William Blattner, May 3, 2022.

122 **In 1987, the prestigious medical journal**: Esther H. Chang et al., "Oncogenes in Radioresistant, Noncancerous Skin Fibroblasts from a Cancer-Prone Family," *Science* 237, no. 4818 (August 1987): 1036–39.

123 **Chang's grant application, submitted to the NIH**: Dr. Esther H. Chang, "The Status of Suppressor Genes in a Cancer-Prone Family," National Institutes of Health grant application, April 1989.

123 **While acknowledging that the application's goal**: NIH "Summary Statement," response to Dr. Chang's grant application, November 24, 1989.

123 **"Maybe I'm naïve"**: Author interview with Dr. Shiv Srivastava, research colleague of Dr. Chang's, July 16, 2021.

124 **Before leaving to join her**: Author interview with Dr. Shiv Srivastava.

124 **"It's un-freaking-believable"**: Author interview with Dr. Kathleen Pirollo, research colleague of Dr. Chang, July 13, 2021.

CHAPTER 22

126   **Then, after double- and triple-checking**: Author interviews with Dr. Stephen Friend and Dr. David Malkin.

126   **Tingling with excitement**: Author interview with Dr. Louise Strong.

126   **First published in 1880,** *Science*: "Science Contributors FAQ," Science, https://www.science.org/content/page/science-contributors-faq#.

127   **He decided to discuss**: Author interview with Dr. Friend.

127   **Friend joined a panel**: *Program and Abstracts Volume*, 41st Annual Meeting, American Society of Human Genetics, October 16–20, 1990, https://www.ncbi.nlm.nih.gov/pmc/articles/PMC1683945/pdf/ajhg00097-0002.pdf.

127   **"Haven't you heard?"**: Author interview with Dr. Shiv Srivastava.

128   **But Chang had a plan**: Author interview with Dr. Chang.

128   **When Friend and his team**: The account of the reaction of Dr. Friend's team after learning of Dr. Chang's p53 research results comes from the author's interviews with Dr. Friend and Dr. Malkin.

128   **Chang, still in Japan, was frantically**: Author interview with Dr. Chang.

CHAPTER 23

130   **The discovery of the long-elusive**: Malkin et al., "Germ Line p53 Mutations in a Familial Syndrome of Breast Cancer, Sarcomas and Other Neoplasms."

130   **The** *New York Times* **recognized**: Natalie Angier, "Researchers Find Genetic Defect That Plays Role in Some Cancers," *New York Times*, November 30, 1990, 1.

131   **The** *Wall Street Journal* **carried**: Michael Waldholz, "Inherited Gene Defect Linked to Cancer," *Wall Street Journal*, November 30, 1990, B1.

131   **"Oh my God"**: Author interview with Christina Li, a sister of Dr. Li's, April 11, 2021.

132   **He was featured in stories**: Author interview with Dr. Malkin.

132   **Similarly, Farideh Zamaniyan Bischoff**: Author interview with Dr. Farideh Zamaniyan Bischoff.

132   **After David Kim returned**: Author interview with Dr. Kim.

132   **Li, known among colleagues**: Author interview with Dr. Malkin.

132   **He also took time to make a phone call**: Author interview with Kelly Kirkpatrick, wife of Darrel Kilius, February 9, 2022.

133   **Louise Strong was exhilarated**: Author interview with Dr. Strong; and MD Anderson Oral History interview with Dr. Louise Strong by Tacey A. Rosolowski, August 2012.

133   **It wasn't published**: Shiv Srivastava et al., "Germ-line Transmission of a Mutated p53 Gene in a Cancer-Prone Family with Li-Fraumeni Syndrome," *Nature* 348 (December 1990): 747–49.

133   **Bert Vogelstein, the cancer genomics pioneer**: Bert Vogelstein, "Cancer: A Deadly Inheritance," *Nature* 348 (December 1990): 681–82.

133   **"If I wasn't so picky"**: Author interview with Dr. Chang.

134   **One of the two dozen experts**: "Summary Statement," in letter to Dr. Chang, November 24, 1989, explaining the decision of the Pathology B Study Section of the NIH convened in October 1989 to turn down her grant application to study p53.

134   **"You were very careful"**: Author interview with Dr. William Blattner.

134   **Researchers were finding that p53 mutations**: Elizabeth Culotta and Daniel E. Koshland Jr., "P53 Sweeps Through Cancer Research," *Science* 262, no. 5142 (December 1993): 1958–61.

134   **Indeed, so central was p53**: D. P. Lane, "P53, Guardian of the Genome," *Nature* 358 (July 1992): 15–16.

CHAPTER 24

137   **This arbitrary pattern could play out:** In a February 17, 2022, interview with the author, Raymond Kilius said he had prostate cancer in his sixties. Given that prostate cancer is common for men that age, and that the odds of having cancer in general increase as people get older, it is likely that his cancer was random rather than related to an inherited p53 mutation; he said he didn't know if he had the mutation, as he wasn't sure if he had taken a genetic test for it.

137   **First cousins Tamera**: The account of the relationship between cousins Tamera (Tammy) Howard Delin and Jennifer Godwin Rivas, and of their decisions regarding getting genetic tests, is based on the author's interviews with Rivas.

138   **Indeed, a Dana-Farber Cancer Institute consent form**: Research Consent Form, Dana-Farber Cancer Institute, December 1997.

138   **This reaction was both surprising**: Author interviews with Dr. Judy Garber, oncologist at Dana-Farber Cancer Institute and a colleague of Dr. Li's.

139   **In the spring of 1991**: Author interviews with Katherine Schneider, genetic counselor at Dana-Farber Cancer Institute, December 26, 2021, and January 5, 2023.

140   **Many families decided not to bother**: Author's December 12, 2021, interview with Jane Gonsoulin Miller, project manager at Dana-Farber Cancer Institute, who worked with Li-Fraumeni syndrome families.

140   **Janette Kilius Godwin, Jennifer's mother**: Author interview with Jennifer Godwin Rivas, Janette's daughter.

140   **Then, in the spring of 1992**: Gerald Howard medical records, June 1992, Torrance Memorial Medical Center, Torrance, California, and author telephone interview with Ronald Vance Jr., half brother of Gerald Howard, November 7, 2020.

141   **A year later, in July 1993**: Jeremy Howard medical records, Long Beach Memorial Medical Center and Bay Shores Medical Group, 1993 and 1994.

141   **But her mother didn't want**: Author's interviews on November 6, 2020; December 7, 2021; and November 28, 2022, with Jaimee Howard Finnell, whose father, Gerald Howard, and brother Jeremy Howard died of brain cancer.

CHAPTER 25

142   **But the biggest prize**: "Basic Information About Breast Cancer," Centers for Disease Control and Prevention, https://www.cdc.gov/cancer/breast/basic_info/.

143   **King had been studying breast cancer**: "Autobiography of Mary-Claire King," September 26, 2018, https://www.shawprize.org/prizes-and-laureates/life-science -and-medicine/2018/autobiography-of-mary-claire-king; and Ushma S. Neill, "A Conversation with Mary-Claire King," *Journal of Clinical Observation* 129, no. 1 (January 2019): 1–3.

143   **She was just twenty-nine**: Mary-Claire King and A. C. Wilson, "Evolution at Two Levels in Humans and Chimpanzees: Their Macromolecules Are So Alike That Regulatory Mutations May Account for Their Biological Differences," *Science* 188, no. 4184 (April 1975): 107–16.

143   **"Why are some families"**: "Q&A with Dr. Mary-Claire King," Breast Cancer Research Foundation, July 7, 2014, https://www.bcrf.org/qa-dr-mary-claire -king/.

143   **With her knowledge of genetics**: Neill, "A Conversation with Mary-Claire King."

144   **"The best way to prove"**: Claudia Dreifus, "A Never-Ending Genetic Quest," *New York Times*, February 10, 2015, D3.

144   **Over time, aided by oncologists**: Mary-Claire King, "'The Race' to Clone BRCA-1," *Science*, 343, no. 6178 (March 2014): 1462–65; and Michael Waldholz, *Curing Cancer: The Story of the Men and Women Unlocking the Secrets of Our Deadliest Illness* (New York: Simon and Schuster, 1999), 45.

145   **King's time slot was 10:30 p.m.**: Jane Gitschler, "Evidence Is Evidence: An Interview with Mary-Claire King," Jane Gitschler, *PLOS Genetics*, September 26, 2013, https://journals.plos.org/plosgenetics/article?id=10.1371/journal.pgen .1003828.

145   **Francis Collins, a renowned scientist**: *Breakthrough: The Race to Find the Breast Cancer Gene* (Hoboken, NJ: Wiley, 1996).

145   **A leading French geneticist, Gilbert Lenoir**: Waldholz, *Curing Cancer*, 52.

145   **Headlined "Some Genetic Pieces"**: Natalie Angier, "Some Genetic Pieces Are Falling into Place in Breast Cancer Puzzle," *New York Times*, December 25, 1990, 38.

145   **A researcher at one of the labs**: "A Conversation with Mary-Claire King," *Journal of Clinical Observation*.

146   **"We're obsessed with finding the gene"**: Natalie Angier, "Scientist at Work: Mary-Claire King; Quest for Genes and Lost Children," *New York Times*, April 27, 1993, C1.

146   **"It was her reason for getting up"**: Natalie Angier, "Fierce Competition Marked Fervid Race for Cancer," *New York Times*, September 20, 1994, C1.

146   **Confident that they were zeroing in**: Natalie Angier, "Vexing Pursuit of Breast Cancer Gene," *New York Times*, July 12, 1994, C1.

146   **Collins likened it to searching**: Waldholz, *Curing Cancer*, 60.

146 **As if that weren't hard enough**: King, "'The Race' to Clone BRCA-1"; and Waldholz, *Curing Cancer*, 88.

146 **King, though disappointed**: Natalie Angier, "Scientists Identify a Mutant Gene Tied to Hereditary Breast Cancer," *New York Times*, September 15, 1994, 1.

147 **This meant he and his team**: Gitschler, "Evidence Is Evidence."

147 **Even so, Skolnick noted**: Angier, "Fierce Competition Marked Fervid Race for Cancer."

147 **The *BRCA* breast cancer gene, like p53**: Y. Miki et al. (including Mark H. Skolnick), "A Strong Candidate for the Breast and Ovarian Cancer Susceptibility Gene BRCA-1," *Science* 266, no. 5182 (October 1994): 66–71.

148 **To the consternation of King and other scientists**: On June 13, 2013, the U.S. Supreme Court unanimously invalidated Myriad's BRCA patent, ruling that "a naturally occurring DNA segment is a product of nature and not patent eligible merely because it has been isolated." Association for Molecular Pathology v. Myriad Genetics Inc., https://supreme.justia.com/cases/federal/us/569/576/.

148 **Adding to King's irritation, she subsequently**: Dreifus, "A Never-Ending Genetic Quest," D3.

CHAPTER 26

150 **Though still in its infancy**: Michael Waldholz, "Some Aim to Fix the Genes Themselves," *Wall Street Journal*, May 6, 1998.

151 **One experiment that got widespread attention**: Lawrence A. Donehower et al., "Mice Deficient for p53 Are Developmentally Normal but Susceptible to Spontaneous Tumours," *Nature* 356, no. 6366 (March 1992): 215–21.

151 **They injected a common type of virus**: Wei-Wei Zhang et al., "High-Efficiency Transfer and High-Level Expression of Wild-Type p53 in Human Lung Cancer Cells Mediated by Recombinant Adenovirus," *Cancer Gene Therapy* 1, no. 1 (March 1994): 5–13.

152 *Science* **magazine anointed p53**: Culotta and Koshland Jr., "P53 Sweeps Through Cancer Research," 1958.

152 **Roth and his colleagues knew**: Unless otherwise noted, the account of the p53 gene therapy treatment on patients in chapter 26 is based on the author's July 18, 2022, interview with Dr. Jack A. Roth, MD Anderson Cancer Center, and email correspondence with him, July 19, 2022.

153 **"The magnitude of the therapeutic responses"**: J. A. Roth et al., "Retrovirusmediated Wild-Type P53 Gene Transfer to Tumors of Patients with Lung Cancer," *Nature Medicine* 2, no. 9 (September 1996): 985–91.

154 **"We will call it a victory"**: Both of Dr. Roth's quotations in this paragraph come from Jeff Lyon and Peter Gorner, *Altered Fates: Gene Therapy and the Retooling of Human Life* (New York: W. W. Norton and Company, 1995), 346 and 323.

154 **"This one little molecule"**: Sharon Begley, "The Cancer Killer: It's Called the p53 Gene. Could It Be the Key to a Cure?" *Newsweek*, December 22, 1996.

CHAPTER 27

155 **Nancy Kilius Gould had little interest**: Unless otherwise noted, the account in chapter 27 of Darrel Kilius's childhood, education, career, cancer diagnoses, and treatment are based on the author's interviews and correspondence with Nancy Kilius Gould, his mother, and Kelly Kirkpatrick, his wife.

156 **It didn't appear to have spread**: Darrel Kilius, "Medical History of Darrel Kilius," self-reported, in Li-Fraumeni Syndrome Family case files at the Dana-Farber Cancer Institute, Boston, Massachusetts.

157 **He got a job at a chemicals company**: U.S. Patent and Trademark Office, Patent No. US-5324755-A, issued June 28, 1994.

157 **"I've heard about false hope"**: Kilius, "Medical History of Darrel Kilius."

158 **They reminded patients that**: Barron H. Lerner, "McQueen's Legacy of Laetrile," *New York Times*, November 15, 2005, F5.

158 **"I suspect because he is looking"**: Kilius, "Medical History of Darrel Kilius."

CHAPTER 28

161 **"Not even his outgoing personality"**: Paul Ingrassia, "Weeks After Dr. Jackson's Surgery, Patient Is Back on the Football Field," *Wall Street Journal*, November 13, 1992, A11.

161 **Still, it had kept growing**: Author interview with Susan Ingrassia, Paul Ingrassia's wife.

162 **"Detecting the tumor six months later"**: Author interview with Pat Massenberg, executive assistant to Paul Ingrassia at Dow Jones Newswires, January 16, 2022.

162 **"Paul needs to take anything"**: Author interview with Susan Ingrassia.

CHAPTER 29

165 **Then, in 1997, she began suffering**: Unless otherwise noted, the accounts in chapter 29 of the cancers and treatment of Janette Kilius Godwin Laule, Jill Godwin, and Tammy Howard Delin come from the author's interviews with Jennifer Godwin Rivas, who is the daughter of Janette Kilius Godwin Laule, sister of Jill Godwin, and cousin of Tammy Howard Delin.

167 **She then developed cancer**: Tamera (Tammy) Howard Delin medical reports, Saddleback Memorial Medical Center, Laguna Hills, California, February 1997 and January 1998, in Li-Fraumeni Syndrome Family case files at the Dana-Farber Cancer Institute, Boston, Massachusetts.

168 **"In the three preceding years"**: Tammy Howard Delin quoted in Barbara Delinsky, *Uplift: Secrets from the Sisterhood of Breast Cancer Survivors* (New York: Washington Square Press, 2003), 130.

168 **"We're clear!"**: Author interview with Darren Delin, Tamera (Tammy) Howard Delin's son, September 21, 2021.

168   **For the better part of a year**: Author interview with Darren Delin.

169   **Years later, he made a request**: Author interview with Darren Delin; and Darren Delin, "My Cancer Story, World Cancer Day 2018," YouTube video, February 4, 2018, https://www.youtube.com/watch?v=a-hA9vHUg3c.

CHAPTER 30

170   **But the article by one of**: Nicholas Wade, "Can the Common Cold Cure Cancer?" *New York Times Magazine*, December 21, 1997, C32.

171   **The first biotech company he joined**: Bernadette Tansey, "The Little Biotech Company That Could: Onyx Finds Success with Cancer Drug, Bayer Partnership," *San Francisco Chronicle*, March 22, 2007.

171   **Despite the demands of life**: Patricia Yollin, "Frank McCormick, Full Throttle at UCSF: Pioneering Biologist Goes Full Throttle in His Passions—Oncology and Fast Cars," *The Chronicle*, June 4, 2010, https://www.sfgate.com/entertainment/article/Frank-McCormick-full-throttle-at-UCSF-3186490.php.

171   **Rather, its goal was defined**: Onyx Pharmaceuticals Inc., 10-K annual report for 1996 filed with the Securities and Exchange Commission, April 1, 1997.

171   **Though Onyx's mission was**: Andrew Pollack, "Onyx Pharmaceuticals Gets Executive Team," *New York Times*, March 17, 1992, D4.

172   **In their initial testing of the idea**: Frank McCormick et al., "An Adenovirus Mutant That Replicates Selectively in p53-Deficient Human Tumor Cells," *Science* 274, no. 5286 (October 1996): 361–66.

172   **Shares of Onyx**: Dow Jones Newswires, "Shares of Onyx Up on Report of Cancer Breakthrough," *New York Times*, October 19, 1996, 39; and Onyx Pharmaceuticals Inc. 10-K annual report for 1996.

173   **"In a couple of patients"**: Eckhardt quoted in Nicholas Wade, "Virus Linked to Colds May Cure Cancer, Scientists Say," *New York Times*, October 18, 1996, A23.

174   **Having conceived and helped launch**: Onyx Pharmaceuticals Inc. 10-K annual report for 1996.

174   **Some of the thirty-two patients**: Onyx Pharmaceuticals Inc. 10-K annual report for 1998 filed with the Securities and Exchange Commission April 2, 1999.

174   **"The kind of results"**: William A. Wells, "Smarter Viruses: Onyx Pharmaceuticals Inc.," *Cell Chemical Biology* 7, no. 12 (December 2000): R223–34.

174   **Some doctors with patients**: Both quotations in this paragraph are from Nicholas Wade, "Genetically Altered Virus Kills Some Cancer Cells in Tests," *New York Times*, May 19, 1998, 18.

175   **Warner-Lambert doubled down**: "General Statement of Acquisition of Beneficial Ownership," Warner-Lambert Co. 13-D filing with the Securities and Exchange Commission, February 28, 2000.

175   **Phase III trials are expensive**: Onyx Pharmaceuticals Inc. 10-Q quarterly report

for period ended September 30, 2002, filed with the Securities and Exchange Commission November 14, 2002.

175 **On September 14, 1999, an eighteen-year-old patient**: Meir Rinde, "The Death of Jesse Gelsinger, 20 Years Later," *Distillations*, June 4, 2019, https://sciencehistory .org/stories/magazine/the-death-of-jesse-gelsinger-20-years-later/; and Sheryl Gay Stolberg, "The Biotech Death of Jesse Gelsinger," *New York Times Magazine*, November 28, 1999, section 6, 37.

176 **Under the glare, the Food and Drug Administration**: Rinde, "The Death of Jesse Gelsinger, 20 Years Later"; Rick Weiss and Deborah Nelson, "Penn Settles Gene Therapy Suit," *Washington Post*, November 4, 2000; and Barbara Sibbald, "Death but One Unintended Consequence of Gene-Therapy Trial," *Canadian Medical Association Journal* 164, no. 11 (May 29, 2001): 1612.

176 **"The biological characteristics"**: Onyx Pharmaceuticals Inc. 10-K annual report for 1999 filed with the Securities and Exchange Commission on March 28, 2000.

177 **The contract manufacturer**: Onyx Pharmaceuticals Inc. 10-K annual report for 2000 filed with the Securities and Exchange Commission on April 2, 2001.

177 **"Enrollment to this trial"**: Onyx Pharmaceuticals Inc. 10-Q quarterly reporting for period ended September 30, 2002, filed with the Securities and Exchange Commission on November 14, 2002.

177 **but the drug didn't work well**: Author interview with Dr. Frank McCormick, July 25, 2022; and Onyx Pharmaceuticals Inc. 10-K annual report for 1998.

177 **Given the many uncertainties, Warner-Lambert**: Onyx Pharmaceuticals Inc. 10-Q quarterly report for period ended September 30, 2002, filed with the Securities and Exchange Commission on November 14, 2002.

177 **This effort would prove**: "Amgen to Acquire Onyx Pharmaceuticals for $125 per Share in Cash," press release, Amgen, August 25, 2013, https://investors.amgen .com/news-releases/news-release-details/amgen-acquire-onyx-pharmaceuticals -125-share-cash.

178 **Like Onyx, Introgen had attracted**: Introgen Therapeutics Inc. prospectus for initial public offering of stock filed October 12, 2000, with the Securities and Exchange Commission.

178 **Then, in 2005, Colgate-Palmolive**: Introgen Therapeutics Inc. 10-Q filing for the quarter ended September 30, 2005, filed with the Securities and Exchange Commission on November 9, 2005.

179 **But the FDA declined to approve**: Introgen Therapeutics Inc. 8-K filing with the Securities and Exchange Commission on December 4, 2008; and "Withdrawal Assessment Report for Advexin," Committee for Medicinal Products for Human Use, European Medicines Agency, October 9, 2009. Dr. Roth said in an interview on July 18, 2022, and subsequent correspondence on February 15, 2023, that he believes Introgen ultimately might have succeeded, but "funding problems" related to the 2008 stock market crash precluded conducting further clinical trials; not receiving FDA approval after early stage trials does not mean "that the drug has no potential for efficacy in subsequent clinical trials." Regarding issues raised by

European Medicines Agency, he said, "Although European regulators cited 'potential risks,' in none of the clinical trials in which I was involved were there any highly serious adverse events." He added that a Chinese company, using similar technology, developed an adenovirus p53 gene therapy drug for head and neck cancer that in 2003 was approved by Chinese regulators, and that has been used to treat patients in many countries, though it is not approved for use in the United States.

179   **"The idea of gene therapy was very compelling"**: Author interview with Dr. Frank McCormick.

CHAPTER 31

180   **What can we do for these families?**: Unless otherwise noted, the account in chapter 31 of Dr. David Malkin's work at SickKids—The Hospital for Sick Children in Toronto, Canada, including research that led to the development of an intensive cancer surveillance program for Li-Fraumeni patients, is based on interviews with Dr. Malkin, May 4, 2021, and November 3, 2022, and with Luana Locke, October 19 and 21, 2022, one of his patients.

186   **By the end of the first stage**: Anita Villani et al., "Biochemical and Imaging Surveillance in Germline TP53 Mutation Carriers with Li-Fraumeni Syndrome: A Prospective Observational Study," *Lancet Oncology* 12, no. 6 (June 2011): 559–67.

187   **In an academic article published in 2011**: Villani et al., "Biochemical and Imaging Surveillance in Germline TP53 Mutation Carriers with Li-Fraumeni Syndrome."

187   **Back at SickKids Hospital**: Anita Villani et al., "Biochemical and Imaging Surveillance in Germline TP53 Mutation Carriers with Li-Fraumeni Syndrome: 11 Year Follow-up of a Prospective Observational Study," *Lancet Oncology* 17, no. 9 (September 2016): 1295–305; and Casey R. Tak et al., "Cost-Effectiveness of Early Cancer Surveillance for Patients with Li-Fraumeni Syndrome," *Pediatric Blood Cancer* 66, no. 5 (May 2019): e27629.

188   **Wyss started by placing a photo**: Speech by Oliver Wyss at the Li-Fraumeni Syndrome Clinical Research Workshop, Bethesda, Maryland, National Institutes of Health, November 2, 2010, https://videocast.nih.gov/summary.asp?Live=9741, from 46:58 to 52:30 in the video recording; Phuong L. Mai et al. (including Oliver Wyss), "Li-Fraumeni Syndrome: Report of a Clinical Research Workshop and Creation of a Research Consortium," *Cancer Genetics*, October 2012.

189   **Tragically, Abella's adrenal gland tumor**: Kara Carlson, "Cancer Nonprofit Becomes Personal When Founders' Kids Diagnosed," *Orange County Register*, July 29, 2014, https://www.ocregister.com/2014/07/29/cancer-nonprofit-becomes-personal-when-founders-kids-diagnosed/.

CHAPTER 32

190   **True to his character**: Author interview with Casey and Michele Grabenstein, friends of Charlie Ingrassia's, July 2, 2021.

191   **"You seem supremely overqualified"**: Author interview with Stacey Mandell, friend and colleague of Charlie Ingrassia's, July 21, 2021.

191 **"You have all this cancer in your family"**: Author interview with Susan Ingrassia, wife of Paul Ingrassia.

192 **"We're still searching for a reason"**: Author interview with Stacey Mandell.

192 **"He still wants to take it slow"**: Email from Charlie Ingrassia to Stacey Mandell, July 28, 2010.

193 **"Not the greatest news on Charlie"**: Email from Susan Ingrassia to Vicki Ingrassia, the author's wife, August 20, 2010.

193 **"As my oncologist put it"**: Email from Charlie Ingrassia to Brandon Thornsvard and other friends, August 20, 2010.

194 **"The good news is that all the scans"**: Email to the author and others from Paul Ingrassia, November 29, 2010.

194 **"I've known you your entire life"**: Author interview with Stacey Mandell.

194 **The mass that doctors removed**: Charlie Ingrassia email to Justin Leinenweber, University of Illinois law school classmate and friend of Charlie's, January 31, 2011.

194 **"We could not have asked"**: Email from Paul Ingrassia to the author, January 4, 2011.

194 **As Charlie later confided in an email**: Charlie Ingrassia email to college classmates and friends, July 4, 2011.

195 **"I'm nervous about the blood counts"**: Email from Susan Ingrassia to Vicki Ingrassia, January 27, 2011.

195 **"I've also been preoccupied"**: Emails from Paul Ingrassia to Stuart Karle, a friend and colleague at Reuters, on February 15 and March 13, 2011.

196 **"I can't express how good it feels"**: Charlie Ingrassia email to Brandon Thornsvard and other friends, July 4, 2011.

CHAPTER 33

197 **Rory wasn't a real person, but a character**: "You've Got to Hide Your Love Away," *Grey's Anatomy*, Season 10, Episode 14, aired March 6, 2014, ABC-TV.

197 **The writer of the episode**: "Local Talent Writes for ABC Television," *Northshore Magazine*, December 20, 2013.

198 **"The part where none of the surgeons"**: Ann Ramer, "Grey's Anatomy and Li-Fraumeni," Living LFS, https://livinglfs.org/greys-anatomy-and-li-fraumeni/.

198 **The *Grey's Anatomy* episode**: "Thursday Final Ratings," TV by the Numbers (former website), Zap2it.com, March 7, 2014.

198 **"Unfortunately I got bad news Friday"**: Paul Ingrassia email to Vicki Ingrassia, the author's wife, December 6, 2014.

198 **My email said, in full**: Author's email to himself, December 8, 2014.

199 **A few weeks later, Paul got back**: Myriad MyRisk genetic result for Paul Ingrassia, December 29, 2014.

199 **"I actually am more relieved"**: Paul Ingrassia email to family members on January 24, 2015.

200 **"You are very lucky"**: Author's email to family members on December 8, 2015.

CHAPTER 34

203 **One of the scientists who found a new variant**: David Malkin et al., "Germline Mutations of the p53 Tumor-Suppressor Gene in Children and Young Adults with Second Malignant Neoplasms," *New England Journal of Medicine* 326 (May 1992): 1309–15; and Tanya Guha and David Malkin, "Inherited TP53 Mutations and the Li-Fraumeni Syndrome," *Cold Spring Harbor Perspectives in Medicine* 7, no. 4 (April 2017): a026187.

203 **The same issue of the *NEJM***: Junya Toguchida et al., "Prevalence and Spectrum of Germline Mutations of the p53 Gene Among Patients with Sarcoma," *New England Journal of Medicine* 326, no. 20 (May 1992): 1301–8.

203 **In 1994, an English research team**: J. M. Birch et al., "Prevalence and Diversity of Constitutional Mutations in the p53 Gene Among 21 Li-Fraumeni Families," *Cancer Research* 54, no. 5 (March 1994): 1298–304.

204 **Yet another paper in 1997 found**: J. M. Varley et al., "Germline Mutations of *TP53* in Li-Fraumeni Families: An Extended Study of 39 Families," *Cancer Research* 57 (August 1997): 3245–52.

204 **By the early 2000s, the number**: J. M. Varley, "Germline TP53 mutations and Li-Fraumeni Syndrome," *Human Mutation* 22, no. 3 (February 2003): 313–20.

204 **The database catalogues included**: Magali Olivier et al. (including Monica Hollstein and Pierre Hainaut), "The IARC TP53 Database: New Online Mutation Analysis and Recommendations to Users," *Human Mutation* 19, no. 6 (May 2002): 607–14.

205 **"You think you found one here?"**: Simone Costa, "'We Saved Many Lives,' Says Doctor Who Tracked Syndrome Linked to Cancer," Universa UOL, August 10, 2022.

205 **Then a group of Brazilian researchers**: Raul C. Ribeiro et al., "An Inherited p53 Mutation That Contributes in a Tissue-Specific Manner to Pediatric Adrenal Cortical Carcinoma," *Proceedings of the National Academy of Sciences* 98, no. 16 (July 2001): 9330–35.

206 *Either I'm overdiagnosing those families*: Dr. Maria Isabel Achatz presentation at the Li-Fraumeni Syndrome Clinical Research Workshop, Bethesda, Maryland, National Institutes of Health, November 2, 2010, from 1:26 to 1:48 in the video recording, https://videocast.nih.gov/summary.asp?Live=9741.

206 **Many of the families with the mutation traced**: Maria Isabel Achatz and Gerard P. Zambetti, "The Inherited p53 Mutation in the Brazilian Population," *Cold Spring Harbor Perspectives in Medicine* 6, no. 12 (2016): a026195.

207 **As many as 1 in every**: Achatz and Zambetti, "The Inherited p53 Mutation in the Brazilian Population"; and "Li-Fraumeni Syndrome Disease at a Glance" (Genetic

and Rare Diseases Information Center, National Institutes of Health https://rarediseases.info.nih.gov/diseases/6902/li-fraumeni-syndrome) estimates that out of a total population of about 330 million, "fewer than 50,000 people" in the United States have LFS.

207 **this particular p53 variant had**: Amanda G. Gilva et al., "Number of Rare Germline CNVs and TP53 Mutation Types," *Orphanet Journal of Rare Diseases* 7, no. 101 (December 2012): 2, https://ojrd.biomedcentral.com/articles/10.1186/1750-1172-7-101#Sec1.

207 **Moreover, they found, people with**: Achatz and Zambetti, "The Inherited p53 Mutation in the Brazilian Population," 2.

208 **While differences in the cancer histories**: Jessica M. Valdez et al., "Li-Fraumeni Syndrome: A Paradigm for the Understanding of Hereditary Cancer Predisposition," *British Journal of Haematology* 176, no. 4 (February 2017): 539–52.

208 **Underscoring the complexities**: "Li-Fraumeni Syndrome," Cancer.net, January 2022, https://www.cancer.net/cancer-types/li-fraumeni-syndrome#; and Katherine Schneider et al., "Li-Fraumeni Syndrome," *Gene Reviews*, January 1, 1999 https://www.ncbi.nlm.nih.gov/books/NBK1311/#.

208 **Depending on the p53 variant**: Valdez et al., "Li-Fraumeni Syndrome"; and Jillian Birch et al., "Cancer Phenotype Correlates with Constitutional TP53 Genotype in Families with the Li-Fraumeni Syndrome," *Oncogene* 17 (September 1998): 1061–68.

208 **Even minor differences in the same p53 variant**: Guha and Malkin, "Inherited TP53 Mutations and the Li-Fraumeni Syndrome," 6.

208 **Hoping to shed light on the interplay**: Author interview with Dr. Arnold Levine; and Chang S. Chan et al. (including Arnold Levine), "Genetic and Stochastic Influences upon Tumor Formation and Tumor Types in Li-Fraumeni Mouse Models," *Life Science Alliance* 4, no. 3 (December 29, 2020), https://www.life-science-alliance.org/content/4/3/e202000952.

210 **"It has been almost 25 years since"**: Kim E. Nichols and David Malkin, "Genotype Versus Phenotype: The Yin and Yang of Germline TP53 Mutations in Li-Fraumeni Syndrome," *Journal of Clinical Oncology* 33, no. 21 (July 2015): 2331–33.

CHAPTER 35

211 **Late one afternoon in the spring of 2014**: Unless otherwise noted, the account in chapter 35 of the family history, genetic testing, and medical treatment of Jaimee Howard Finnell and her family members is based on the author's interview with Finnell.

214 **For moral support, her cousin Darren**: Author interview with Darren Delin, a cousin of Jaimee Howard Finnell's.

214 **"LFS has taken out everyone"**: Jaimee Howard Finnell post on Facebook, May 6, 2014.

214 **"My 4 and 6 year old are also mutants"**: Jaimee Howard Finnell post on Facebook, June 4, 2014.

215 **The risk for LFS patients, in fact**: Author interview with Dr. Arnold Levine; Gaëlle Bougeard et al., "Revisiting Li-Fraumeni Syndrome from TP53 Mutation Carriers," *Journal of Clinical Oncology* 33, no. 21 (July 2015): 2345–52; and "*BRCA* Gene Mutations," Centers for Disease Control and Prevention," https://www.cdc.gov /cancer/breast/young_women/bringyourbrave/hereditary_breast_cancer/brca _gene_mutations.htm#.

215 **"I feel like this is a shit storm"**: Jaimee Howard Finnell post on Facebook, May 6, 2014.

CHAPTER 36

217 **On October 8, 2015, the *Journal***: Lisa M. Abegglen et al. (including Carlo C. Maley and Joshua C. Schiffman), "Potential Mechanisms for Cancer Resistance in Elephants and Comparative Cellular Response to DNA Damage in Humans," *Journal of the American Medical Association* 314, no. 17 (November 2015): 1850–60.

217 **The study was the brainchild**: Unless otherwise noted, the account of Dr. Joshua Schiffman's personal history, early career, and research into elephant p53 is based on the author's interview with Dr. Schiffman, August 23, 2022.

219 **and they found something surprising**: Abegglen et al., "Potential Mechanisms for Cancer Resistance in Elephants and Comparative Cellular Response to DNA Damage in Humans."

219 **"It's as if the elephants said"**: Dr. Joshua Schiffman, "Why Don't Elephants Get Cancer," video, University of Utah, October 12, 2015.

219 **Another research group working independently**: Michael Sulak et al. (including Vincent Lynch), "TP53 Copy Number Expansion Is Associated with the Evolution of Increased Body Size and an Enhanced DNA Damage Response in Elephants," eLife 5:e11994 (September 19, 2016); and Vivian Callier, "Solving Peto's Paradox to Better Understand Cancer," *Proceedings of the National Academy of Sciences* 116, no. 6 (February 2019): 1825–28.

220 **Not only would the article become**: Statistics compiled by Almetric, a data science company that tracks online mentions of published academic research, https: //jamanetwork.altmetric.com/details/4601305#score.

220 ***Newsweek* ran a cover story**: Alexander Nazaryan, "Elephants Don't Get Cancer: And Scientists Think They Know Why," *Newsweek*, October 8, 2015; and Jackie Judd, "Elephant Genes Hold Big Hopes for Cancer Researchers," aired February 22, 2016, *PBS NewsHour*, PBS.

221 **"I don't promise my patients"**: Quoted in Judd, "Elephant Genes Hold Big Hopes for Cancer Researchers."

221 **In 1999, researchers at pharmaceutical giant**: Barbara A. Foster et al., "Pharmacological Rescue of Mutant p53 Conformation and Function," *Science* 286, no. 5449 (December 24, 1999): 2507–10; Ori Hassan and Moshe Oren, "Drugging p53 in Cancer: One Protein, Many Targets," *Nature Reviews/Drug Discovery* 22, suppl. 15 (October 2022): 127–44; and Thomas M. Rippin et al., "Characterization of the

p53-Rescue Drug CP-31398 in Vitro and in Living Cells," *Oncogene* 21 (April 2002): 2119–29.

222   **In 2002, they reported promising test tube**: Vladimir J. N. Bykov et al., "Restoration of the Tumor Suppressor Function to Mutant p53 by a Low-Molecular-Weight Compound," *Nature Medicine* 8, no. 3 (March 2002): 282–88.

222   **A group dedicated to p53 research**: "18th International p53 Workshop," Weizmann Institute of Science, May 22–25, 2022, https://conferences.weizmann .ac.il/P53W2020/18th-international-p53-workshop.

223   **As a result, the number of clinical trials**: Hassan and Oren, "Drugging p53 in Cancer: One Protein, Many Targets," 130.

223   **"That's a depressing thing"**: Author interview with Dr. Arnold Levine.

CHAPTER 37

224   **"Just occurred to me that this"**: Email exchange between the author and his brother, Paul Ingrassia, January 26, 2017.

224   **At times, he had taken drugs**: Email exchange between the author and his brother, Paul, February 1, 2017.

225   **"The full-body MRI I had"**: Paul Ingrassia email to the author, March 3, 2017.

225   **While still on the flight**: Emails between Paul Ingrassia and his wife, Susan, March 13, 2017.

226   **The tumor was small and confined**: Author's email to family members March 15, 2017.

226   **In early April, while out running**: Email from Charlie Ingrassia to friends, May 15, 2017.

226   **A month later, while walking home**: Paul Ingrassia eulogy at Charlie's funeral Mass, February 21, 2019.

226   **Visibly upset, Charlie was crying**: Eulogy by Austin Bartlett, law firm colleague of Charlie Ingrassia, at Charlie's funeral Mass, February 21, 2019.

227   **Ever the optimist, Charlie told friends**: Charlie Ingrassia email to friends, May 15, 2017.

227   **Paul, though worried, wrote**: Paul Ingrassia email to family and friends, April 25, 2017.

227   **The tumor in his hip**: Paul Ingrassia email to family and friends, July 18, 2017.

228   **"All part of Li-Fraumeni"**: Paul Ingrassia email to the author, July 18, 2017.

228   **As the day of the surgery approached**: Paul Ingrassia email to family and friends, October 20, 2017.

229   **More than the rest of us**: Paul Ingrassia email to family and friends, October 31, 2017.

229   **"Losing the leg is tough"**: Email from Charlie Ingrassia to friends, November 1, 2017.

229   **Then, while Charlie was doing rehab**: Paul Ingrassia phone conversation with the author in early February 2018; emails to his former colleagues at Reuters, February 14 and 27, 2018; and emails to family members, April 5, 2018.

229   **In early May, he walked**: Paul Ingrassia email to family members, May 17, 2018.

230   **"There aren't many options left"**: Susan Ingrassia email to Vicki Ingrassia, the author's wife, July 11, 2018.

230   **"We need a miracle"**: Paul Ingrassia email to the author, September 15, 2018.

230   **The tumor was potentially life-threatening**: Paul Ingrassia email to author, November 22, 2018.

231   **But feeling they couldn't wait for an answer**: After Charlie died, the insurer approved the appeal for Keytruda and reimbursed Paul and Susan.

231   **In early February, he told a cousin**: Mark Ahrens, a first cousin of Paul Ingrassia's and the author's.

CHAPTER 38

232   **"It will take me a very long time"**: Email from Paul Ingrassia to Alix Freedman and Michael Williams, colleagues and friends at Reuters, March 15, 2019.

233   **"I call it my Rip van Winkle trip"**: Paul Ingrassia email to the author, Vicki Ingrassia, and Susan Ingrassia, April 19, 2019.

233   **"Just down the street from the Confederate Monument"**: Paul Ingrassia email to the author, Vicki Ingrassia, and Susan Ingrassia, April 17, 2019.

233   **The top of the article had a sobering line**: Ayham Deeb, Sulsal-Ul Haque, and Olugbenga Olowokure, "Pulmonary Metastasis in Pancreatic Cancer, Is There a Survival Influence?," *Journal of Gastrointestinal Oncology* 6, no. 3 (June 2015): E48–E51.

234   **"Definitely encouraging," I emailed him**: Email exchange between the author and Paul Ingrassia, June 16, 2019.

234   **"My PET scan at Columbia"**: Email from Paul Ingrassia to family and friends, June 18, 2019.

234   **"It's unclear just what the origin"**: Email from Paul Ingrassia to family and friends, June 28, 2019.

234   **We were all alarmed**: Email from Paul Ingrassia to Alix Freedman, Reuters colleague and friend, June 25, 2019.

234   **He sent friends a photo of himself**: Paul Ingrassia email to colleagues at Reuters, July 3, 2019.

235   **The next morning, Paul had coffee**: Author interview with Stephen Adler, former editor in chief of Reuters, August 27, 2021.

236   **Upset with the delay, he wrote**: Paul Ingrassia email to the author, July 30, 2019.

237   **"I want you to know that"**: Author interview with Pat Massenberg.

CHAPTER 39

239   **"One of the major advances we've had"**: Sabrina Tavernese, "The Condition Cancer Research Is In," *New York Times*, March 30, 2015, D4.

239   **Hereditary syndromes**: Gina R. Brown et al., "A Review of Inherited Cancer Susceptibility Syndromes," *Journal of the American Academy of PAs* 33 (December 2020): 10–16.

239   **Since 2011, at least 5,000 new articles**: PubMed search results for "p53," National Library of Medicine, National Institutes of Health, https://pubmed.ncbi.nlm.nih .gov/?term=p53.

240   **Moreover, these new therapies**: "Global Oncology Trends 2018," IQVIA, May 24, 2018, https://www.iqvia.com/insights/the-iqvia-institute/reports/global-oncology -trends-2018.

240   **Cancer is still a dread and deadly disease**: See "Five-Year Cancer Survival Rates in the U.S.," a chart credited to the *Journal of the National Cancer Institute*, in "The New Age of Oncology Drugs," n.d., Optum.com, https://cancerhistoryproject.com /research-milestone/deciphering-cancer/; and Lasker Foundation, "Deciphering Cancer," Cancer History Project, May 20, 2021, https://cancerhistoryproject.com /research-milestone/deciphering-cancer/.

241   **"Since 1970, there's maybe 50 percent"**: Ruth Reader and Alex Pasternack, "A Cancer Genius Died from Cancer. His Startup Is Getting Revenge," *Fast Company*, December 13, 2021.

242   **"Any singles here who have dealt"**: Jason Axelrod, Facebook post on Li-Fraumeni Syndrome Support Group, December 30, 2022.

242   **"Does anyone understand the genetic"**: Sonal Anand, Facebook post on Li-Fraumeni Syndrome Support Group, October 20, 2020.

242   **"LFS is robbing me of my family"**: Julie Fuller, Facebook post on Li-Fraumeni Syndrome Support Group, October 15, 2020.

243   **"I just received confirmation"**: Jody Sanders, Facebook post on Li-Fraumeni Syndrome Support Group, January 9, 2019.

243   **"Does anyone else have a hard time"**: Danielle Hake, Facebook post on Li-Fraumeni Syndrome Support Group, August 3, 2023.

243   **"We were told today"**: Rochaun Essi Lopez, Facebook post on Li-Fraumeni Syndrome Support Group, August 3, 2023.

243   **"Does anyone have positive LFS stories?"**: Hannah Leigh, Facebook post on Li-Fraumeni Syndrome Support Group, December 2, 2022.

244   **"When I was 28, I had an astrocytoma"**: Rebecca Conrad Ross, Facebook post on Living LFS—Li-Fraumeni Syndrome, December 2, 2022.

244   **"I'm 51, I have had 2 cancers"**: Jody Sanders, Facebook post on Li-Fraumeni Syndrome Support Group, December 2, 2022.

244   **"My mother LFS, 70 years old"**: Vanessa, who requested that only her first name

be used, Facebook post on Li-Fraumeni Syndrome Support Group, December 2, 2022.

244 **"Despite my circumstances"**: Brandy Emerson Kohler, Facebook post on Li-Fraumeni Syndrome Support Group, June 27, 2021.

CHAPTER 40

245 **Jennifer Doudna, an American, and Emmanuelle Charpentier**: Martin Jinek et al. (including Jennifer Doudna and Emmanuelle Charpentier), "A Programmable Dual RNA-Guided DNA Endonuclease in Adaptive Bacterial Immunity," *Science* 337, no. 6096 (June 2012): 816–21.

246 **The *New York Times*, which typically**: In a search for "CRISPR" and "Doudna" on nytimes.com, the first reference is "A Powerful New Way to Edit DNA," Andrew Pollack, *New York Times*, March 4, 2014, D1. Pollack, who covered biotechnology, confirmed that it was the first story in the *New York Times* about CRISPR in a LinkedIn message exchange with the author, February 21, 2023.

246 **In 2020, in recognition of CRISPR's importance**: "Genetic Scissors: A Tool for Rewriting the Code of Life: The Nobel Prize in Chemistry 2020," https://www.nobelprize.org/uploads/2020/10/popular-chemistryprize2020.pdf.

247 **"It's kind of a profound thing"**: Alexandra Wolff, "Jennifer Doudna: The Promise and Peril of Gene Editing," *Wall Street Journal*, March 11, 2016.

247 **In time, she has said**: Jennifer Doudna, "Doudna Discusses the Ethics of Germline Editing," Innovative Genomics Institute, November 30, 2015, https://innovativegenomics.org/multimedia-library/doudna-discusses-ethics/.

247 **The efficiency of early CRISPR therapies**: Gregorio Alanis-Lobato et al., "Frequent Loss of Heterozygosity in CRISPR-Cas9-edited Early Human Embryos," *Proceedings of the National Academy of Sciences* 118, no. 22 (April 2021): e2004832117.

248 **Its experimental medicine was designed**: Bart P. Leroy et al., "Leber Congenital Amaurosis Due to CEP290 Mutations—Severe Vision Impairment with a High Unmet Medical Need," *Retina* 41, no. 5 (May 2021): 898–907.

248 **Of fourteen patients undergoing treatment**: Jocelyn Kaiser, "Groundbreaking CRISPR Treatment for Blindness Only Works for Subset of Patients: Company Sponsoring Landmark Trial Will Seek Partner to Keep Developing the Therapy," *Science/Science Insider*, November 17, 2022; and "Editas Medicine Announces Clinical Data Demonstrating Proof of Concept of EDIT-101 from Phase 1/2 BRILLIANCE Trial," Press Release, Editas Medicine, November 17, 2022.

249 **While encouraging, "a major caveat"**: Hassan and Oren, "Drugging p53 in Cancer: One Protein, Many Targets," 140.

249 **"Overall, these results highlight"**: James Tran, "Generating Isogenic Models of Li-Fraumeni Syndrome and Restoring p53 Using CRISPR" (PhD thesis, Department of Medical Biophysics, University of Toronto, 2020).

CHAPTER 41

251 **"I have never forgotten your sister"**: Email to author from Dr. Gershon Locker, Angela Ingrassia's oncologist, June 28, 2022.

252 **"I was a basket case"**: Author interview with Dr. Gershon Locker, June 30, 2022.

253 **His poignant reply**: Email to the author from Michael Nystuen, Gina Ingrassia's husband, July 22, 2020.

Acknowledgments

On many a late afternoon after I began working on this book, my phone would ring. "Hi, Larry, this is Joe. How are things?"

It was Dr. Joseph Fraumeni Jr., touching base in case I had any questions he could help me with. He was cheerful, curious, thoughtful, and patient. In his late eighties, his memory for details from half a century ago was remarkable; and even though he was retired, he always knew about the latest research on hereditary cancers. No wonder, I marveled, that he was so well liked and respected in the competitive world of cancer research and that he never got discouraged during the many years he traversed the scientific wilderness with Dr. Frederick Li while they searched for the cause of the clusters of family cancers they had stumbled upon many years earlier.

Thank you, Dr. Fraumeni, not only for sharing your knowledge but for devoting your career to helping families like mine. I wish I had met Dr. Li, who died in 2015, but would like to thank him for his dedication, as well as his wife, Dr. Elaine Shiang, and his sisters, Virginia Li, Angela Li-Scholz, and Christina Li, who offered me insight into him and why he felt compelled to pursue his research for decades. Thanks also to the many other doctors who helped me, including Esther Chang, Judy Garber,

David Malkin, Joshua Schiffman, Stephen Friend, Louise Strong, Gershon Locker, William Blattner, Arnold Levine, and Mark Stoopler. And special thanks to Holly Fraumeni, Dr. Fraumeni's niece and vice president of the Li-Fraumeni Syndrome Association, which is devoted to furthering research into LFS and helping affected families; Holly provided invaluable assistance throughout my journey. My literary agent, Eric Lupfer, encouraged me to write this book, when I initially wasn't sure if there was a book to write; and I thank my editors at Henry Holt, Sarah Crichton, Tim Duggan, and Anita Sheih, as well as my copy editor, Jenna Dolan, who collectively provided the suggestions and support that every author needs.

This book wouldn't have been possible without members of families with Li-Fraumeni syndrome telling their stories. "Family A," the extended Kilius-Stansberry family, generously shared their memories, even though it was at times painful, and granted me access to family medical records at Dana-Farber Cancer Institute, which made it possible for me to turn back the clock more than half a century and recount the early years of research and the family's heartbreaking medical history. Especially helpful were Nancy Kilius Gould, who went through what no wife and mother should have to; Kelly Kirkpatrick, the wife of Darrel Kilius; Jennifer Rivas, who like me lost her siblings and her mother to cancer, and told me when I met her, "You are one of few who understands what it feels like to lose your entire family"; and Jaimee Finnell, the latest generation of her family with LFS to battle cancer.

Thanks also to the many friends and colleagues who have been part of this long journey with me—the journey of life and the journey of this book. Laura Landro, who wrote about her own experience surviving cancer and urged me to write about my family; Michael Waldholz, medical writer par excellence who shared his insight into the early years of genomic research; my cousin Dr. Frank LoGerfo, for reading the manuscript with a keen medical eye; colleagues and friends John Bussey, Bill Grueskin, Tara Parker-Pope, Jenny Anderson, Joe Nocera, Paula Dwyer, Kevin Helliker, Ron Suskind, Rich Gelfond, Charles Duhigg, Helene

Cooper, Matthew Rose, Adam Bryant, Anne Plechner, and Mike Dwyer, who counseled and encouraged me along the way; Anita Borsdorf Messerschmidt, my sister Angela's best friend; my brother Paul's many pals and colleagues, including Stephen Adler, Alix Freedman, and Michael Williams; my nephew Charlie's college and work friends, especially Stacey Mandell; and my friend Richard Gray, who helped me sharpen the old and often fading family photos that appear in this book.

Above all, a heartfelt thank-you to my sister-in-law Susan Ingrassia, a loving mother and wife who spent so much of her life caring for her son Charlie and husband Paul; my many relatives for sharing with me their memories of our extended family and for showering us with love throughout our travails, including my aunt Dot Coppola and uncle Tony Ingrassia before they died, and my aunt Marion Smith; my brother-in-law Michael Nystuen, for opening his heart about my sister Gina and offering her diaries to me. And my wife, Vicki, who lived through it all, sharing many tears but always providing unstinting love and support, while also being a critical reader and sounding board.

More than anything, this is a book about family, and we've been truly blessed, with our son Nicholas and his wife, Sarah, and their four boys, Charlie, Mason, Nate, and Riley; and our daughter Lisa and her husband, Chris Slevin, and their daughter, Georgina, and son, Sam. As a father and grandfather, my greatest wish is that they all live long, healthy, and happy lives.

Illustration Credits

21. Karen Ceifets

22. Mary Levin, University of Washington

23. Courtesy of Esther Chang

24. Courtesy of Imagion Biosystems Ltd.

25. Courtesy of Creighton University

26. M. Hanley

27. Nancy Gould

28. Courtesy of General Motors

29. © Copyright Newsweek Publishing Inc. 1996

30. Courtesy of Jennifer Godwin Rivas

31. Courtesy of Jennifer Godwin Rivas

32. Courtesy of Jennifer Godwin Rivas

33. Courtesy of Jennifer Godwin Rivas

34. Published with "Soft-Tissue Sarcomas, Breast Cancer, and Other Neoplasms: A Familial Syndrome?" by Frederick P. Li and Joseph F. Fraumeni Jr., *Annals of Internal Medicine*, October 1969

Index

abdominal cancer, 55, 202, 242
Abel, I. W., 46
Academy of Sciences, Humanities, and Arts
    (Lyon), 21
A.C. Camargo Cancer Center, 205–6
Achatz, Maria Isabel, 205–7
acute myeloid leukemia, 9–12
adenocarcinoma, 115, 162, 225
adenovirus, 151, 170, 172–78, 220
Adler, Stephen, 235
adrenal cortical carcinoma (*aka* adrenocortical
    cancer), 184, 205, 206
adrenal gland tumors, 86, 184, 186, 188, 189, 205
aging, 27–28
alcohol, 239
Allergan, 248
American Cancer Society, 23, 117
American Society of Human Genetics, 41, 127, 142,
    144–45
Amgen, 177
Amherst College, 88
Anderson, David E., 60
aniridia, 18
Annals of Internal Medicine, 37, 64
anti-angiogenesis drugs, 240
antibodies, 178–79, 221
anti-oncogene (cancer suppressor gene), 92,
    94–95, 116
apoptosis, 219
Aprea Therapeutics, 222

Archives of Internal Medicine, 41
Arizona, 25
Armour, Debra Daugherty, 56–57, 84
Armour, George Robert, 84
Arseneau, James, 174–75
arsenic, 105
asbestos, 105
Atomic Bomb Casualty Commission (Japan), 17
atrial septal defect, 39
autosomal dominant, 136
Aventis, 178

Baltimore, 10, 11, 18, 26, 27, 30, 31, 116, 158
Bartlett, Austin, 226–27
basal cell carcinomas, 54
Baylor College of Medicine, 132, 151
Bellevue Hospital, 13, 15
benzene, 105
beryllium, 105
beta thalassemia, 248
Bethesda Oak Hospital (Cincinnati), 31
bilaterals, 51
biotech companies, 171–78
Birch, Jillian, 203
birth defects, 18
Bishop, J. Michael, 88–91
bladder cancer, 134
Blattner, William, 121–22, 127, 134
blood cancer, 28. *See also* leukemia
Boland, C. Richard, 42–43

bone cancer, 25, 28, 109, 181, 184, 197, 209, 226–28, 230, 249. *See also* osteosarcoma.
Bonner, Susan, 76
Borsdorf, Anita, 72–73, 75, 77–78
Boston, 16, 46, 68–69, 107–8, 117, 126, 128, 166–67
bowel cancer, 25, 64
brain tumor, 64, 67, 108, 121, 141, 181, 186, 188, 197, 218. *See also* choroid plexus carcinoma; glioblastoma multiforme; gliomas.
Brazil, 205–8
BRCA genes, 145–49, 181, 183, 215, 239
breast cancer, 1, 21–22, 33, 35–36, 38, 61, 63–64, 68, 75, 83–84, 86, 91, 141–47, 165, 180–81, 197, 202, 207, 215, 240, 242, 249
Britain, 51
British Parliament, 22
Broca, Pierre Paul, 22, 63
Bueno, Jeanne Stillinger Kilius Durand, 32, 58

California Institute of Technology (Caltech), 49–50
Canadian Broadcasting Corporation, 132
Canadian National Health Care System, 183
"Cancer Family Syndrome in Twenty-four Kindreds, A" (Li et al.), 96, 140
Cancer Medicine, 86
"cancerous fraternities," 41
Cancer Research Institute (University of California, San Francisco), 173–74
cancer. *See also* Ingrassia family; Kilius family; Li-Fraumeni syndrome; *and specific types*
aging and, 27–28
cancer-causing genes and, 92
causes of, 18, 21–23, 28, 90, 238
complexity of, 239
deaths caused by, 22, 46
early detection and treatment and, 23, 182, 186, 240
funding for, 22, 46–47
history of, 21–24
Knudson studies on genetics and, 49–51
Lynch studies on genetics and, 40
p53 gene linked to, 90–91, 115–16, 134–35
rates of, by county, 68
viruses and, 19–21, 48, 90
war on, 46, 48, 59, 241
"Cancer—The Great Darkness" (article), 22–23
Cancer Therapy and Research Center (San Antonio), 173
carcinoembryonic antigen test (CEA), 195
Carleton College, 143
Cell, 90

cell mutations, 28, 50, 52–53, 90. *See also* genetic mutations
Celsus, Aulus Cornelius, 21
cervical cancer, 134
Chang, Esther Hwei-Ping, 120–24, 127–29, 133–34, 239
Charles S. Mott Prize, 135
Charpentier, Emmanuelle, 245–47
cheek cancer, 79–80, 202
chemical exposure, 21, 47, 64, 68, 75–76, 105, 219, 239, 253
chemotherapy, 9–10, 13, 46, 55, 75–77, 81, 179, 195, 240
Chiang Kai-shek, 14
Chicago Sun-Times, 71
Children's Hospital (Philadelphia), 92
Chimney Sweepers Act (Britain, 1788), 22
chloroform, 105
choroid plexus carcinoma, 186, 188
chromosome 17, 144–46
chromosomes, 92, 94–95
Chua, Gina, 235
Ciafardone, Joyce Kilius, 26, 30, 32–35, 38, 57, 84, 165
Citizens' Committee for the Conquest of Cancer, 46
Cleveland, 30
CNBC, 225, 236
cobalt radiation treatment, 55
codons, defined, 118
Colgate-Palmolive, 8, 178
Collins, Francis, 145–46
colon cancer, 38, 43, 46, 91, 95, 134, 146
colonoscopy, 192, 193, 202, 228
colorectal cancer, 41, 43, 116, 193, 208, 227–28
Columbia Medical School, 50, 89
Columbia University, 47
  Medical Center, Cancer Genetics Program, 198–99
congenital anomalies, 14, 50
Constitution, USS (frigate), 107
copper smelting, 68
Coppola, Dorothy "Dot," 2
CRISPR technology, 246–50
Crohn's disease, 192
cystic fibrosis, 150, 247

Daily Illini, 71
Damon Runyon Cancer Research Foundation, 44
Dana-Farber Cancer Institute, 46, 68–69, 108, 110, 138–39, 166
Daugherty, Berneda. *See* Ernst, Berneda Daugherty

Daugherty, Debra. *See* Armour, Debra Daugherty

Daugherty, Henry, 30, 56

Daugherty, James, 56

Daugherty, Sena Stansberry, 31, 56

Daugherty branch, 25, 56, 84

DDT, 105

Delin, Darren, 167–69, 214

Delin, Patrick, 168

Delin, Tamera Howard "Tammy," 33, 137–38, 167–69, 212, 214

de novo mutations, 188, 201, 207

Depression, 40

diesel exhaust, 105

diet, 90, 238

dioxin, 105

disseminated liposarcoma, 73–75

DNA, 93–94, 117–18, 246–47

Doudna, Jennifer, 245–48

Dow Jones Newswires, 160, 237

Dryja, Thaddeus, 94, 95

Duke University School of Medicine, 16

dwarfism, 50

ear, cancer of, 35

Eckhardt, S. Gail, 173

Editas medicine, 248

Ed's Typewriter Service, 26

Egypt, ancient, 21

elephants, 218–21

Eleven Blue Men (Roueché), 24

environmental factors, 22–23, 25, 27, 36–37, 44, 47, 50, 60, 65, 68, 90, 105, 143, 208–9, 238–39

EP53 (elephant p53), 221

epidemiology, 13, 17, 24, 37, 60–61, 106, 135

Ernst, Berneda Daugherty, 56

Ernst branch, 25

ethylene, 105

eye cancer. *See* retinoblastoma

Facebook, 214, 215, 241, 242

Family A, 36. *See also* Kilius family

Family B, 36

Family C, 36

Family D, 36

Family G, 42

Family M, 41–42

Family N, 41–42

Farber, Sidney, 46

Federwisch, Anne Ingrassia, 235

fibroblasts, 112–13, 122

fibrous histiocytoma, 186

Finnell, Gracee, 213–16

Finnell, Jaimee Howard, 141, 211–16

Finnell, Sean, 213

Finnell, Taylin, 211–16

Florida, 2, 59, 61, 101, 113, 225, 229, 248, 254

Food and Drug Administration (FDA), 173, 176–77, 179

forensic investigations, 24

formaldehyde, 3, 105

Fortune, 22–23

Fraumeni, Joseph, Jr.

awarded Charles S. Mott Prize, 135

background and education of, 15–18, 24

cancer studies with Miller and, 18, 25, 35

Chang paper on *raf* and, 122

childhood rhabdomyosarcomas and, 28, 80

environmental studies and, 36–37, 68

Genetics of Human Cancer conference and, 61, 63–65

heredity-cancer link and, 48, 66–70, 90

Kilius family studies and, 15, 18, 24–39, 44, 54, 56–58, 61, 64–70, 83–86, 121, 201, 203, 238

Knudson and, 53

LFS genetic mutation and, 95–97

LFS named for Li and, 86–87

LFS workshop of 2010 and, 189

NCI and, 17, 48

p53 gene therapy and, 154

p53 genetic mutation in LFS and, 108, 126–27, 130–31

p53 testing and, 138–40

Persons at High Risk of Cancer conference and, 59–61

Strong and, 113–14

treats families with cancers across generations, 66–67

work not widely known among clinical oncologists, 105

Freedman, Alix, 235

Friend, Stephen H., 92–95, 107–10, 114–15, 117–19, 121, 124–32, 134, 142, 203, 239

gallbladder, 20

Gallo, Robert C., 62

Garber, Judy, 138

Gargon, Gloria (wife of mother's cousin), 4

Gelsinger, Jesse, 175–76, 177

"Genealogy of Cancer in a Family" (Blattner et al.), 121

Genentech, 171

genes. *See also* genetic mutations; *and specific genes*

chimpanzees and, 143

retinoblastoma and, 91–95

gene sequencing, 94, 109–10, 113, 117, 122, 124, 206

gene therapy, 150–52, 170–79, 220–21
genetic counseling, 139–40, 184, 200
"Genetic Factors" (Fraumeni), 86
"Genetic Markers and Cancer" (King), 63
genetic mutations. *See also* p53 genetic mutation
  breast cancer and, 63
  cancer and, 21–23, 47–49, 91, 95–96, 122, 142
  CRISPR and, 245–49
  germline type, 91–92
  Knudson on eye cancer and, 49–53
  Li-Fraumeni studies implicate, 31, 37–38, 96–97
  Lynch studies and, 39–44
  NCI funding and, 48
  sporadic, spontaneous, somatic, 92
  Varmus, Bishop, Levine, and Lane studies on, 91
Genetics and Disease (Knudson), 23, 49, 50
genetic screening, 240–41
Genetics of Human Cancer conference (1975, Orlando), 61–65
Gerald, Park S., 62–63
germline mutation, 91, 130, 188, 203–4, 249, 250
Gettysburg College, 88
Ghana, 170
Glen Ellyn, IL, 79
glioblastoma multiforme, 141
gliomas, 84, 186
Godwin, Janette Kilius. *See* Laule, Janette Kilius Godwin
Godwin, Jennifer. *See* Rivas, Jennifer Godwin
Godwin, Jill, 57–58, 84–85, 166, 169
Godwin, John B. (father), 34, 57, 84–85
Godwin, John C. (son), 38, 54, 57, 84, 85, 137, 165
Godwin family, 25
Gould, Nancy Kilius, 8–12, 26, 33, 155–58
Grey's Anatomy (TV show), 197
growth signal inhibitors, 240
Gustafson, Einar, 46

Hainaut, Pierre, 206
Hartwell, Leland, 241
Harvard University, 16, 62, 89, 121, 133
  Medical School, 69, 88, 89
  School of Public Health, 17
head and neck cancers, 173
health insurance, 138, 148, 230–31, 242, 249
hematoma, 79
hereditary angioedema, 248
hereditary factors, 22–23, 31, 36–44, 48–53, 60–61, 63, 65–68, 70, 86, 90–91, 105, 108, 121, 134–35, 138, 142, 145, 147–48, 181, 198, 200, 212, 238–39, 248, 253
"Hereditary Factors in Cancer" (Lynch et al.), 41–42

Hippocrates, 21
Hirschhorn, Kurt, 65
Hodgkin's disease, 13, 217
Hogle Zoo, 219, 220
Holland, 51
Hospital for Sick Children, 108, 180, 184, 187
Howard, Gerald "Jerry," 33, 137, 140–41, 166–67, 211
Howard, Jaimee. *See* Finnell, Jaimee Howard
Howard, Jeremy, 141, 166–67, 211
Howard, Joan Kilius. *See* Vance, Joan Kilius Howard
Howard, Michael C. (son), 26–27, 30, 33, 38, 80, 137, 141, 169, 212
Howard, Michael G. (father), 169
Howard, Tamera "Tammy." *See* Delin, Tamera Howard
Howard family, 25
Huntington's disease, 247

Iacono, Elizabeth (author's maternal grandmother), 3, 4, 5, 77, 255
Iacono, Josephine "Joie" (mother's sister), 5
Iacono, Salvatore (author's maternal grandfather), 77
ileostomy, 194–96
immune system, 50
  gene therapy and, 178–79
immunogenicity, 220–21
immunotherapy, 230, 236, 240
Imperial Cancer Research Fund (London), 90
Indiana University, 92
Ingrassia, Adam, 72, 74, 252
Ingrassia, Angela (author's sister), 1, 3, 6, 72–78, 80, 98, 159–60, 200–202, 251–52, 255–56
Ingrassia, Angelo (author's father), 1–3, 5–6, 75–78, 105, 252, 255–56
Ingrassia, Charlie (Paul and Susan's son), 72, 79–83, 159–61, 163, 190–96, 199, 201–2, 213, 226–33, 235, 240
Ingrassia, Daniel (Paul and Susan's son), 72, 79, 161, 202, 229, 252–53
Ingrassia, Gina (author's sister), 1, 3, 5–6, 72, 74, 76–78, 97–106, 159–60, 162, 199–202, 253, 255–56
Ingrassia, Lisa (author's daughter), 80, 228
Ingrassia, Marianna (author's paternal grandmother), 4, 255
Ingrassia, Nicholas (author's son), 72, 81
Ingrassia, Paul (author's brother), 1, 3, 71, 159–64, 191–98, 202, 224–37, 255–56
  Charlie and, 79, 82, 160–61, 193–96, 227, 228–31
  death of, 237, 240, 252

death of Angela and, 78
death of Charlie and, 231–33, 235
death of father and, 77
death of Gina and, 103–5
education and career of, 71–72, 79, 160–61
Gerald Loeb Lifetime Achievement award, 254
last visit with, 254
LFS test and, 198–201, 224
marries Susan Rougeau, 72, 74
Pulitzer Prize, 160
revisits Laurel, 232–33
Scottish golf trip and, 163–64, 224–25
Ingrassia, Regina Iacono (author's mother), 1–7,
    71, 74, 75, 98, 105, 159, 160, 201, 202, 215, 252,
    253, 256
Ingrassia, Susan Rougeau (Paul's wife), 72, 79–82,
    161–62, 191–95, 225–27, 230–31, 234, 237,
    251
Ingrassia, Vicki Johnson (author's wife), 72, 74,
    80, 98, 103, 163, 195, 233, 253–56
Ingrassia family, 160
International Agency for Research on Cancer
    (Lyon), 145
International p53 Workshop, 222–23
Introgen Therapeutics, 171, 178–79
in vitro fertilization (IVF), 213
Ironside, Joseph, 153–54

Japan, 61, 128
Javits, Jacob, 47
Jimmy Fund, 46
Johns Hopkins Hospital, 10, 17, 25, 158
Johns Hopkins University, 19
    Medical School, 116
Johnson, Florence (born Lily Mae Stansberry),
    30–31, 56
Journal of Medical Genetics, 86
Journal of the American Medical Association, 121,
    217, 220

Karolinska Institutet, 222
Kennedy, Robert F., 6
Keytruda, 230, 240
Khuri, Fadlo, 175
kidney cancer, 18, 38, 142, 146, 151, 177
Kilius, Charles, 26, 30, 33–34, 58, 84, 136, 165, 212
Kilius, Cora Stansberry, 30–31, 56, 212
Kilius, Darrel, 8–13, 15, 19, 25–27, 30, 32–33,
    37–38, 54–55, 80, 132, 137, 155–58
Kilius, Edward "Ned" (son) 8–13, 15, 18–19, 25–26,
    30–33, 54, 137, 155
Kilius, Edward W. (father), 26, 29–30, 32, 54–56,
    136–37, 156

Kilius, Iola. *See* Kingsley, Iola Kilius
Kilius, Irma Cser. *See* Swan, Irma Cser Kilius
Kilius, Janette. *See* Laule, Janette Kilius
    Godwin
Kilius, Jeanne. *See* Bueno, Jeanne Stillinger
    Kilius Durand
Kilius, Joan. *See* Vance, Joan Kilius Howard
Kilius, Joyce. *See* Ciafardone, Joyce Kilius
Kilius, Nancy (Ned's wife). *See* Gould, Nancy
    Kilius
Kilius, Raymond, 32, 137
Kilius, Robert, 32, 137
Kilius, Walter, 31–32
Kilius family
    cancer history, 9, 12, 28–35, 53–59, 215
    Li and Fraumeni build medical history of, 24–31,
        61, 64–65, 85, 109
    p53 discovery and, 136–42
    psychological toll on, 57
    Southerland family and, 121
    tissue and blood samples of, 33–36, 85, 108
    two-hit hypothesis and, 53
Kim, David, 117, 118, 124–25, 132
King, Martin Luther, Jr., 6
King, Mary-Claire, 61, 63, 142–47, 148
Kingsley, Iola Kilius, 30, 136–37
Kingsley family, 25
Kirkpatrick, Kelly, 156, 157, 158
Kleiner Perkins, 171
Knudson, Alfred G., Jr., 23, 49–53, 59–61, 90–92,
    111, 131
Koprowksi, Hilary, 62
Krush, Anne, 41, 43–44

laetrile, 158
Landers, Ann, 45
Lane, David, 90–91, 115, 135, 187
larynx cancer, 56, 64, 67, 134
Lasker, Albert, 45–46
Lasker, Mary, 45–47
Laule, Janette Kilius Godwin, 34, 38, 57, 84–85,
    137, 140, 165–67
Laurel, Mississippi, 1–2, 105, 232–33
Lawrence, Mary Wells, 46
Leber congenital amaurosis type 10 (LCA10),
    248
Lederer, Eppie ("Ann Landers"), 45
leiomyosarcoma, 55, 156–57
Lenoir, Gilbert, 145
leukemia, 9–12, 14, 30, 46, 50, 54, 66, 68, 86, 108,
    137, 184, 217–18
Levine, Arnold, 90–91, 115, 187, 209, 223
Li, Christina, 131

Li, Frederick Pei
background and education of, 13–15, 24, 120
cancers among blood relatives, and hope offered
    by, 85–86
Charles S. Mott Prize and, 135
childhood rhabdomyosarcomas and, 28, 80
Genetics of Human Cancer conference and, 61,
    63–65
hereditary and cancer and, 66–68, 90
Kilius family studies and, 13–16, 18, 24–39, 44,
    54–58, 61, 64–70, 80, 83–86, 96, 121, 155, 201,
    203, 238
Knudson and, 53
LFS gene mutation studies and, 95–97, 108–10,
    114–15
LFS named for Fraumeni and, 86–87
LFS patients cancer screening and, 183–84
Malkin and, 108
NCI and, 13–15, 48
NCI Dana-Farber family cancer studies and,
    68–70
p53 gene therapy experiments and, 154
p53 genetic mutation for LFS and, 117, 126–27,
    130–32
p53 genetic testing and, 138–40, 166
Persons at High Risk of Cancer conference and,
    59
Strong and, 113–14
Tokyo symposium on cancer research and,
    95–96
work not widely known among clinical
    oncologists, 105
world tour of public health agencies and, 15
Li, Virginia, 14
Li-Fraumeni-like syndrome (LFL), 208
Li-Fraumeni syndrome (LFS)
age of contracting cancer and, 137
Brazil and, 205–7
coping with, 169, 202–3, 238, 241–44
CRISPR and, 249–50
decision whether to have children and, 213
Facebook support group for, 214, 241–43
Friend and Malkin's research on genetic
    mutation in, 108–10
future of, 245–46, 250
gene therapy and, 179
Grey's Anatomy and, 197–98
health insurance and, 242
Ingrassias fail to see news about, 160, 162–63,
    227
intensive screening and, 189
interplay of external and genetic factors and,
    208–9

LF spectrum vs., 208
Li talk in Tokyo on, 96
Locke and, 181
Malkin's screening studies for patients with,
    180–89
NCI and, 212
NIH workshop on, 187–89
p53 gene and, 115–18, 126–27, 130–33, 142, 148,
    151, 160, 162–63, 180, 217–19, 239
p53 genetic testing and counseling and, 137–40
p53 variants and, 208
Paul tests positive for, 198–99
preventive surgery and, 183
rarity of, 239
relatively unknown, 198
Schiffman's research on, 217–19
scientific achievement and, 238
term coined, 86–87, 203
tissue cultures and fibroblasts studies and,
    111–14
liposarcoma, 25
liver, 20
liver cancer, 134
Locke, Juliet, 186
Locke, Luana, 180–82, 184–85, 204
Locke, Lucas, 182, 184–86
Locker, Gershon, 75, 251–52
Los Angeles Times, 160
lung adenocarcinomas, 115, 162
lung cancer, 23, 26, 30, 35, 56, 59, 64, 67, 99–106,
    134, 153–54, 162–63, 197, 202, 240
lupus, 50
lymphocytes, 19
lymphoid tumors, 116
lymphoma, 14, 217
lymphosarcomas, 13
Lynch, Henry T., 39–44, 59–63, 90, 95
Lynch, Jane, 43, 61
Lynch, Patrick, 43, 61
Lynch syndrome, 239

macrobiotic diet, 102
Magee, Johnny, 233
Maley, Carlo, 218
Malkin, David, 108–10, 116–19, 124–26, 128, 132,
    180–89, 203, 210, 218, 249
Mandell, Stacey, 191–92, 194
Mao Zedong, 14
marijuana, 101
Marinol (synthetic marijuana), 101
Martin, Richard, 71
Masonite Corp., 2–3
Massachusetts Eye and Ear Infirmary, 94

Massachusetts General Hospital, 16, 107, 121
Massachusetts Institute of Technology (MIT), 92
Massenberg, Pat, 237
Mayo Clinic, 60
McCormick, Frank, 170–74, 177, 179
McQueen, Steve, 158
MD Anderson Cancer Center, 42, 50–52, 60–61,
    111, 113, 126, 132–33, 144, 151–54, 171, 175,
    224–25
Meadows, Anna, 59, 61, 92
"Medical Genetics in Nebraska" (Lynch et al.),
    39–40
Memorial Hospital (New York), 50
Memorial Sloan Kettering Cancer Center, 17
metastasis, 177
mice studies, 113, 115–16, 151–52
Miller, Robert, 17–18, 24–25, 35, 48, 53
molecular biology, 41, 88, 93–94, 110, 142, 144, 150,
    170–71, 240
Mormon families, 61, 147
Mount Desert Island Biological Laboratory, 218
MRI scans, 184, 186
multiple myeloma, 13
Mulvihill, John, 61–62
"Mutation and Cancer: Statistical Study of
    Retinoblastoma" (Knudson), 52–53
myelodysplastic syndromes, 222
myotonia dystrophica, 39
Myriad Genetics, 147–48

Nader, Ralph, 143
nanoparticles, 220–21, 223
Napolitano, Tia, 197–98
National Cancer Act (1971), 45, 47
National Cancer Institute (NCI), 9, 48–49, 120,
    212, 239, 241, 250
  cancer-prone family questionnaire, 68
  Clinical Center, 66
  Clinical Genetics program, 62
  creation of, 23
  database of childhood cancers, 18
  epidemiological study on breast, ovarian, and
      uterine cancer, 143–44
  epidemiology department, 13, 15, 17–18
  Fraumeni hired by, 17
  Kilius family studies and, 25–26, 34–35
  Li hired by, 13–17, 25
  Persons at High Risk of Cancer conference and,
      61–62
  Rauscher heads, 65
  Special Virus Cancer Program, 23, 48
national cancer registry, 62
national childhood cancer mortality registry, 36

National Institutes of Health (NIH), 44, 55,
    88–90, 123–24, 134, 145, 173
  Clinical Center, 66
  Hospital, 121
  LFS Syndrome Workshop, 187
  National Center for Human Genome Research,
      145
  RAC and, 153
National Lancers, 16
National Panel of Consultants on the Conquest of
    Cancer, 46–47
Nature, 90, 116, 129, 133, 151
NBC, 146
Nebraska, 39–42, 44
Nebraska State Medical Journal, 39
neuroblastoma, 197
Nevada, 25
New England Journal of Medicine (NEJM), 18, 203
New Mexico, 25, 84
Newsweek, 154, 220
New York Daily News, 160
New Yorker, 17, 24, 48
  Annals of Medicine, 24
New York Times, 95, 130–31, 145–46, 160, 175,
    246, 253
  Magazine, 170
New York University, 65
Nixon, Richard, 46–48, 241
Nobel Prize
  Bishop and, 90
  Doudna and Charpentier and, 246–47
  Rous and, 19–21, 89
  Varmus and, 90, 239
Northwestern Memorial Hospital, 228
Northwestern University, 132, 156
nose cancer, 35
Nystuen, Michael, 76–77, 97–98, 100–101, 103–6,
    253

Ohio, 56
Omaha Veterans Administration Hospital, 41
oncogene, 89–90, 115, 122
oncogenic virus, 25, 60
Onyx-015, 173–77, 179
Onyx Pharmaceuticals, 170–78
oral chemotherapy, 177
osteogenesis imperfecta, 39
osteosarcoma, 66, 68, 116, 197
ovarian cancer, 134, 140, 143, 165, 168, 215, 223

p53 gene (TP53), 90–91, 115–17, 222–23, 239–40
  elephants and, 217–20
  experiments on mice born without, 151

p53 gene (*TP53*) (*cont'd*)
as guardian of the genome, 135
as "Molecule of the Year," 152
as tumor suppressor gene, 116, 123, 134–35, 147,
150–51, 171–72, 178, 181, 218
p53 gene mutation, 158, 203
autosomal dominant, 136
Brazilian cases and, 205–8
cancer-fighting powers turned off by, 116
CRISPR and, 249–50
decision to have children and, 212–13
de novo, 201
discovery of link to LFS, and race to publish,
115–19, 124–37, 142, 144
family members and, 187–89
gene therapy prospects and, 135, 149–54, 171–72,
178–79, 221–22, 235
genetic counseling and, 139–42
genetic testing and, 137–39, 163, 165–67, 182–83,
199–201, 212–16, 218, 240–42
germline, 204
Grey's Anatomy and, 197
hot spots or codons and, 116, 118, 125, 132,
181–82, 206
Ingrassias fail to see news on, 160, 163
Malkin's testing and screening program and,
180–88
new variants of, 203–10
noninherited somatic, 134
number of, 223
p53-related drugs and, 180, 223
rarity of, 148
somatic, 204
Pacific Lutheran University, 156
pancreatic cancer, 35, 56, 165, 197, 225–27, 240
PBS News Hour, 220
Peel Therapeutics, 221
Perkin Elmer 480 machine, 109
Persons at High Risk of Cancer conference and,
59–60
Peyrilhe, Bernard, 21–22
Pfizer, 221–22
Pirollo, Kathleen, 124
PMV Pharma, 223
Poisson distribution, 52
polio, 19, 47
"Potential Mechanisms for Cancer Resistance in
Elephants" (Schiffman), 217
Pott, Percivall, 22
PRIMA-1 or APR-246, 222
Princeton University, 90
Prine, Phyllis Ernst, 56
Prine, Thomas, 84

Prine family, 25
Proceedings of the National Academy of Sciences,
49
"Programmable Dual RNA-Guided DNA
Endonuclease in Adaptive Bacterial
Immunity, A" (Doudna and Charpentier), 246
prostate cancer, 55, 64, 134, 142, 191, 198, 223–24,
233, 240
prostate-specific antigen (PSA), 191, 198

Quirks and Quarks (TV show), 132

rabbit studies, 20
radiation, 47, 122, 128, 239
radiation therapy, 81, 82
raf oncogene, 122
Rainbow Babies and Children's Hospital, 79–80
ras gene, 120, 123
rat sarcoma tumor cells, 120
Rauscher, Frank, 48, 65
Rauscher leukemia virus, 48
Rb tumor suppressor gene, 94–95, 107, 109–10,
115–17, 126, 131, 134, 142
Reader's Digest, 9
Recombinant DNA Advisory Committee (RAC),
152–53
referral bias, 36
Reno, Nevada, 30, 33
respiratory acidosis, 11–12
retinoblastoma (eye cancer), 49–53, 91–95, 109,
134
retrovirus, gene therapy and, 153, 220
Reuters, 195–96, 235–36
Revs Institute, 225
rhabdomyosarcoma, 10–12, 26–28, 54–55, 79–82,
105, 116
Ringling Bros. and Barnum and Bailey Circus, 219
Rivas, Jennifer Godwin, 57–58, 84–85, 137–38,
140–41, 165–68
Rivas, Rudy, 166, 167
Rockefeller, Laurance, 46
Rockefeller Institute for Medical Research, 19
Rome, ancient, 21
Roth, Jack, 150–54, 171
Rous, Peyton, 19–22, 49, 89
Rous sarcoma, 89–90
Runyon, Damon, 44
Russia, 61

Salk vaccine, 47
Salvation Army missing person program, 166
San Diego State University, 8
Santo André, Brazil, 205

sarcoma, 20, 86, 109, 181, 203
SBLA syndrome (*later* Li-Fraumeni syndrome), 86
Schiffman, Joshua, 217–21
Schmidt, Benno, Sr., 46
Schneider, Katherine, 139–40
Schoenberg, Bruce S., 60
Schroeder, Avi, 220–21
Science, 122, 126–33, 143, 145–46, 148, 152, 172, 220, 246
Securities and Exchange Commission, 176
selection bias, 70
Shiang, Elaine, 69
sickle-cell anemia, 50, 247–48
silica dust, 105
Skelton, Red, 9
skin biopsies, 82
skin cancer, 28, 29, 54, 134, 142, 166, 209
skin cancer gene, 146
Skolnick, Mark, 61, 145–48
soft-tissue sarcoma, 20, 28, 36, 68, 75
"Soft-Tissue Sarcomas, Breast Cancer and Other Neoplasms: A Familial Syndrome?" (Li and Fraumeni), 37
somatic mutations, 92, 134, 204, 250
Southerland family, 121–24, 127–28
Southern, Edwin, 93
Southern blot analysis, 93–94, 117
Southern Illinois University, 120
Spiegelman, Sol, 47–48
spinal tumor, 57, 66
Srivastava, Shiv, 123–24, 128, 133
Stanford University, 117, 132, 217–18
Stansberry, Lily Mae. *See* Johnson, Florence
Stansberry, Minnie Mefford, 31, 35
Stansberry, Thomas, 35
Stansberry family, 25, 31, 35, 121
Stevens, Amy, 235
St. Mary's Hospital (Reno), 33
stomach cancer, 134
Stoopler, Mark, 199
Strong, Louise, 37–38, 61, 111–13, 118, 126–27, 133, 135, 144–45, 189
sulfuric acid, 105
Sun Yat-sen, 120
Swan, Irma Cser Kilius, 11, 26–27, 29–35, 44, 54–56, 84, 132, 136, 155–57

Tainsky, Michael, 111–13
testicular cancer, 197
three-visit model, 139–40
thyroid cancer, 64, 134
tobacco, 23, 59, 68, 153, 239
Toronto, 115

Toronto Protocol, 187, 218, 226
TP53 gene, 90
Traité des tumeurs (Broca), 22
Traitor Within, The (video), 23
transthyretin-mediated amyloidosis cardio myopathy, 248
Tucker, Margaret, 69–70
tumors. *See also specific types*
  cell mutations and, 50
  malignant vs. benign, 21
tumor suppressor genes, first identified, 92, 94–95, 116. *See also* p53 gene; *Rb* tumor suppressor gene
Tumor Suppressor Genes panel, 127
Turner syndrome, 32
"Two Families with the Li-Fraumeni Cancer Family Syndrome" (Li and Fraumeni), 86
two-hit hypothesis, 52–53, 59, 91

Uniformed Services University of the Health Sciences, 120–21
U.S. Congress, 23, 45, 46, 47
U.S. Marine Hospital, 10
U.S. Navy, 40
U.S. Public Health Service Hospital, 10, 25–26
U.S. Supreme Court, 148
U.S. surgeon general, 23
University of California, Berkeley, 61, 63, 143, 148, 171
University of California, Los Angeles (UCLA), 9, 26
University of California, San Francisco (UCSF), 88, 89
  Cancer Research Institute, 173–74
  Medical School, 143
University of Chicago, 76
University of Denver, 40
University of Illinois, 71, 74, 76, 190
University of Maryland Medical Center, 158
University of Miami, 17
University of Michigan, 41–42, 145
University of Minnesota, 100, 104
University of Nebraska College of Medicine, 39, 40, 42
University of New York, Stony Brook, 111
University of Oklahoma, 40
University of Pennsylvania, 175–76
University of Rochester Medical School, 14–15
University of Southern California, 34
  Medical Center, 200
University of Texas, Galveston, 40
University of Texas, Houston, 111
University of Texas Medical School, 37

University of Utah, 61, 146, 217
  Huntsman Cancer Institute, 218
University of Washington, 148
Utah, 147, 185, 217–18
uterine cancer, 56

Vance, Joan Kilius Howard, 26, 33–34, 38, 57, 84,
  137, 141, 165, 169, 212
Varmus, Harold E., 88–91, 239
Vietnam War protests, 6, 47
Vincent, Susan Boone, 233
vinyl chloride, 105
viruses, 27, 238
  ability to modify, 150
  as cause of cancer, 23, 33–34, 36, 47–48, 50, 60,
    239
  Genetics of Human Cancer conference and, 62
  Levine studies of p53 gene and, 91
  ras gene and, 120
  Rous studies of, 20–21, 23
  used to deliver drugs, 175
  Varmus and Bishop turn cancer research away
    from, 89–90
Vogelstein, Bert, 116–18, 133–34, 187

Wall Street Journal, 71–72, 79, 103, 131, 160,
  194–95, 235, 253
Warner-Lambert, 173, 175, 177
Warthin, Aldred, 41–42
Washington Post, 160
Wasserman, Lewis, 46
Weinberg, Robert, 92–95, 109, 131
Wellesley College, 69
Whitehead Institute for Biomedical Research, 92
Williams, Michael, 235
Wilms tumor, 18, 38, 108
Wilson, Allan, 143
World War II, 40
Wynder, Ernst, 59
Wyss, Abella, 188–89
Wyss, Hudson, 188
Wyss, Jamie, 188
Wyss, Oliver, 187–89, 241

X-rays, 57, 99, 156, 162, 184, 227

Yale School of Medicine, 42

Zamaniyan Bischoff, Farideh, 111–14, 132

About the Author

Lawrence Ingrassia is a former deputy managing editor at the *New York Times*, having previously spent twenty-five years at the *Wall Street Journal*. He also served as managing editor of the *Los Angeles Times*. The coverage he directed won five Pulitzer Prizes as well as Gerald Loeb Awards and George Polk Awards. He lives in the Seattle area.